PEDIATRIC DERMATOLOGY AND DERMATOPATHOLOGY

PEDIATRIC DERMATOLOGY AND DERMATOPATHOLOGY

A CONCISE ATLAS

Ruggero Caputo MD

Professor and Chairman
Istituto di Scienze Dermatologiche
Università di Milano
IRCCS Ospedale Maggiore
Milan, Italy

Carlo Gelmetti MD

Associated Professor
Istituto di Scienze Dermatologiche
Università di Milano
IRCCS Ospedale Maggiore
Milan, Italy

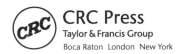

CRC Press
Taylor & Francis Group
Boca Raton London New York

CRC Press is an imprint of the
Taylor & Francis Group, an **informa** business

CRC Press
Taylor & Francis Group
6000 Broken Sound Parkway NW, Suite 300
Boca Raton, FL 33487-2742

First issued in paperback 2019

ISBN-13 978-1-84184-120-   bk
ISBN-13 978-0-367-3967 -6 pbk

i it t e Ta or   ra ci   e ite at
tt :   ta ora d ra ci com

a d t e   re   e ite at
tt :   crc re   com

CONTENTS

PREFACE

It is almost ten years since the first volume of *Pediatric Dermatology and Dermatopathology* was published. The original, four-volume textbook represents the synthesis of the clinical experience of the Milan school of pediatric dermatology and the unrivalled expertise of US dermatopathologists. This landmark text built on the tradition of the late Professor Ferdinando Giannotti; and Bernard Akerman and his co-workers, among whom we would like to mention Evita Sison-Torre and Giorgio Annessi, made an invaluable contribution providing all the histological images.

At present, pediatric dermatology is a fast-growing specialty, and there is a real need for educational resources. It is with this in mind that we have decided to bring together a concise edition of *Pediatric Dermatology and Dermatopathology* in one single, accessible volume. The text has been revised to take account of the latest developments in the field, some of the old chapters have been deleted and new ones have been added. The illustrations have been selected to offer a comprehensive distillation of the original textbook.

Ruggero Caputo
Carlo Gelmetti

ACKNOWLEDGEMENTS

We would like to thank Gianluca Tadini for revising the chapters on genodermatosis. In particular, our thanks go to Bernard Ackerman for his generosity in allowing us to use his unique collection of histological images. We also wish to thank Dr R. Gianotti for the new histological slides, Professor G.H. Findlay and Dr L. Smith, who provided clinical photographs of black children, and Professor Y.K. Zhao, who contributed all the pictures of Asian children.

ACANTHOSIS NIGRICANS

Acanthosis nigricans manifests itself as dark, soft plaques with papillated surfaces. It has a predilection for the flexures. It may develop *de novo* or in response to a variety of systemic disorders.

EPIDEMIOLOGY

Acanthosis nigricans is rare in children and usually develops after infancy.

CLINICAL FINDINGS

The earliest change – tan, dark brown or black pigmentation with accentuation of skin markings – typically affects the axillae, the back and sides of the neck (Fig. 1.1), the groin (Fig. 1.2), the perineum and the antecubital fossae. The plaques may be studded by acrochordon-like excrescencies of different sizes. Acanthosis nigricans involves the oral cavity in nearly half of the patients; more rarely it involves the anogenital mucosa (see Fig. 1.2).

LABORATORY FINDINGS

Children with acanthosis nigricans may have overt diabetes.

HISTOPATHOLOGICAL FINDINGS

All forms of acanthosis nigricans are characterized by marked papillomatosis (see Figs 1.3 and 1.4) (i.e. dermal papillae that project above the surface of the contiguous normal skin). The epidermis is thinned rather than acanthotic, and it is usually only slightly hyperpigmented.

ETIOLOGY AND PATHOGENESIS

Acanthosis nigricans is probably caused by activation of receptors for specific growth factors (e.g. insulin-like growth factors, epidermal growth factors) on the surface of keratinocytes. The traditional subdivision of acanthosis nigricans into a 'benign' form (not associated with any other disorder and occasionally familial), a 'malignant' form (paraneoplastic acanthosis nigricans), a 'syndromal' form (associated with endocrine disorders), a 'pseudo' form (in obese people) and a 'drug-induced' form is as incorrect pathophysiologially as it is morphologically. In fact, all forms of acanthosis nigricans have the same clinical and histopathological features.

COURSE

The course of acanthosis nigricans depends entirely on whether there is an underlying disease and, if there is, on its nature.

MANAGEMENT

The treatment is symptomatic. Underlying disorders should be treated as appropriate.

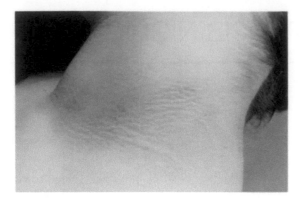

Figure 1.1
Acanthosis nigricans. Grey–brown papillated lesions situated between accentuation of normal skin creases on the neck.

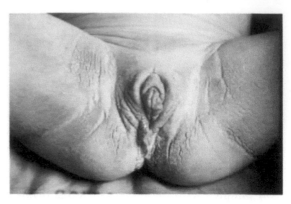

Figure 1.2
Acanthosis nigricans. Seip–Lawrence syndrome (generalized lipodystropy, diabetes mellitus, muscular hypertrophy, acromegaloid facies and early bone maturation). Prominent, brownish, confluent papillations accentuate the normal skin markings. The clitoris is hypertrophied.

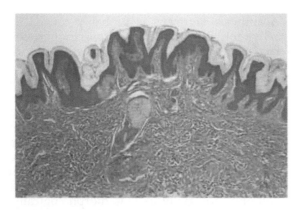

Figures 1.3 and 1.4
Acanthosis nigricans. Thin papillations are covered by cornified cells in a 'basket-weave' configuration. They are further characterized by thinned epidermis, thinned elongated dermal papillae and slight epidermal hyperpigmentation.

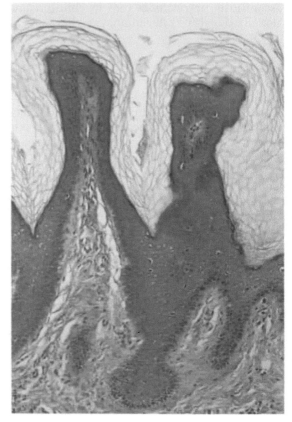

Figure 1.4

ACNEIFORM DISORDERS

Acne is an extremely common disorder of the folliculosebaceous unit. It may occur in the first year of life (acne neonatorum and acne infantum), but it is predominantly a disease of the second decade of life (acne vulgaris). Less frequent acneiform disorders are acne fulminans, drug-induced acne and chloracne.

ACNE VULGARIS

CLINICAL FINDINGS

The lesions of acne are polymorphic:

- comedones may be open ('blackheads') or closed ('whiteheads') (Fig. 2.1);
- papules with or without inflammation (Fig. 2.2);
- pustules caused by suppurative folliculitis (see Fig. 2.2, Fig. 2.3);
- nodules that develop after rupture of comedones or follicular cysts (see Fig. 2.3).

One type of lesion may predominate.
The face, back, chest and shoulders are common sites.

COMPLICATIONS

Complications of acneiform disorders include:

- scars, which may be depressed or hypertrophic;
- excoriations induced by emotional factors;
- coalescence of nodules, cysts and abscesses with formation of interconnecting channels and sinus tracts (acne conglobata);

- post-inflammatory hyperpigmentation.

ETIOLOGY AND PATHOGENESIS

The clinical variety of lesions that typify acne result from an interplay of factors, such as:

- altered cornification of follicular infundibula;
- increased and altered secretion of sebum;
- proliferation of bacteria within infundubula;
- increased androgen activity.

COURSE

The course of acne is unpredictable. The lesions usually begin to decline at about the age of 20 years.

HISTOPATHOLOGICAL FINDINGS

Open comedones are follicular infundibula that have become widely dilated because of plugging with a markedly increased number of orthokeratotic cornified cells (Fig. 2.7).

Closed comedones are tiny infundibular cysts that are filled with cornified cells, sebum and micro-organisms (Fig. 2.8).

Pustules are collections of neutrophils that fill widened follicular infundibula.

Inflammatory papules and nodules are suppurative granulomatous inflammation resulting from ruptured infundibular cysts (Fig. 2.9).

MANAGEMENT

Topical therapy

Topical treatments include:

- benzoyl peroxide (2.5%, 5% or 10%);
- retinoids (mainly for comedonic acne);
- antibiotics (clindamycin or erythromycin);
- azelaic acid.

Systemic therapy

Systemic treatments include:

- isotretinoin (0.5–1 mg/kg per day for 4–6 months for severe cases; 0.5 mg/kg per day for the first week of the month for 4–6 months for moderate cases);
- antibiotics (tetracycline, doxycycline, minocycline or erythromycin).

ACNE NEONATORUM AND ACNE INFANTUM

Acne neonatorum occurs before the third month of life.

The eruption of acne neonatorum and acne infantum is usually limited to a few comedones, papules or pustules, but in infants the lesions may be numerous (Fig. 2.4).The condition is believed to result from stimulation of fetal sebaceous glands by maternal hormones.

ACNE FULMINANS

Acne fulminans is seen exclusively in teenage boys. It is characterized by an explosive onset of large, reddish, exquisitely tender papules and nodules on the back and chest (Fig. 2.5). Ulceration ensues rapidly. The youth is febrile and complains of pain in the muscles or joints. Osteolytic lesions are sometimes present at sites of tenderness. Systemic corticosteroids and antibiotics must be initiated immediately if the process is to be brought under control.

DRUG-INDUCED ACNE

Topical and systemic corticosteroids, androgens, iodides, bromides, rifampicin (rifampin), isoniazid, phenobarbital, diphenylhydantoin and lithium carbonate have all been reported as causes of acneiform eruptions. The lesions in drug-induced acne consist of reddish papules and small pustules. Comedones and cystic nodules are rare.

CHLORACNE

Children exposed to dioxin for short periods develop only a few comedones, whereas those exposed for longer periods develop keratotic papules, large pustules, nodules and cysts, especially on the face (Fig. 2.6). Histopathologically, the lesions of chloracne show infundibula and eccrine ducts plugged by cornified cells and typical features of a suppurative folliculitis (Fig. 2.10).

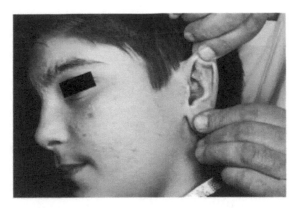

Figure 2.1
Acne vulgaris. There are numerous comedones on the ear, cheek, forehead and nose.

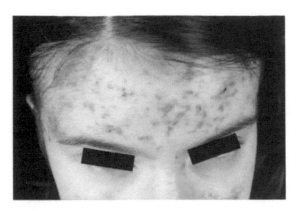

Figure 2.2

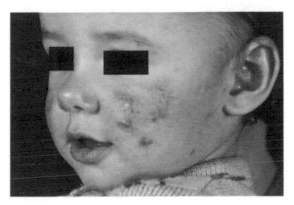

Figure 2.4
Acne infantum. Reddish papules and pustules coexist with atrophic scars.

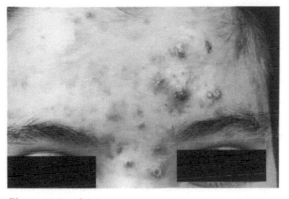

Figures 2.2 and 2.3
Acne vulgaris. The foreheads of the two girls are covered by typical lesions (comedones and pustules), on which are yellowish and hemorrhagic crusts.

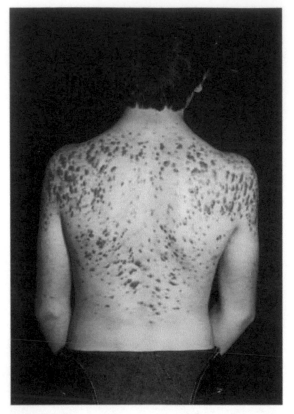

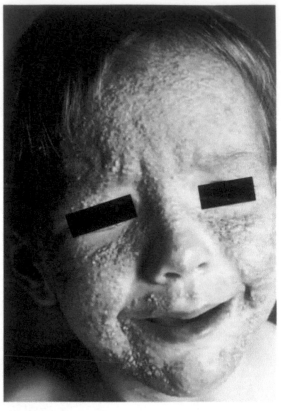

Figure 2.5
Acne fulminans. Widespread reddish papules and nodules are located in zones where sebaceous glands are most numerous. Each large lesion represents suppurative granulomatous inflammation in response to rupture of an infundibular cyst.

Figure 2.6
Chloracne. Diffuse involvement of comedones, papules and pustules, many of which are topped by crusts.

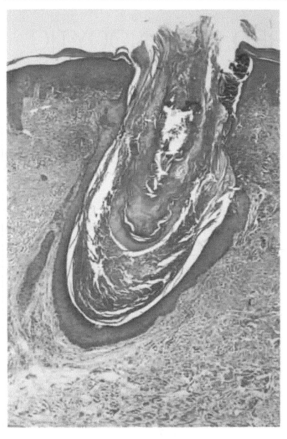

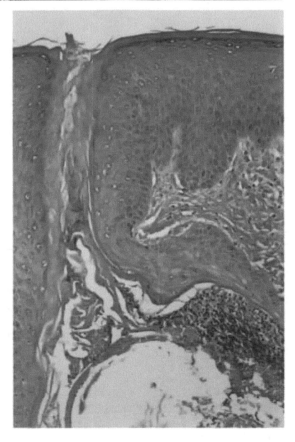

Figure 2.7
Acne vulgaris. Open comedones are simply follicular infundibula that have become widely dilated because of plugging by a markedly increased number of orthokeratotic cornified cells, which are arranged in laminated and compact fashion.

Fig. 2.9
Acne vulgaris showing suppurative folliculitis. There is an abscess within the dilated follicular infundibulum, with rupture of the infundibular epithelium.

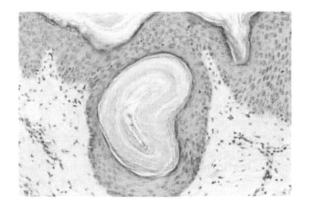

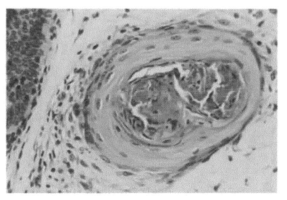

Figure 2.8
Acne vulgaris. Closed comedones are tiny infundibular cysts filled by cornified cells and sebum.

Figure 2.10
Chloracne. An eccrine dermal duct plugged by cornified cells.

3

ACQUIRED MELANOCYTIC NEVI

UNNA'S NEVI

CLINICAL FINDINGS

Unna's nevi are skin-colored or brown, soft, pedunculated or sessile lesions. They are sometimes papillomatous excrescences (Fig. 3.1). They often cannot be differentiated clinically from acrochordons. They are uncommon in children.

HISTOPATHOLOGICAL FINDINGS

Histology shows pedunculated or sessile lesion with nests, cords and strands of melanocytes within a markedly thickened exophytic papillary dermis. Some nests of melanocytes may be present at the dermoepidermal junction.

MIESCHER'S NEVI

CLINICAL FINDINGS

Miescher's nevi are globoid, smooth-surfaced, skin-colored or tan papules. They are almost always found on the face. Like Unna's nevi, they are uncommon in children.

HISTOPATHOLOGICAL FINDINGS

Histology shows dome-shaped nevi. They are usually intradermal but they may be compound. A wedge-shaped array of usually small, round melanocytes extend into the reticular dermis and occasionally into the subcutaneous fat (Fig. 3.2).

SPITZ'S NEVI

CLINICAL FINDINGS

Spitz's nevi are dome-shaped, smooth, firm, hairless, nodules. They are usually less than 10 mm in diameter. They are usually pink or red in color, but they may be tan, brown or even black. Spitz's nevi are usually solitary and favor the face, but they may occur anywhere on the integument (Figs 3.3 and 3.4). One-third of patients are aged under 10 years.

HISTOPATHOLOGICAL FINDINGS

Spitz's nevi are characterized by melanocytes with large nuclei and usually with abundant amphophilic cytoplasm and round, oval, polygonal or spindle shapes. Multinucleated or mononuclear giant melanocytes are commonly seen. Spitz's nevi evolve through junctional compound and intradermal stages. Junctional and compound types may show hyperkeratosis, hypergranulosis and the presence of dull, pink globules (Kamino bodies) within the epidermis (Figs 3.5 and 3.6).

CLARK'S NEVI

CLINICAL FINDINGS

Clark's nevi are often small, symmetrical, well-circumscribed macules or papules. They usually have a relatively uniform dark brownish color centrally with a lighter brown color peripherally. Occasionally they may be large (more than 10 mm in diameter), asymmetrical with scalloped or notched borders and variegated in shades of brown. Sites of predilection are the trunk and proximal part of extremities. Clark's nevi are the commonest type of acquired nevi (Fig. 3.7).

HISTOPATHOLOGICAL FINDINGS

Clark's nevi may be junctional, compound or intradermal. In junctional nevi, there are nests of melanocytes at the dermoepidermal junction. In compound nevi, nests of melanocytes at the dermoepidermal junction extend for some rete ridges beyond nests of melanocytes in the papillary dermis. In intradermal nevi, nests of melanocytes are in a thickened papillary dermis. Melanocytes tend to be small and oval and monomorphous (Fig. 3.8).

SUTTON'S NEVI

CLINICAL FINDINGS

Sutton's nevi (or halo nevi) are simply a distinctive variant of Clark's nevi around which a rim of depigmentation begins and extends centrifugally. The nevus is centrally located and eventually tends to disappear (in months or years) Sutton's nevi occur mainly on the trunk (Fig. 3.9).

HISTOPATHOLOGICAL FINDINGS

Histology shows a junctional or compound nevus surrounded by a lymphocytic infiltrate (Fig. 3.10).

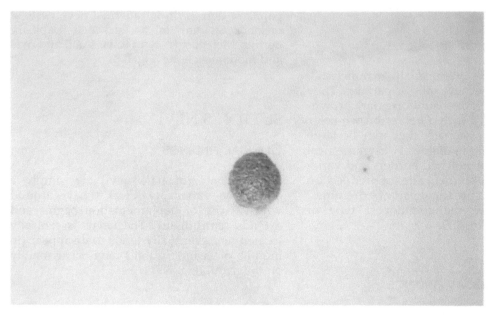

Figure 3.1
Unna's nevus. This papillomatous lesion is composed largely of nests, cords and strands of melanocytes in the dermis.

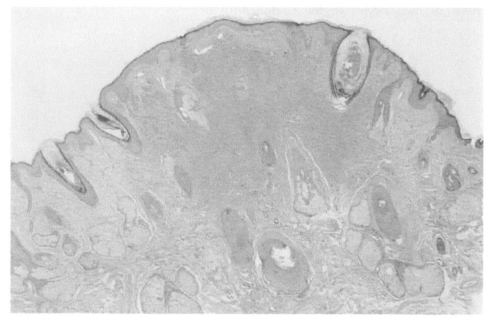

Figure 3.2
Miescher's nevus. This domed nevus is characterized by orderly nests, cords and strands of melanocytes that extend throughout the reticular dermis.

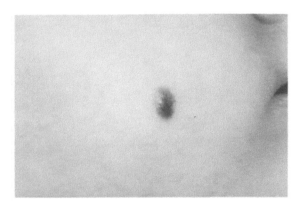

Figure 3.3
Spitz's nevus. The lesion is small, symmetrical, well circumscribed, smooth-surfaced and uniformly brown–red in color.

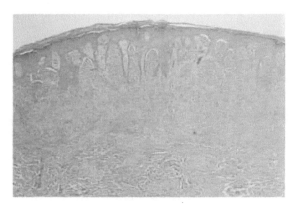

Figure 3.5

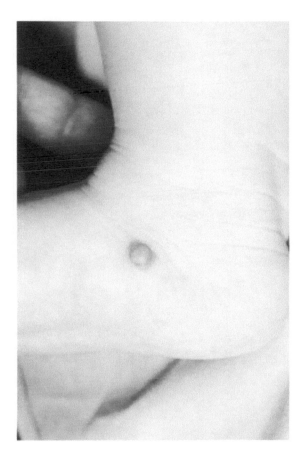

Figure 3.4
Spitz's nevus. The lesion is small, and the central dome-shaped portion is symmetrical. It is relatively well circumscribed, slightly scaly and pinkish red in color.

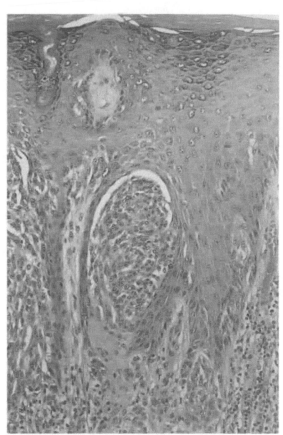

Figures 3.5 and 3.6
Spitz's nevus, compound type. In addition to epidermal and dermal oval-shaped melanocytes with relatively large nuclei, there is hyperkeratosis, hypergranulosis, irregular epidermal hyperplasia, clefts between elongated nests of melanocytes and surrounding keratinocytes, and dull pink globules (Kamino bodies) within the epidermis.

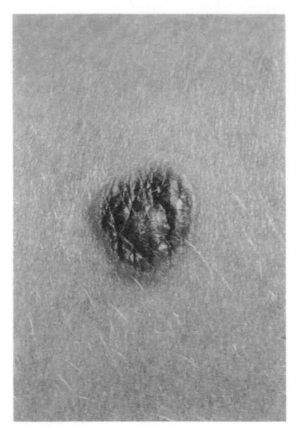

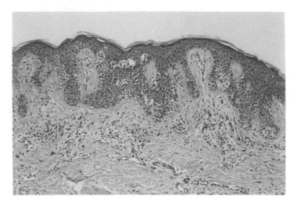

Figure 3.8
Clark's nevus, compound type. This nevus is characterized by nests of melanocytes at the dermoepidermal junction and in a thickened papillary dermis.

Figure 3.7
Clark's nevus. This lesion is benign because it is relatively small, symmetrical and well circumscribed, and its skin markings are preserved. Note a tan rim around a darker centre. These are the clinical features of a very common type of nevus, a 'dysplastic' nevus.

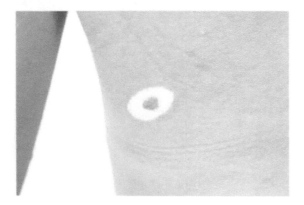

Figure 3.9
Sutton's nevus. In the center, a pigmented Clark's nevus is surrounded by a zone of depigmentation. This constellation of features is that of a 'halo' nevus.

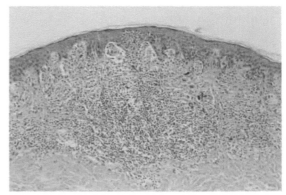

Figure 3.10
Sutton's nevus. This is a Sutton's nevus because of the dense infiltrate of lymphocytes that obscures much of the nevus.

4

ACRODERMATITIS ENTEROPATHICA

Acrodermatitis enteropathica is a rare autosomal-recessive disease caused by a deficiency of zinc. It is characterized by protean signs, including orificial and acral dermatitis, diarrhea and alopecia. These symptoms become evident during infancy by the time the child is weaned.

CLINICAL FINDINGS

The earliest signs of acrodermatitis enteropathica in an infant are lack of interest in feeding, apathy and irritability. Typically, there are crops of vesicles and pustules that often appear around body orifices. In time, these become reddish, psoriasiform plaques covered by scaly crusts (Fig. 4.1). Concurrent with these signs are alopecia of the eyebrows, eyelashes and scalp (Fig. 4.2), severe persistent diarrhea and cachexia. Nail changes include irregular transverse ridges, onychodystrophy, onycholysis and paronychia that becomes chronic. Blepharitis, conjunctivitis and photophobia may also occur.

LABORATORY FINDINGS

Low plasma zinc levels (less than 500 mg/dl) are found in acrodermatitis enteropathica.

HISTOPATHOLOGICAL FINDINGS

Features of well-established lesions are parakeratosis, hypogranulosis, marked ballooning of keratinocytes in the upper part of the epidermis and a sparse, superficial perivascular infiltrate of lymphocytes (Figs 4.3 and 4.4).

ETIOLOGY AND PATHOGENESIS

Acrodermatitis enteropathica results from a poor absorption of zinc from the intestine. The cause of the malabsorption is not yet known. It may be due to an inadequate pancreatic secretion of a ligand that binds to zinc in the intestinal lumen and transports the zinc into the mucosa. The cutaneous and systemic features of the disease are the consequence of the zinc deficiency, since zinc is an indispensable constituent of more than 200 metalloenzymes.

MANAGEMENT

Elemental zinc, 5 mg/kg per day, given as zinc sulfate, zinc gluconate, or zinc dipicolinate, produces a dramatic disappearance of the signs and symptoms of acrodermatitis enteropathica. Diarrhea stops within 1 day. The child's mood improves in 1–2 days. Skin lesions clear in 1–2 weeks. Within 1 month, there is marked improvement in body growth and hair growth.

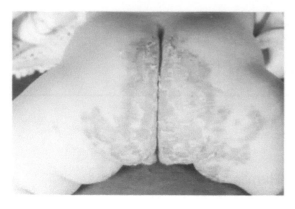

Figure 4.1
Acrodermatitis enteropathica. Discrete violaceous papules and well-circumscribed, brownish plaques are covered by prominent scales and crusts. The lesions are psoriasiform and typically located around body orifices.

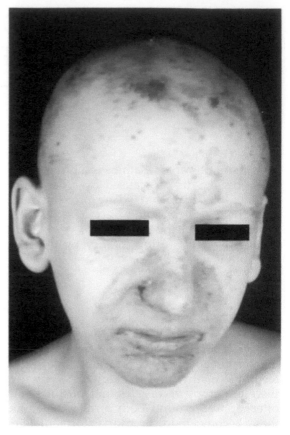

Figure 4.2
Acrodermatitis enteropathica. Pustules, erosions, scales and crusts are present around the nose and the mouth. Note the extensive blepharitis and patchy alopecia.

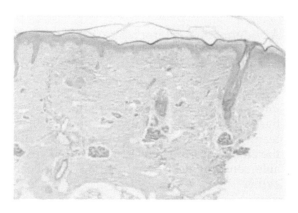

Figure 4.3

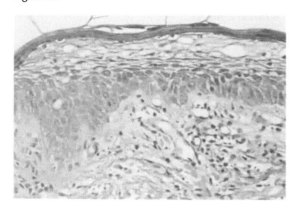

Figure 4.4

Figures 4.3 and 4.4
Acrodermatitis enteropathica. The characteristic features consist of marked ballooning of keratinocytes and slight spongiosis in the upper half of the epidermis, associated with epidermal necrosis. The severe ballooning causes reticular alteration, a net-like appearance of the epidermis formed by membranes of swollen necrotic cells.

ACUTE HEMORRHAGIC EDEMA OF INFANCY

Acute hemorrhagic edema of infancy (AHEI) (Finkelstein's disease) is a distinctive expression of leukocytoclastic vasculitis. It is characterized by tender edema and rosette-shaped purpuric lesions that resolve without treatment.

CLINICAL FINDINGS

The onset of AHEI is acute and marked by fever, exquisitely tender symmetric edematous foci on the face and extremities (Figs 5.1 and 5.2), and, subsequently, the rapid development of a characteristic purpuric eruption within areas of pre-existing edema. Lesions begin as edematous papules with central petechiae that expand centrifugally to form three distinct zones – a central hemorrhagic crust surrounded by a pale palpable annulus which, in turn, is rimmed by redness that blanches on pressure. These rosette-like lesions may become confluent to form purpuric patches and plaques that assume nummular, arciform or polycyclic shapes. Lesions appear in crops and, at any given time, they may be in different stages of development. Sites of predilection are the face, the upper part of the trunk and the arms.

The infant seems to be in great distress and may cry incessantly. Aside from warmth caused by fever and the skin lesions, the physical examination is normal. Despite the impressive lesions, the course is uneventful; and resolution occurs spontaneously in 1–3 weeks, with post-inflammatory pigmentary changes. Recurrences have never been reported.

Age of onset

AHEI is a rare disease of newborns, but children up to 2 years of age may be affected. The disease occurs mostly during winter, after an upper respiratory tract infection.

LABORATORY FINDINGS

Elevated erythrocyte sedimentation rate, leukocytosis (lymphocytic or polymorphonuclear) and elevated alpha-2 globulin may be present. There is no hematuria.

HISTOPATHOLOGICAL FINDINGS

Early in the course of the disease, there is a superficial and deep, perivascular and interstitial infiltrate composed mostly of neutrophils and of abundant nuclear 'dust' (Figs 5.3 and 5.4). Later, the neutrophil infiltrate becomes denser, and deposits of fibrin are present in the walls of some venules. In sum, the histological changes of AHEI are those of leukocytoclastic vasculitis.

ETIOLOGY AND PATHOGENESIS

The cause of AHEI is unknown. The increased frequency of the disease during winter and its association with upper respiratory tract infections (and also vaccinations) suggest that this special expression of leukocytoclastic vasculitis is mediated by immune complexes generated in response to infectious agents.

MANAGEMENT

No treatment is required.

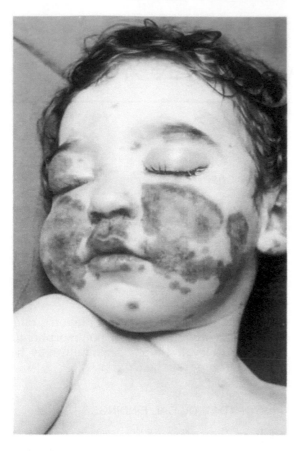

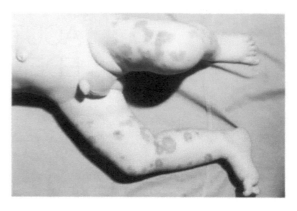

Figure 5.2
Acute hemorrhagic edema of infancy. Rust-colored macules, papules and plaques are present on the legs. Some of the plaques have an arciform configuration, others are arranged in concentric sign and still others have a scalloped appearance. The rust color is a consequence of extravasation of erythrocytes in the upper part of the dermis.

Figure 5.1
Acute hemorrhagic edema of infancy. Papules and plaques with slightly elevated, scalloped borders have a deep red and purple color. The eyelids are edematous.

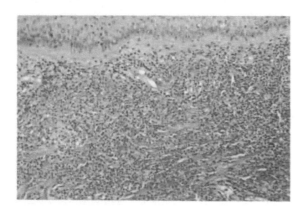

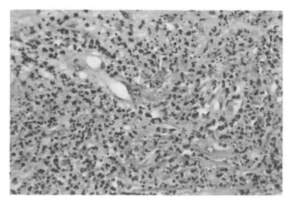

Figure 5.3   **Figure 5.4**

Figures 5.3 and 5.4
Acute hemorrhagic edema of infancy. Photomicrographs illustrating a fully developed lesion of leukocytoclastic vasculitis.

ALOPECIA AREATA

Alopecia areata is a common disorder characterized by well-circumscribed patches of hair loss from any part of the body, but especially from the scalp (Fig. 6.1). If there is loss of hair from the entire scalp, the condition is called alopecia totalis (Fig. 6.2), and is there is loss of hair from the entire body, it is called alopecia universalis. The disease usually begins at about 4–5 years of age. A positive family history is obtained in 10–20% of patients (see Fig. 6.2).

CLINICAL FINDINGS

The onset of alopecia areata is sudden. There are no symptoms other than loss of hair. Lesions consist of well-circumscribed, round or oval patches that are either completely devoid of hair or have little of it. The lesions are usually situated on the scalp, but they may be present on any part of the body that bears hair. The skin in these zones is smooth and, in Caucasians, ivory–white. A feature considered pathognomonic for alopecia areata is 'exclamation point' hairs. These are short stumps of hair that are broad at their distal end and very narrow at their proximal end (hence the analogy to an exclamation point). Exclamation point hairs are found most readily at the margins of lesions.

Alopecia areata may be estimated to be active if, when hairs are pulled at the margin of a lesion, more than five or six hairs come out in one tug. The initial patch of alopecia areata may remain solitary and enlarge centrifugally, or new patches may appear and become confluent.

Ophiasis refers to a clinical form of alopecia areata that occurs mainly in children and consists of a patch of alopecia that begins in the occipital region and extends in a band around the base of the scalp.

When the hair regrows, usually in the center of the patches, new hairs are thin and often white or gray. Recurrences are frequent. Dystrophy of the nail plate is seen in 10–20% of patients.

Associations

Autoimmune diseases such as vitiligo, pernicious anemia, Hashimoto's thyroiditis, diabetes mellitus, and Addison's disease are more common in patients with alopecia areata than in the rest of the population

LABORATORY FINDINGS

There is increased likelihood of detecting thyroid microsomal and thyroglobulin antibodies as well as antibodies against gastric parietal cells and smooth muscle cells in patients with alopecia areata.

HISTOPATHOLOGICAL FINDINGS

Early in the course of alopecia areata there are infiltrates of lymphocytes around hair follicle bulbs in the anagenic phase. Later, whorls of collagen bundles that contain degenerated glassy membranes appear at sites where follicular papillae have been bared during catagen or at its onset (Figs 6.3 and 6.4).

ETIOLOGY AND PATHOGENESIS

The cause of alopecia areata is not known. The increased incidence of autoimmune disorders in association with alopecia areata suggests that it is an autoimmune disease sustained by antibodies against the hair bulbs.

MANAGEMENT

No curative treatments are currently available. The most popular agents for management of alopecia areata are corticosteroids. Children with very localized alopecia can be treated with topical corticosteroids applied twice a day. Intralesional injections must be avoided. If there is no response to this therapy or the disease is widespread, an induction of allergic contact dermatitis with diphencyprone or squaric acid dibutylester may be attempted. Psychotherapy may be a very important support.

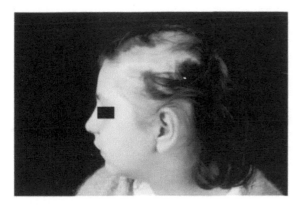

Figure 6.1
Alopecia areata. Patches have become confluent as a consequence of extreme involvement of the scalp. The circular patch of the occiput helps to differentiate this condition from trichotillomania. Note that the eyelashes and eyebrows are present.

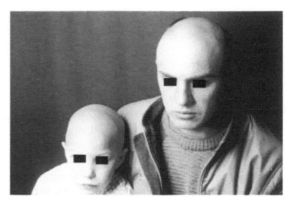

Figure 6.2
Familial alopecia totalis. All the hairs are missing from the scalp of this father and son. The eyebrows are present in both, but the eyelashes are missing in the son.

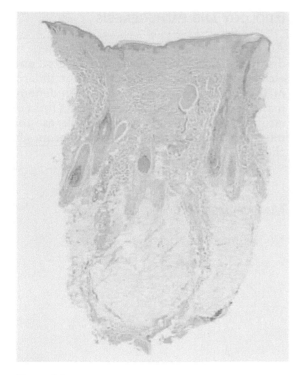

Figure 6.3

Figure 6.4

Figures 6.3 and 6.4
Alopecia areata. There are hair follicles in both anagen and catagen. The follicles are thinned and situated wholly in the dermis rather than rooted in the normal position for follicles on the scalp, namely in the subcutaneous fat. Fibrous tracts are present beneath the follicles in catagen, and a moderately dense lymphohistiocytic infiltrate is present around the bulbs. The latter is a *sine qua non* for diagnosis of active lesions of alopecia areata.

ANETODERMA

Anetoderma is a specific type of cutaneous atrophy that develops secondary to inflammatory processes. It is marked by circumscribed areas of thin, soft, wrinkled skin that usually bulge above the regular surface of the skin, although they may be slightly depressed (Fig. 7.1).

EPIDEMIOLOGY

Anetoderma is rare and may be familial. The onset is usually in the first or second decade of life.

CLINICAL FINDINGS

The typical lesions vary in size from less than 1 mm to a few centimeters (see Figs 7.1, 7.2). The number, site and distribution of the lesions depend on the nature of the primary process. The sites most commonly involved are the arms, the neck, the chest and the upper part of the back. The atrophic skin does not ulcerate. Anetoderma persists once it has developed.

HISTOPATHOLOGICAL FINDINGS

The dominant pathological findings are a focal alteration and loss of collagen (Fig. 7.3) and the absence of elastic fibers (Fig. 7.4) in the middle and upper parts of the reticular dermis.

ETIOLOGY AND PATHOGENESIS

Anetoderma is an end-stage of a variety of disorders that cause loss of collagen and elastic tissue. Release of enzymes from inflammatory cells seems to be the common denominator for development of this distinct form of atrophy. Acne vulgaris and varicella are the most frequent causes of anetoderma in children.

MANAGEMENT

No treatment has been successful.

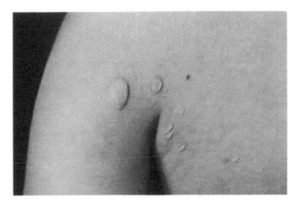

Figure 7.1
Anetoderma. These skin-colored papules and plaques are herniated easily into the subcutaneous fat by slight pressure. This process doubtlessly began as an inflammation, but its precise nature cannot be defined.

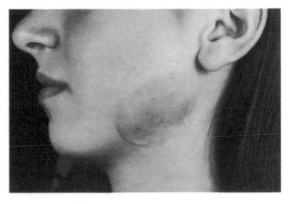

Figure 7.2
Anetoderma. This sagging plaque fulfils the criteria for cutaneous atrophy because the skin wrinkles easily in both the hypopigmented and the hyperpigmented areas, and it is covered by numerous telangiectases. An atrophic lesion such as this was once a long-standing inflammatory plaque.

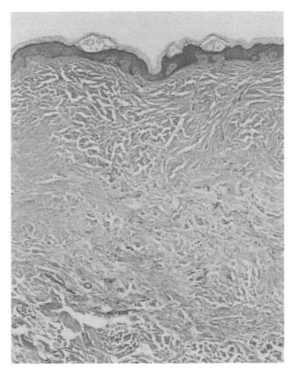

Figure 7.3
Anetoderma. The collagen in the middle part of the reticular dermis is different from the normal skin in terms of thickness and orientation. The collagen bundles are thinner and less parallel to the skin surface. (Hematoxylin and eosin stain.)

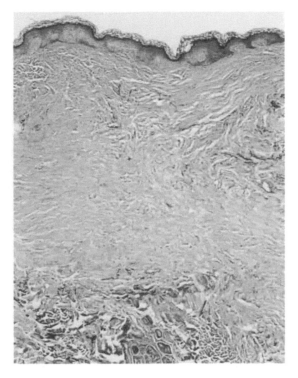

Figure 7.3
Anetoderma. This section stained with elastic tissue stain confirms that the abnormal zone is in the middle part of the reticular dermis, where the elastic fibers are markedly decreased in number.

8 ANGIOBLASTOMA

Cutaneous angioblastoma of Nakagawa is a rare, benign, vascular neoplasm composed mostly of immature endothelial cells.

EPIDEMIOLOGY

Angioblastoma is an uncommon tumor that chiefly affects prepubertal children.

CLINICAL FINDINGS

The earliest sign of angioblastoma is a poorly demarcated pink or red macule or patch. This soon evolves into a deep red, blue or purple indurated plaque (Fig. 8.1) or a cluster of nodules and tumors of similar color. Lesions are often painful. Tenderness is acknowledged by about 90% of patients. The neoplasm is almost always solitary, and the sites of predilection, in descending order of frequency, are the neck, trunk, extremities and head. The neoplasm neither metastasizes nor regresses without treatment, but it usually persists. The well-being of the patient is unaffected.

HISTOPATHOLOGICAL FINDINGS

Lobules of plump oval cells are aligned along pre-existing vascular plexuses in the dermis and sometimes in the subcutaneous fat. Many of these cells surround tiny lumina of vessels that resemble capillaries (Figs. 8.2 and 8.3).

MANAGEMENT

Complete surgical excision is the best treatment. Therapy with soft X-rays has also been reported to be effective.

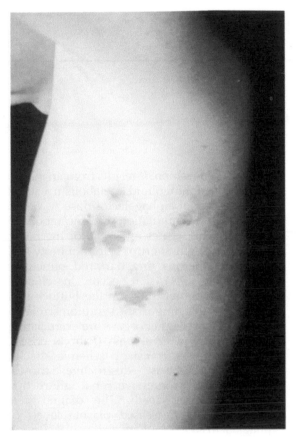

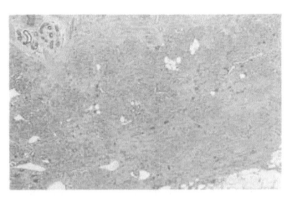

Figure 8.2

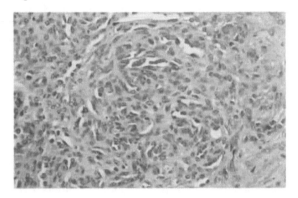

Figure 8.3

Figure 8.1
Angioblastoma. Numerous red plaques of various sizes with shapes and scalloped borders can be seen.

Figures 8.2 and 8.3
Angioblastoma. In the lower half of the dermis and in the upper part of subcutaneous fat there are clusters of numerous, closely crowded, small blood vessels lined by plump oval endothelial cells.

ANGIOKERATOMA

Angiokeratomas are vascular lesions with keratotic elements. They appear clinically as dark red to black papules covered by scales. Angiokeratomas may be subdivided into localized types (angiokeratoma of Mibelli, angiokeratoma of Fordyce, angiokeratoma circumscriptum) and widespread types (Fabry's disease).

CLINICAL FINDINGS

Angiokeratoma of Mibelli consists of typical red to purple, keratotic, asymptomatic papules of 2–5 mm diameter, situated over bony prominences such as the dorsa of fingers and toes (Fig. 9.1), elbows and knees. This rare type of angiokeratoma begins in childhood or early adolescence and persists for life. It occurs mostly in females.

Angiokeratoma of Fordyce is the commonest of all the angiokeratomas. It is characterized by dome-shaped reddish–purple papules of 2–4 mm in diameter, situated on the scrotum (Fig. 9.2) or vulva. If traumatized, angiokeratomas of Fordyce may bleed profusely because the venules that they comprise are superficial.

Angiokeratoma circumscriptum is the least common type of all the angiokeratomas. It presents as a large, solitary, linear, unilateral plaque composed of verrucous dark red to black papules that have become confluent (Fig. 9.3). Half of the lesions reported on have had their onset in infancy, and some were present at birth. With age, angiokeratoma circumscriptum tends to increase in size and become increasingly keratotic. There is no tendency to involution.

Angiokeratoma corporis diffusum (Fabry's disease) is a rare genetic disorder transmitted in an X-linked fashion. It results from an inborn error of glycophingolipid metabolism caused by a deficiency of alphagalactosidase A, which leads to an accumulation of uncatabolized ceramide in all tissues and cells of the body. Skin lesions begin to erupt before puberty and consist of numerous, tiny, dark red, punctuate papules (Fig. 9.4) that occur in clusters distributed symmetrically on the buttock and thighs. In males, important symptoms related to involvement of other organs are excruciating episodic crises of acral pain (Fabry's crises), acral paresthesias, transient ischemic attacks, systemic thrombosis, destructive corneal dystrophy and progressive renal failure that ultimately causes death. The diagnosis is confirmed from decreased plasma levels of alphagalactosidase A.

HISTOPATHOLOGICAL FINDINGS

The common denominators of the angiokeratomas (Fig. 9.5) are:

- focal compact orthokeratosis of variable degree;
- widely dilated, thin-walled, endothelium-lined blood vessels in the upper part of the dermis;
- a thin zone of collagen that separates the dilated blood vessels from the epidermis.

MANAGEMENT

Angiokeratomas may be treated by laser, cryosurgery, electrodesiccation with curettage, or surgical excision.

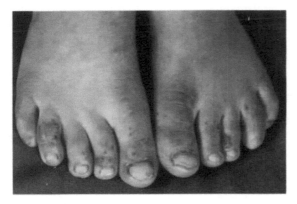

Figure 9.1
Angiokeratoma of Mibelli. Discrete reddish papules are situated on the toes. Some of the papules have become confluent and formed plaques.

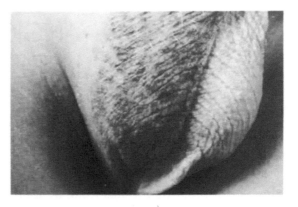

Figure 9.2
Angiokeratoma of Fordyce. Innumerable discrete and confluent, tiny reddish–purple macules and papules cover half of the scrotum.

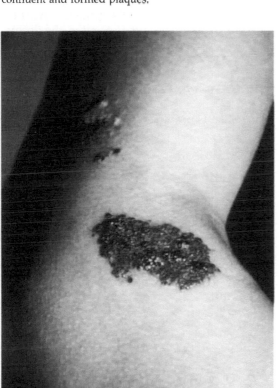

Figure 9.3
Angiokeratoma circumscriptum. This multicolored plaque has scalloped borders and is studded with pink, purple and black papules covered by scales. The combination of vascular proliferation and scales makes this an angiokeratoma.

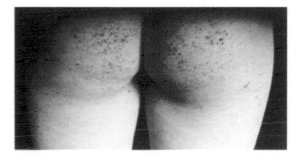

Figure 9.4
Angiokeratoma corporis diffusum (Fabry's disease). The buttocks are covered with rust colored and red–black macules and papules, each of which is an individual angiokeratoma. The distribution of lesions is typical.

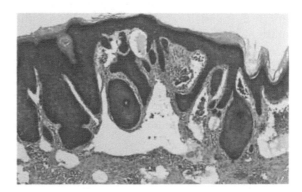

Figure 9.5
Angiokeratoma. The neoplasm is well circumscribed and is composed of widely dilated, blood-filled vessels. The epidermis is focally hyperplastic, hypergranulotic and hyperkeratotic.

10 ANGIOLYMPHOID HYPERPLASIA

Angiolymphoid hyperplasia is a distinctive vascular disorder that results from an arteriovenous shunt. It is often accompanied by infiltrates of lymphocytes and eosinophils.

EPIDEMIOLOGY

The condition may occur in young children and adolescents. Three-quarters of the patients are female.

CLINICAL FINDINGS

Angiolymphoid hyperplasia may consist of a single lesion (as it does in 80% of patients) or of many lesions. The lesions are dome-shaped, shiny, pink, purple or reddish–brown papules and nodules (Fig. 10.1), that are most commonly situated on the face, especially around the ears, and on the scalp. The lesions tend to persist. The general health of the patient is unaffected.

LABORATORY FINDINGS

Peripheral eosinophilia is present in less than 20% of patients.

HISTOPATHOLOGICAL FINDINGS

The lesion is well circumscribed and consists of widely dilated, thick-walled blood vessels lined by plump endothelial cells that protrude prominently into the lumens (Figs 10.2 and 10.3). Inflammatory cells (mostly lymphocytes) are nearly always present in the dermis.

ETIOLOGY AND PATHOGENESIS

The cause is not known.

MANAGEMENT

Injection of corticosteroids directly into lesions may be beneficial by causing them to resolve at least partially. If that fails, surgical excision is the treatment of choice. Other modalities, including cryotherapy, radiation therapy and laser therapy, have not been successful.

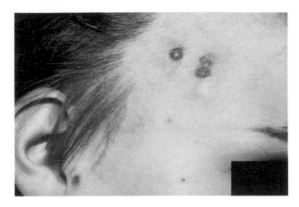

Figure 10.1
Angiolymphoid hyperplasia. Well-circumscribed, smooth-surfaced, pink–orange papules situated on the face.

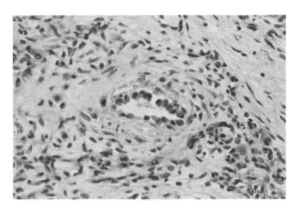

Figure 10.3   **Figure 10.2**

Figures 10.2 and 10.3
Angiolymphoid hyperplasia. Throughout the dermis there is an increased number of widely dilated, thick-walled blood vessels. Endothelial cells protrude far into the lumens.

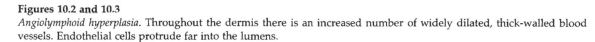

APLASIA CUTIS CONGENITA

Aplasia cutis congenita is a localized absence of skin. It is present at birth and occurs in about 1 in 10,000 newborns.

CLINICAL FINDINGS

Aplasia cutis congenita consists at first of one or more well-circumscribed ulcers with granulation tissue at the base (Fig. 11.1). The individual lesions may be round, oval or triangular. The commonest site is the midline of the scalp, usually near the vertex. The second commonest site is a lower limb. Any site, however, may be involved. Upon healing, defects are replaced by smooth white, gray or yellowish scars (Fig. 11.2).

Associations

Aplasia cutis congenita may be found in association with other developmental defects.

HISTOPATHOLOGICAL FINDINGS

Aplasia cutis congenita consists of ulcers that involve the dermis and sometimes the subcutaneous fat. The ulcers heal with scarring.

ETIOLOGY AND PATHOGENESIS

The cause of this disorder has yet to be established. Various factors, such as intrauterine injury, effects of a drug and viral diseases in the mother, have been implicated, but none has been proven to be a cause.

MANAGEMENT

Every attempt should be made to avoid trauma to the involved site. Local cleanliness can prevent secondary infection. If there is neither trauma nor secondary infection, the defects of the skin and of the underlying skull should heal in a few months.

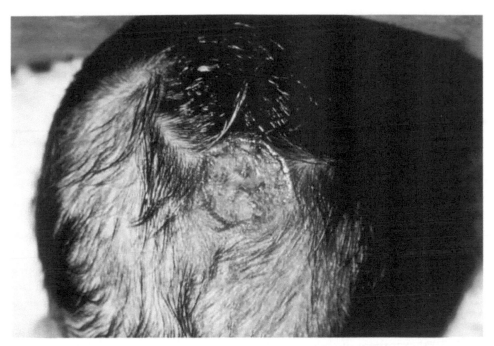

Figure 11.1
Aplasia cutis congenita. In a newborn, there is a round, sharply marginated ulcer surrounded by an elevated border.

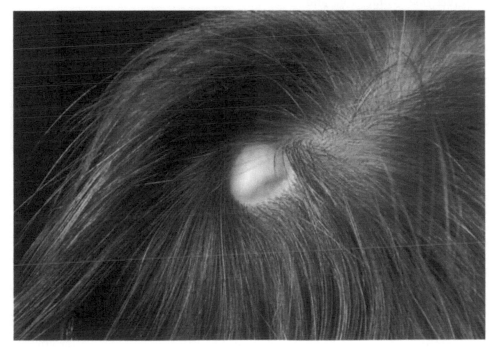

Figure 11.2
Aplasia cutis congenita. This smooth alopecic yellow–white scar can be determined to be long-standing because of these features and also because of the absence of pinkness.

12 ASYMMETRICAL PERIFLEXURAL EXANTHEM OF CHILDHOOD

Asymmetrical periflexural exanthem of childhood is an exanthem of unknown etiology that typically involves one axillary fold with central spread – this explains the term 'unilateral laterothoracic exanthem of childhood', which is used by some authors.

CLINICAL FINDINGS

Asymmetrical periflexural exanthem of childhood appears as either a maculopapular scarlatiniform eruption or an eczematiform dermatitis that involves one axillary fold and spreads centrally on to the thorax and proximal part of the corresponding arm (Figs 12.1 and 12.2). In a minority of patients, initial lesions develop around the antecubital or popliteal flexures; onset around distal flexures or on the face is rare.

The lesions tend to be confluent around the fold and become more sparse distally. Individual lesions can be purpuric. After 5–10 days, similar but smaller lesions appear on the contralateral side, and rarely the exanthem becomes more diffuse, with minor lesions elsewhere. The disease does not affect the general health but can be moderately pruriginous. Mild ipsilateral lymphadenopathy can be found in about 50% of cases.

Resolution with mild hyperpigmentation or pityriasis desquamation is noted in about 1 month.

The age of the patients is typically between the ages of 1 and 4 years, although adults can also be affected. The presence of small epidemics has been noted, and the condition is often associated with prodromal symptoms of an upper respiratory tract or digestive tract infection.

HISTOPATHOLOGICAL FINDINGS

Skin biopsy usually is non-contributory. Histology is non-specific, showing areas of epidermal spongiosis accompanied by exocytosis of mononuclear cells, while a moderate perivascular and periappendageal lymphohistiocytic infiltrate is present in the dermis.

ETIOLOGY AND PATHOGENESIS

The cause of asymmetrical periflexural exanthem of childhood is presently unknown. However, the features in favor of a viral origin for the condition are numerous – the age of the patients, the presence of small epidemics, the frequency of associated prodromes, the spontaneous resolution in a few weeks, the regional lymphadenopathy, the lack of response to antibiotics and topical corticosteroids. The possible causative role of parvovirus B19 is anecdotal.

MANAGEMENT

Treatment is not necessary is most instances. Symptomatic oral antihistamines and nonsteroidal lenitive creams can be prescribed when necessary. Topical corticosteroids are not effective.

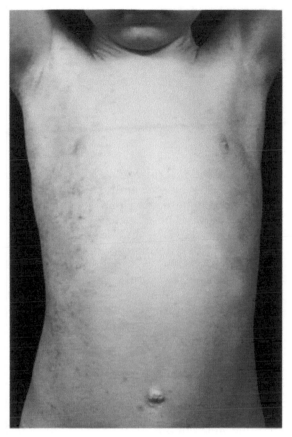

Figure 12.1
Asymmetrical periflexural exanthem of childhood. A maculopapular scarlatiniform eruption involves the right axillary fold of this child, with spread on to the thorax and proximal inner part of the correspinding arm. A cluster of lesions is also present on the hip.

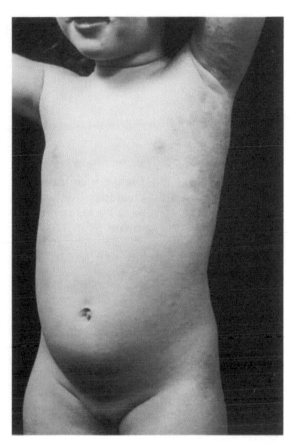

Figure 12.2
Asymmetrical periflexural exanthem of childhood. In this infant the rash is more eczematiform and involves the left side of the body. It affects the same sites as the patient shown in Fig. 12.1.

13   ATOPIC DERMATITIS

Atopic dermatitis is a disease of children with personal or family histories of allergic urticaria, allergic rhinitis or allergic asthma. It results from severely pruritic skin.

EPIDEMIOLOGY

Atopic dermatitis is a common disorder that affects about 3% of all infants. Symptoms of the disease may be noted shortly after birth and they appear by the first year in 60% of patients.

CLINICAL FINDINGS

Findings in atopic dermatitis vary with age. Acute skin lesions consist of erythematous patches of intensely pruritic papules and hints of vesicles that ooze and become crusted (Figs 13.1, 13.2 and 13.3). These lesions may appear first on the face, with sparing of the perioral and perinasal skin (see Fig. 13.1); later the extremities, dorsa of the hands (see Fig. 13.2) and flexures (see Fig. 13.3) are involved.

Chronic skin lesions consist of thickening of the skin with accentuation of skin markings (lichenification) as a consequence of persistent rubbing (Figs 13.4, 13.5 and 13.6). These lesions usually affect children over the age of 3 years. They often involve the popliteal and antecubital fossae, the ankles, the wrists and the sides of the neck.

Stigmata of atopic dermatitis include dry skin and characteristic creases on the lower eyelids (Dennie–Morgan sign). Special features are represented by pityriasis alba and juvenile plantar dermatosis. Pityriasis alba is characterized by several round, asymptomatic, hypopigmented patches covered by subtle scales. These patches are mainly confined to the face and limbs (Fig. 13.7). Juvenile plantar dermatosis is characterized by redness, scaling and painful fissures on weight-bearing parts of the feet (Fig 13.8).

Atopic dermatitis is long-lasting with exacerbations and remissions. A spontaneous, more or less complete remission during childhood is the rule.

Associations

Asthma and allergic rhinitis occur in about 30% of patients, cataract in 10%, ichthyosis vulgaris and keratosis pilaris in 5%. Alopecia areata and defective polymorphonuclear chemotactic activity each occur in less than 1% of patients.

COMPLICATIONS

The most common complication is secondary infection by *Staphylococcus aureus* and herpes simplex virus (eczema herpeticum).

LABORATORY FINDINGS

Between 60 and 70% of patients with atopic dermatitis have elevated serum levels of immunoglobulin E. About 40% have hypereosinophilia. A few have a deficiency of T lymphocytes.

HISTOPATHOLOGICAL FINDINGS

In very early lesions, intraepidermal intercellular edema, spongiosis are seen (Fig. 13.9). Later, characteristic features of lichen simplex chronicus (hyperkeratosis, hypergranulosis, irregular acanthosis and dermal lymphohistiocytic infiltrate) appear (Fig. 13.10).

ETIOLOGY AND PATHOGENESIS

The cause of atopic dermatitis is unknown. Elevated levels of serum immunoglobulin E and the fact that these tend to correlate with the severity of atopic dermatitis have been interpreted to suggest that hypersensitivity reactions may be responsible for most of the manifestations of the disease. It has been demonstrated that epidermal Langerhans cells possess high-affinity immunoglobulin E receptors, through which eczema-like reaction could be triggered.

MANAGEMENT

The single most important step in management of atopic dermatitis is prevention of pruritus. Educating the patient to avoid rubbing and scratching, to prevent dry skin and to wear cotton clothes is very important. Treatments that are helpful in managing pruritus and inflammatory lesions of atopic dermatitis include:

- oral antihistamines for pruritus;
- oral antibiotics to cure staphylococcal infections;
- topical emollients to prevent xerosis;
- topical non-steroidal anti-inflammatory agents, which may be the treatment of choice;
- topical corticosteroids when necessary (long-term use must be avoided);
- ultraviolet B and ultraviolet A phototherapy, which may be effective;
- systemic corticosteroids, or cyclosporin, which should be reserved for patients with important life-threatening problems and used only for short courses.

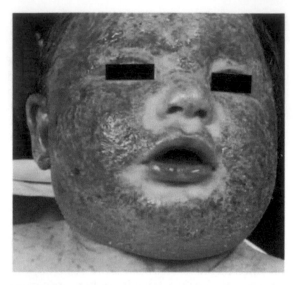

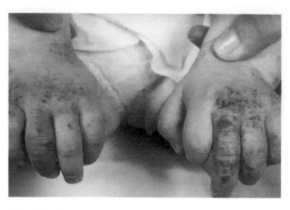

Figure 13.2

Atopic dermatitis. There are many erosions, hemorrhagic crusts and lichenified papules. Hemorrhagic crusts are the consequence of vigorous scratching, and lichenified papules are the result of persistent rubbing.

Figure 13.1

Atopic dermatitis. Weeping lesions are eroded and crusted. The crusts are both serous and hemorrhagic. Observe the sparing of the skin around the nose and the lower lip.

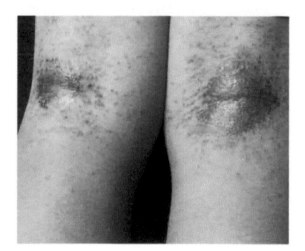

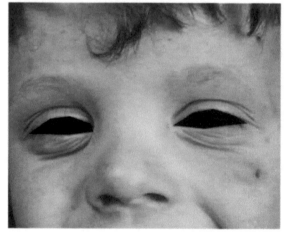

Figure 13.3

Atopic dermatitis. Numerous eroded papules in the popliteal fossa have become confluent. These lesions have been secondarily denuded by vigorous scratching.

Figure 13.4

Atopic dermatitis. The periorbital skin of both eyelids is markedly thickened, reddish and scaly. The skin markings of the lower eyelids are accentuated and the eyebrows are partially alopecic. These changes do not develop spontaneously but are the consequence of prolonged external trauma.

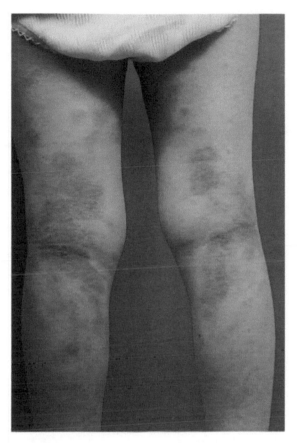

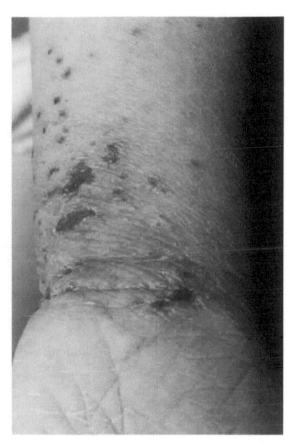

Figure 13.5
Atopic dermatitis. Popliteal fossae are a site of predilection
in children over 3 years of age.

Figure 13.6
Atopic dermatitis. Hemorrhagic crusts, ulcerations and
erosions are the consequence of vigorous scratching, and
lichenification is the result of persistent rubbing.

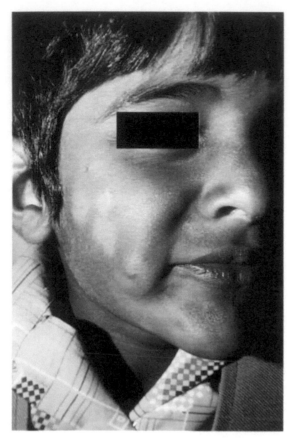

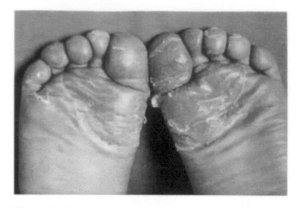

Figure 13.8
Juvenile plantar dermatosis. This term is given to scales on top of shiny skin in the area affected by atopic dermatitis. Symmetrical lesions such as these could conceivably be a manifestation of atopic dermatitis, but this a mere supposition.

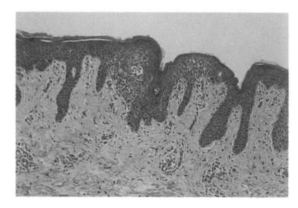

Figure 13.7
Pityriasis alba. The hypopigmented nummular lesions in this Indian boy represent post-inflammatory hypopigmentation.

Figure 13.9
Atopic dermatitis. Foci of spongiosis are evident within the epidermis.

Figure 13.10
Atopic dermatitis. Lichen simplex chronicus. The indubitable signs of chronic persistent rubbing are seen here. These signs are orthokeratosis, hypergranulosis, irregular acanthosis and dermal lymphohistiocytic infiltration.

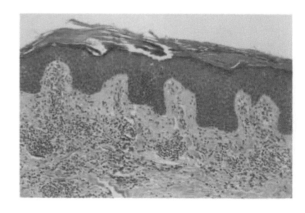

BASAL CELL CARCINOMA

Basal cell carcinoma is a poorly differentiated malignant neoplasm composed of basaloid cells that arise from basal cells of the epidermis or epithelial structures of adnexa. Basal cell carcinoma is extremely rare in children and may be either a solitary neoplasm or one of numerous neoplasms in the nevoid–basal cell carcinoma syndrome.

SOLITARY BASAL CELL CARCINOMA

CLINICAL FINDINGS

Basal cell carcinomas in children have the same clinical features as in adults. They evolve as smooth, skin-colored or opalescent, shiny, roundish, asymptomatic papules that in time may develop rolled margins covered by telangiectases and central ulcers (Fig. 14.1). The neoplasms vary in size from millimeters to many centimeters in greatest diameter. Sites of predilection are the face, particularly the nose, cheeks and eyelids, the neck and the shoulders. The trunk and extremities may also be involved.

Various morphological expressions of basal cell carcinomas seen in adults are also noted in children (i.e. superficial, nodular, ulceronodular, pigmented, fibroepithelial, adenoid, adenoid cystic, and sclerodermoid or morpheiform) (Fig. 14.2). These tumors are mostly seen in the second decade of life.

HISTOPATHOLOGICAL FINDINGS

Basal cell carcinomas are characterized by asymmetrical aggregations of basaloid cells.

The peripheral cells of these aggregations are arranged in palisades and are separated from the surrounding altered stroma by clefts (Figs 14.5 and 14.6).

ETIOLOGY AND PATHOGENESIS

No cause is known for basal cell carcinomas in children who have received little exposure to sunlight.

MANAGEMENT

Surgical excision is the treatment of choice. Mohs surgery is indicated in certain locations, such as the central area of the face and around the ears. Small lesions can be treated with laser therapy or electrosurgery.

NEVOID–BASAL CELL CARCINOMA SYNDROME

Nevoid–basal cell carcinoma syndrome (NBCS) is a genetic disorder characterized by numerous basal cell carcinomas, pits in the palms of the hand and soles of the feet, cysts in the jaw, skeletal anomalies and ectopic calcifications.

EPIDEMIOLOGY

NBCS has an autosomal-dominant inheritance. It usually begins during childhood.

CLINICAL FINDINGS

Children afflicted with NBCS develop numerous basal cell carcinomas, which appear as translucent skin-colored or pigmented papules and nodules with or without ulcers (Figs 14.3 and 14.4). The lesions are located on the face, neck and upper trunk. In addition, 60% of patients have numerous irregularly shaped pits, 1–3 mm in diameter, on the palms and of the hands and the soles of the feet. Patients continue to develop basal cell carcinomas with increasing frequency throughout life.

Associations

Among the more common anomalies associated with the NBCS are skeletal defects such as cysts of the jaws (in 80% of patients), neural defects such as calcification of the falx cerebri (in 80%), anomalies of the vertebrae (in 65%), abnormalities of the ribs (in 60%) and cysts of the long bones and phalanges (in 45%). Ophthalmological defects include hypertelorism (in 30% of patients), strabismus (in 25%), and congenital blindness (in 5%).

HISTOPATHOLOGICAL FINDINGS

The basal cell carcinomas seen in the NBCS seem to be virtually identical histopathologically to nearly all varieties of solitary basal cell carcinomas described above (Figs 14.5 and 14.6).

ETIOLOGY AND PATHOGENESIS

The cause of NBCS is not known.

MANAGEMENT

Because basal cell carcinomas in NBCS are usually so numerous and tend to behave in a benign manner, not every basal cell carcinoma must be removed. Palmar and plantar pits do not require treatment as long as there is no clinical evidence of carcinoma at those sites.

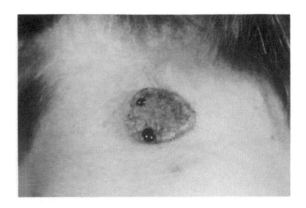

Figure 14.1
Basal cell carcinoma. Sharply circumscribed elevated borders characterize this lesion in a 14-year-old girl. Note the central ulcer covered by blood and crusts.

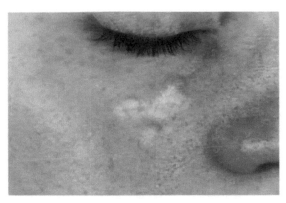

Figure 14.2
Morpheiform basal cell carcinoma. White zones surrounded by pink rims characterize this irregularly shaped plaque. A lesion such as this is exceptional in an adolescent.

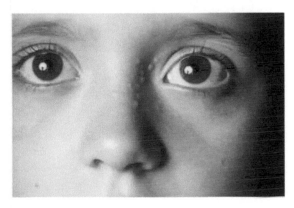

Figure 14.3
Nevoid–basal cell carcinoma syndrome. Each skin-colored papule shown here is a basal cell carcinoma. The face is a site of predilection.

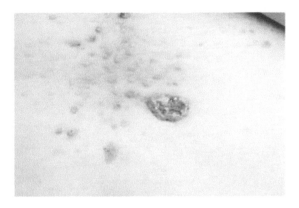

Figure 14.4
Nevoid–basal cell carcinoma syndrome. Basal cell carcinoma in a patient with NBCS. The lesions consist of sharply elevated borders and an ulcer covered by a hemorrhagic crust in the center. Around this lesion there are numerous skin-colored smaller lesions evolving into basal cell carcinomas.

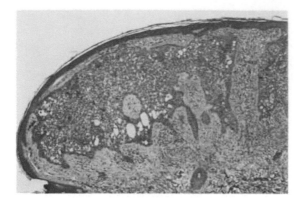

Figure 14.5

Figures 14.5 and 14.6
Nevoid–basal cell carcinoma syndrome. The neoplasm consists of basaloid cells with cribriform and cystic arrangements separated by clefts from the surrounding dermis.

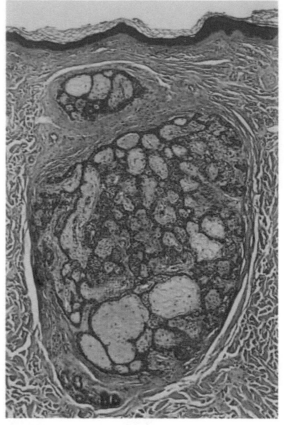

Figure 14.6

15

BECKER'S NEVUS

Becker's nevus is a cutaneous hamartoma that manifests itself clinically as a unilateral hyperpigmented patch covered more or less by coarse dark hairs.

EPIDEMIOLOGY

Becker's nevus is a common condition. It is more common in boys than girls. It usually appears in the first decade of life.

CLINICAL FINDINGS

Becker's nevus usually consists of a unilateral, localized, brownish patch or a plaque that is so slightly elevated that it is barely discernible. The color ranges from tan to dark brown and is usually uniform except at the periphery, where it may be uneven. The outline is irregular, but the margins are sharply circumscribed. The sites of predilection are the shoulders (Fig. 15.1), the anterior chest and the scapular region. A patch may be as large as 200 mm or more in greatest diameter. In time, sometimes as long as 2 years after onset, hypertrichosis develops in over half of cases. The hairs in the patch are coarser and darker than those on other parts of the body. Few other changes occur to the lesion during the patient's life. The lesion is totally benign.

HISTOPATHOLOGICAL FINDINGS

The epidermis is hyperpigmented with oblong rete ridges that have a flat base. There is an increase number of terminal hair follicles and an increased number of muscles of hair erection (Fig 15.2)

MANAGEMENT

Excision is usually not possible because the lesion is too large. Some patients elect to have the hairs within the lesion removed by laser therapy or electroepilation.

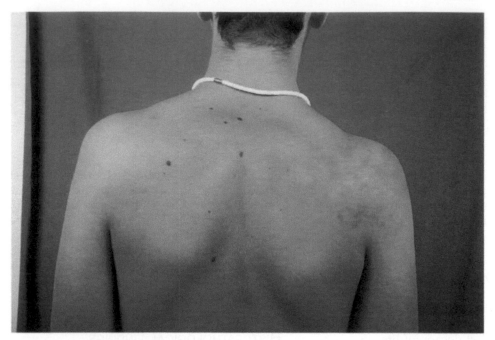

Figure 15.1
Becker's nevus. This browinsh patch covered by hairs is typical. Note the ill-defined borders of the lesion. The shoulder is a site of predilection.

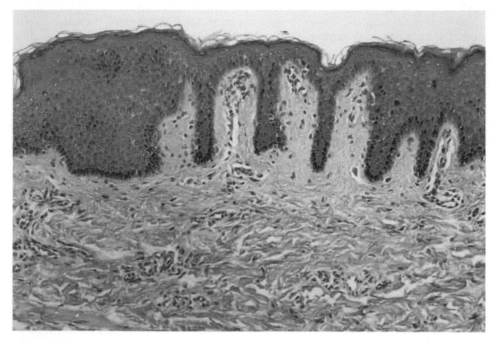

Figure 15.2
Becker's nevus. The lesion can be seen to be a Becker's nevus because the hyperpigmented rete ridges are elongated and some of them have a flattish bottom. Moreover, two terminal hair follicles are in close proximity.

16 BENIGN CEPHALIC HISTIOCYTOSIS

Benign cephalic histiocytosis (BCH) is a self-healing, non-Langerhans cell, non-lipid, cutaneous histiocytosis of children. It usually involves the head.

CLINICAL FINDINGS

BCH begins during the first 3 years of life as an eruption of asymptomatic, yellow to red–brown macules or papules, 2–5 mm in diameter (Figs 16.1 and 16.2). The initial number of lesions varies considerably from a few to more than 100. The individual lesions are slightly raised or flat-topped. The lesions are situated first on the upper part of the face. In time, papules come to cover the entire head and the neck. A few papules may appear on the arms and shoulders and, uncommonly, on the buttocks and thighs. The mucous membranes, palms and soles, and viscera are spared. Spontaneous regression occurs on average 2 years after the onset.

HISTOPATHOLOGICAL FINDINGS

Papules consist of well-circumscribed lymphohistiocytic infiltrates situated immediately beneath the epidermis (Fig. 16.3). Most of the histiocytes have pleomorphic nuclei and abundant, pale, eosinophilic cytoplasm (Fig. 16.4). The histiocytes are S100- and CD1a- and do not contain Langerhans granules

MANAGEMENT

No treatment is necessary because the disease is benign and self-limiting.

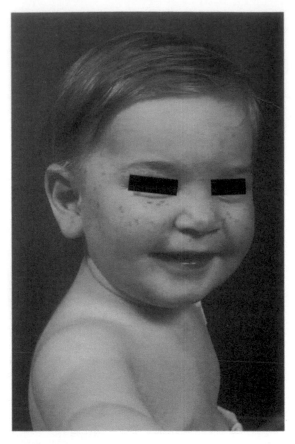

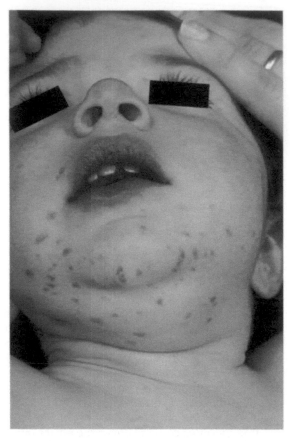

Figure 16.1
Benign cephalic histiocytosis. The papular eruption involves the face exclusively.

Figure 16.2
Benign cephalic histiocytosis. Many brownish papules are scattered beneath the chin and the cheeks, and most of them are discrete.

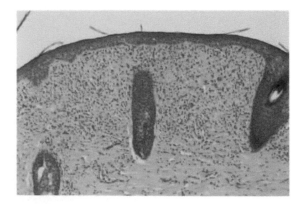

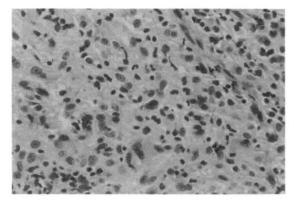

Figure 16.3

Figure 16.4

Figures 16.3 and 16.4
Benign cephalic histiocytosis. This domed lesion is characterized by a dense diffuse infiltrate of histiocytes, many of them with abundant, pale, eosinophilic cytoplasm.

17

BLUEFARB–STEWART SYNDROME

Bluefarb–Stewart syndrome consists of purplish nodules on a limb as a consequence of an underlying arteriovenous malformation. The syndrome is one of several that in the past have been designated 'pseudo-Kaposi's sarcoma' because the cutaneous lesions resemble those seen in the plaque stage and sometimes in the nodular stage of Kaposi's sarcoma.

EPIDEMIOLOGY

The syndrome is rare and the lesions may start as early as the first or second decade of life.

CLINICAL FINDINGS

The lesions of Bluefarb–Stewart syndrome begin as violaceous macules or patches. They develop slowly into soft, smooth, non-tender, reddish to purple papules and nodules (Fig. 17.1). These papules have a predilection for the first three toes of the foot, particularly the second toe. Other sites on the dorsal aspect of the foot or the leg may be involved. The first clue of an underlying arteriovenous malformation may be increased pulses distal to the skin lesions. The affected limb may be warmer than the other limb, even in the absence of signs of cellulitis. The prognosis depends on complications that may arise.

COMPLICATIONS

Lesions are prone to become infected recurrently and to bleed. Intense pain or physical deformity or also cardiac failure of a high output type may cause severe functional disability.

LABORATORY FINDINGS

Definitive diagnosis is accomplished by echo-color Doppler scan and by angiography, both of which reveal numerous large arteriovenous malformations in the area.

HISTOPATHOLOGICAL FINDINGS

Skin lesions in Bluefarb–Stewart syndrome are characterized by a markedly increased number of closely crowded, thick-walled blood vessels in the dermis. These vessels are lined by plump endothelial cells, extravasated erythrocytes (which resemble those present in skin which has been affected by severe stasis), innumerable siderophages, and often by fibrosis (Figs 17.2 and 17.3).

ETIOLOGY AND PATHOGENESIS

The skin changes are due to the underlying arteriovenous malformation of unknown cause.

MANAGEMENT

Lesions should be managed conservatively with measures such as elevation of the leg, bandages applied with pressure, maintenance of good hygiene, prevention of trauma, use of antibiotics, and meticulous attention to ulcers if they develop. The vascular malformations are too diffuse to be removed by surgery. If life-threatening complications develop, amputation of the limb may be the only treatment.

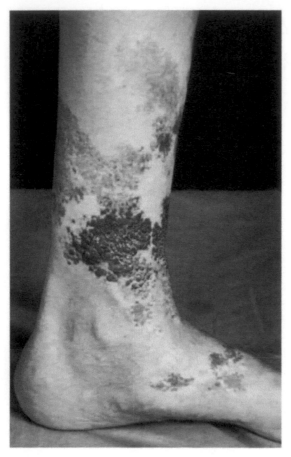

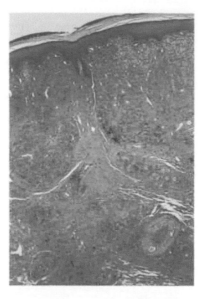

Figure 17.2

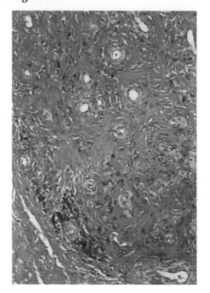

Figure 17.1
Bluefarb–Stewart syndrome. There are irregularly shaped, poorly circumscribed tannish patches and dark brown patches with scalloped borders. The surfaces of the plaques are papillated. These lesions may simulate Kaposi's sarcoma, but they are unrelated to it.

Figure 17.3

Figures 17.2 and 17.3
Bluefarb–Stewart syndrome. This lesion is characterized by a proliferation of small blood vessels throughout the dermis nearly to the subcutis. Unlike the situation in Kaposi's sarcoma, the vessels are normal and oval in shape and they are lined by plump endothelial cells. Furthermore, newly formed, thin-walled vessels are not present around the venules of the pre-existing plexus. Siderophages may be seen in both conditions but are not required for the diagnosis of either.

18

BLUE NEVI

Blue nevus is a congenital or acquired benign neoplasm that is characterized clinically by a bluish hue and histopathologically by proliferation of pigmented melanocytes, at least some of which are dendritic. Blue nevi may occur as patches (in nevus of Ota and Mongolian spots), or as macules, papules, plaques or nodules.

EPIDEMIOLOGY

Nevus of Ota is relatively rare, whereas Mongolian spots are by far the commonest birthmarks noted in neonates: nearly 95% of black infants, 45% of Hispanic infants and nearly 10% of white infants are born with Mongolian spots.

CLINICAL FINDINGS

Nevus of Ota (also known as nevus fusco-caeruleus ophthalmomaxillaris of Ota) is a bluish patch situated on skin and mucous membranes that are supplied by branches of the trigeminal nerve. It is usually solitary, unilateral (Fig. 18.1) and distributed along a dermatome innervated by the ophthalmic and maxillary branches of the trigeminal nerve. It therefore usually occurs on the forehead, the temple, the malar area, or the ala nasi. The upper lip and nasolabial folds are almost always spared. Some mottled brownish coloration may be seen within the bluish patch. Hyperpigmentation of mucous membranes commonly affects the pharynx, the oral mucosa, the nasal mucosa, the ear canal and the tympanic membrane.

The eye is often affected in nevus of Ota (Fig. 18.2). In about two-thirds of afflicted patients, an ipsilateral ocular hypermelanosis involves the sclera, iris and conjunctiva. If there is ocular involvement, a bluish–gray discoloration of the sclera on the ipsilateral side can be seen. Vision is not impaired as a result of the ocular findings. Nevus of Ota may change color during the patient's life.

The major complication in nevus of Ota is an increased incidence of cutaneous and ocular melanomas within the nevus itself. There are many reports about nevus of Ota affecting the central nervous system.

Nevus of Ota is present at birth in about 60% of affected children. In the rest, this distinctive form of blue nevus becomes apparent near puberty. About 80% of affected children are girls, most commonly Asians and Africans, but a person of any race may be affected. Rarely, nevus of Ota may be familial.

Mongolian spots are bluish-gray patches that are mostly situated in the sacrogluteal region (Fig. 18.3). The condition occurs usually as a demarcated patch that ranges in size from a few millimetres to 100 mm. In one-quarter of patients, a Mongolian spot is found on extrasacrogluteal locations, especially the shoulders and the upper limbs. Mongolian spots are usually present at birth, but they may appear any time in the first 2 years of life. Mongolian spots change color until puberty, when they begin to fade.

Macules, papules and nodules of blue nevi usually make their appearance in the second decade of life as well-demarcated, bluish-gray to blue lesions (Fig. 18.4). These forms of blue nevi are extremely rare in children aged younger than 10 years. Papular, plaque and nodular expressions of blue nevi may be located on any anatomic site.

HISTOPATHOLOGICAL FINDINGS

In patches of blue nevi, markedly pigmented dendritic melanocytes are scattered as solitary units throughout the dermis (Figs. 18.5 and 18.6), but especially the upper half of the dermis, although they are not uncommonly seen in the lower part of the dermis even in the upper part of the subcutaneous fat. Melanophages are present in addition to melanocytes. The lesions look blue clinically because melanin is present in melanocytes and macrophages in the middle and lower parts of the dermis. In papular, plaque and nodular forms of blue nevi, oval melanocytes may predominate over dendritic ones. The collagen may be entirely unaffected or strongly thickened (collagenized).

ETIOLOGY AND PATHOGENESIS

It is thought that melanocytes of blue nevi are a consequence of arrest during migration during embryonic life. The factors responsible are not known. The various neurological abnormalities in patients with nevus of Ota suggest that this nevus may be a cutaneous manifestation of a neurocutaneous syndrome.

MANAGEMENT

Nevus of Ota and Mongolian spots are usually too large to be excised surgically. Management is therefore limited to cover with cosmetics. Laser therapy can be helpful in selected cases. Papular and nodular forms of blue nevi may be excised.

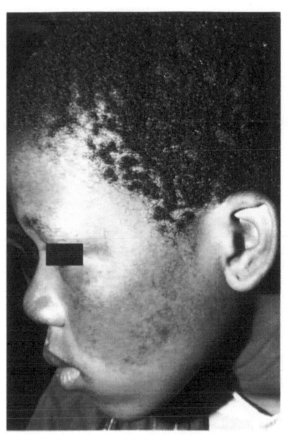

Figure 18.1
Nevus of Ota with scleral involvement. The broad blue–gray patch pictured here is mottled and extends into the sclera.

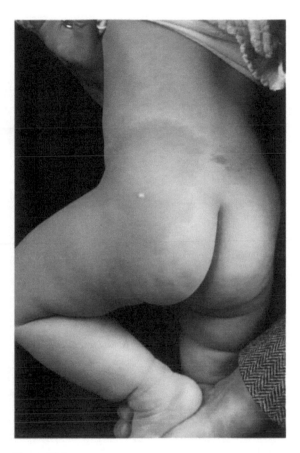

Figure 18.3
Mongolian spot. This lesion on the thigh, buttock and waist is analogous to a nevus of Ota. A Mongolian spot such as the one shown here tends to lighten with time.

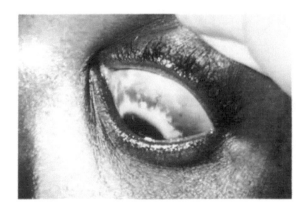

Figure 18.2
Nevus of Ota with scleral involvement. The sceral changes of nevus of Ota are analogous to those in the skin, namely, those of a patch of blue nevus.

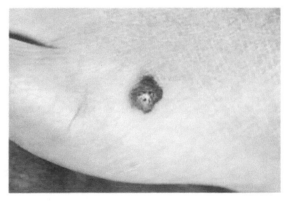

Figure 18.4
Blue nevus. This lesion is benign because is small and well circumscribed; it is a blue nevus because of its bluish hue.

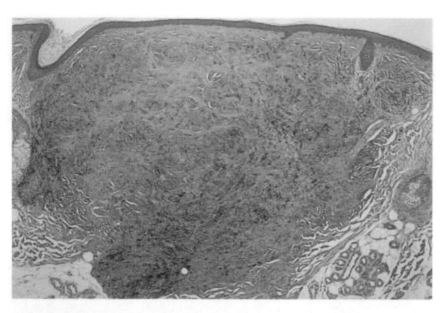

Figure 18.5

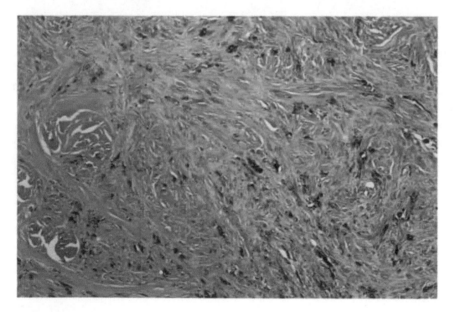

Figure 18.6

Figures 18.5 and 18.6

Blue nevus with collagenization. This relatively small, well-circumscribed lesion fills the dermis and extends into the subcutaneous fat. It is characterized by a proliferation of dendritic and oval-shaped melanocytes. There are also numerous melanophages in addition to melanocytes. The lesions look blue clinically because melanin is present in melanocytes, and collagen bundles are markedly thickened. The latter phenomenon, collagenization, occurs in blue nevi when dendritic melanocytes are scattered among bundles of collagens, and never when they are arranged cohesively in parallel. In papular nevi, dendritic melanocytes are scattered among bundles of collagen and never arranged cohesively in parallel.

19   BLUE RUBBER-BLEB NEVUS SYNDROME

The blue rubber-bleb nevus syndrome (Bean syndrome) is a peculiar angiomatosis characterized by numerous cavern-like hemangiomas that involve the skin, mucous membranes and other parts of the body.

EPIDEMIOLOGY

The syndrome is rare and not usually familial. There is also no predilection for any race or either sex.

CLINICAL FINDINGS

Typical skin lesions of blue rubber-bleb nevus syndrome consist of soft, blue papules that resemble rubber nipples (Fig. 19.1). The lesions are often detected at birth or in early infancy. They are easily compressible and refill promptly when the pressure is released. The lesions often are multiple, sometimes numbering hundreds, and are scattered randomly on the trunk and limbs. The blebs can be painful, both when pressed and without pressure. The pain in these hemangiomas becomes manifest at puberty and is said by patients to be most troublesome at night. In about 90% of patients, numerous hemangiomas are also found in the gastrointestinal tract, most commonly in the small bowel. Lesions may be situated on mucous membranes of the lips, oral cavity (Fig. 19.2), glans penis and nasopharynx. The lungs, urinary tract, liver, spleen, brain, meninges, and heart may be involved by the angiomatosis, although this is rare. New lesions may appear and old ones may continue to grow well into adulthood. The lesions are persistent and prognosis depends on severity of complications.

Complications

Angiomas in the gastrointestinal tract may bleed, with consequent hematemesis, melena, severe iron-deficiency anemia and even death.

LABORATORY FINDINGS

Iron-deficiency anemia is common in blue rubber-bleb nevus syndrome. X-rays may reveal many polypoid filling defects throughout the length of the bowel. These defects may also be visualized easily by fiberoptic endoscopy. Computed tomography scans and magnetic resonance imaging often help to determine the full extent of involvement by the angiomatosis.

HISTOPATHOLOGICAL FINDINGS

The features consist of very widely dilated vein-like structures in the dermis and the subcutaneous fat, some of which may thrombose and become organized (Fig 19.3), and of cavern-like hemangiomas together with some changes of angiokeratoma that affect the lamina propria and submucosa in the gastrointestinal tract.

ETIOLOGY AND PATHOGENESIS

The cause of blue rubber-bleb nevus syndrome is a mutation in the gene situated in the chromosome 9p.

MANAGEMENT

Cutaneous lesions that are particularly troublesome may be excised surgically. Laser therapy has been used to provide excellent results in removal of the vascular nevi. Hemorrhage from the gastrointestinal tract may be controlled endoscopically.

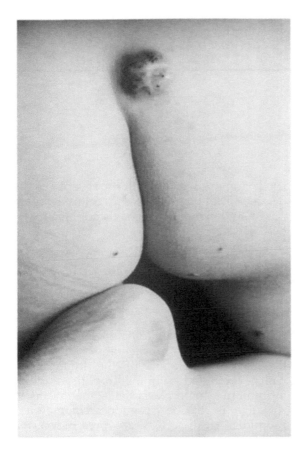

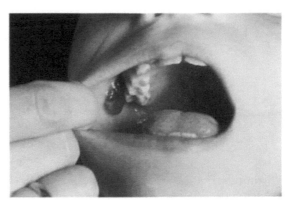

Figure 19.2
Blue rubber-bleb nevus syndrome. The nodule on the buccal mucosa is benign because is well circumscribed and symmetrical. It has a mahogany hue and it glistens.

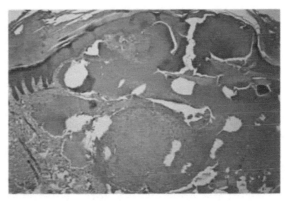

Figure 19.1
Blue rubber-bleb nevus syndrome. There are several papules and nodules. The nodule above and to the right of the intergluteal fold is gray–black. The nodule behind the malleolus is slightly bluish. Such a lesion is easily herniated by gentle pressure and is not painful to pressure.

Figure 19.3
Blue rubber-bleb nevus syndrome. With scanning magnification, a striking vascular malformation can be seen extending from the subcutaneous fat to immediately beneath the thinned epidermis.

20

BROMODERMA

Bromoderma is a skin eruption caused by ingestion of bromides. It is similar to eruptions caused by other halogens such as iodides and fluorides.

EPIDEMIOLOGY

Bromoderma is now rare in children. It has no predilection for any race or for either sex.

CLINICAL FINDINGS

The clinical lesions of bromoderma vary with the stage of the disease. The earliest lesions are often papules that quickly become pustular and resemble those seen in acne vulgaris. As the process evolves, vesicles and bullae tend to form, which may leave large residual ulcers when they rupture. The ulcers often develop crusts in their centers (Fig. 20.1) and pustules along their peripheries.

Vegetations are seen mainly in adolescents as reddish-blue, heaped-up crusts that are most prominent on the lower legs (Fig. 20.2). The mucous membranes, hair and nails are not usually affected. The lesions persist unless exposure to halogens is terminated.

LABORATORY FINDINGS

Blood levels of halogens may be elevated, but levels do not correlate with the severity of the disease. The total leukocyte count is often raised, and extremely high eosinophilia (68%) has been noted.

HISTOPATHOLOGICAL FINDINGS

The inflammatory process of bromoderma primarily affects hair follicles (Figs 20.3 and 20.4). The affected follicles are characterized by marked dilatation of the infundibula, which are filled with neutrophils, and by infundibular hyperplasia that sometimes is so striking as to be 'pseudocarcinomatous'. Prominent scaly crusts are present on the surfaces of some lesions. A dense, mixed inflammatory cell infiltrate (composed mostly of neutrophils, but also of lymphocytes and histiocytes) is present in the upper part of the dermis.

ETIOLOGY AND PATHOGENESIS

The exact manner in which halogens induce the eruptions is not known.

MANAGEMENT

The offending halogen must be withdrawn. Compresses followed by powerful topical corticosteroids are adjuncts to termination of the halogen.

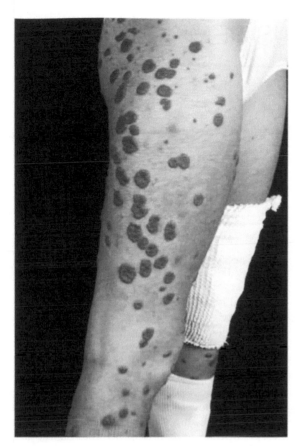

Figure 20.1
Bromoderma. There are many roundish papules and plaques, and the borders of the plaques are partially elevated. At this stage the lesions consist mostly of hemorrhagic and purulent crusts.

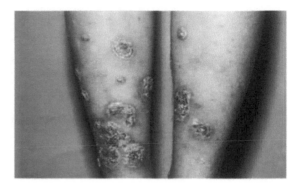

Figure 20.2
Bromoderma. Many plaques are covered by vegetations and are surrounded by rims of dusky erythema. The vegetations consist of both scales and crusts.

Figures 20.3 and 20.4
Bromoderma. This papillated lesion is characterized by widely dilated follicular infundibula plugged by ortho-keratotic and parakeratotic cells and filled by abscesses. Polymorphonuclear leukocytes are present, mostly within hyperplastic follicular infundibula but also within the dermis and within the scaly crusts.

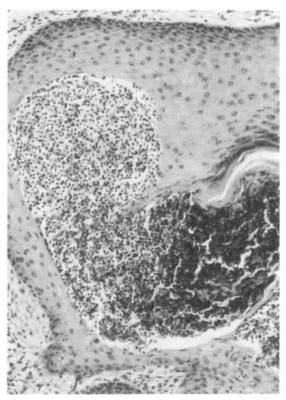

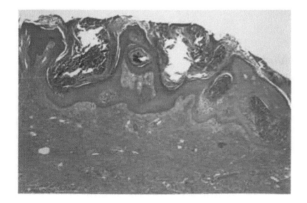

Figure 20.3

Figure 20.4

21

BULLOUS PEMPHIGOID

Bullous pemphigoid is a blistering disorder characterized by tense subepidermal vesicles and bullae.

EPIDEMIOLOGY

Bullous pemphigoid is rare in children. The onset is usually in the first decade of life.

CLINICAL FINDINGS

The disease presents first as urticarial papules and plaques and then as tense, discrete vesicles and bullae (Figs 21.1 and 21.2). The blisters cannot be extended centrifugally by pressing against their edges (Nikolsky's sign). Furthermore, urticarial plaques do not always result in blisters. The lesions of bullous pemphigoid usually affect the flexural areas and the lower part of the abdomen. Erosions in the mouth secondary to rupture of blisters are rare but are more frequent in children than in adults with the disease. The erosions in the oral cavity may be painful. At times, cutaneous bullae are hemorrhagic.

LABORATORY FINDINGS

Direct immunofluorescence reveals deposits in linear array of immunoglobulin G at the basement membrane zone in nearly all patients (Fig. 21.3). Indirect immunofluorescence reveals circulating immunoglobulin G antibodies directed against basement membrane zone in about 70% of patients who have active disease.

HISTOPATHOLOGICAL FINDINGS

Urticarial lesions are characterized by a superficial perivascular and interstitial infiltrate of lymphocytes and eosinophils. Numerous eosinophils are present within the upper part of the edematous dermis, and some of them may even be present in the epidermis, where spongiosis of variable extent is seen. The blister that develops in the lamina lucida is subepidermal and contains eosinophils (Fig. 21.4). Papillae at the base of the blister are usually preserved.

ETIOLOGY AND PATHOGENESIS

The source of the autoantibodies that are thought to be responsible for the disease is unknown.

MANAGEMENT

The agents of choice for treating bullous pemphigoid in children are systemic corticosteroids. Prednisone (1–2 mg/kg per day) almost always controls the disease. The dose should be tapered and discontinued as quickly as possible. Dapsone is an effective adjuvant, which may exert an effect that permits less use of corticosteroids.

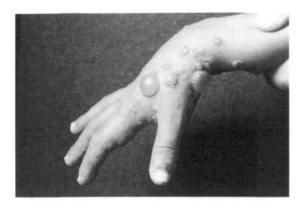

Figure 21.1
Bullous pemphigoid. Tense vesicles and bullae of different sizes and shapes contain straw-colored fluid.

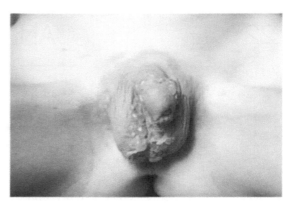

Figure 21.2
Bullous pemphigoid. Numerous tense vesicles, some of them confluent, are situated on dusky-red plaques.

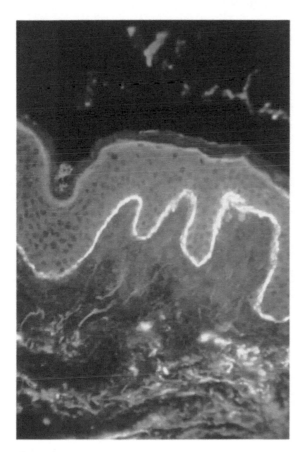

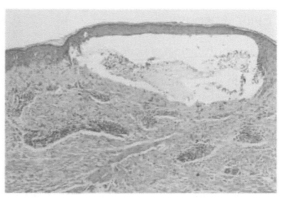

Figure 21.4
Bullous pemphigoid. Subepidermal blisters contain numerous eosinophils.

Figure 21.3
Bullous pemphigoid. Direct immunofluorescence. There are deposits of immunoglobulin G in a linear pattern at the basement membrane zone.

22

CANDIDIASIS

Candidiasis results from proliferation of yeasts of the genus *Candida*, usually *Candida albicans*, in the cornified cells of the skin and mucous membranes and, rarely, in internal organs.

EPIDEMIOLOGY

Oral candidiasis has been said to occur in less than 1% of children to about 20%. Familial chronic mucocutaneous candidiasis is a rare autosomal-recessive disorder.

CLINICAL FINDINGS

Cutaneous candidiasis

Candidiasis of the skin mostly involves the intertriginous regions, where it presents as reddish, eroded patches with small pustules at the margins. The commonest cutaneous site in infants is the diaper (nappy) area (Fig. 22.1). Other sites of involvement are the axillae, the webs of the fingers and toes and occasionally the skin of the face (Fig 22.2). The penile shaft or the vulva may be involved in older children. Candidal paronychia and onychosis consist of redness and swelling of the nail fold associated with thickening of the nail plate (Fig. 22.3). Congenital cutaneous candidiasis is a rare form in which neonates develop extensive lesions at birth (see Fig. 22.2). The face, palms and soles are often involved but the diaper area is characteristically spared.

Oral candidiasis

Candidiasis in the oral cavity manifests itself as patches and plaques of whitish 'cheesy' material (Fig. 22.4). The infection may extend to the region around the lips or the angles of the mouth.

Chronic mucocutaneous candidiasis

Long-term recurrent candidiasis is most commonly seen in people with congenital immunologic disorder (e.g. T-cell deficiency) or an endocrinologic defect (e.g. hypoparathyroidism, hyperparathyroidism, diabetes mellitus). Cutaneous lesions consist of papules, pustules, nodules, granulomas and abscesses (Fig 22.5).

HISTOPATHOLOGICAL FINDINGS

The diagnostic feature is the presence of candidal pseudohyphae in the cornified cells of the epidermis and epithelium of the mucous membranes (Figs 22.6 and 22.7).

LABORATORY FINDINGS

The diagnosis of candidiasis is confirmed when examination of scrapings of cornified cells in preparations treated by potassium hydroxide reveal abundant hyphae.

ETIOLOGY AND PATHOGENESIS

There are nearly 20 species of the genus *Candida*. Most infections are caused by *Candida albicans*; *Candida tropicalis* is the second commonest cause. Predisposing conditions, such as prematurity, immunosuppression and various endocrine syndromes, are very important in determining the capacity for candidal infection.

MANAGEMENT

An essential step in the treatment of cutaneous and mucous candidiasis is to remove any predisposing cause. Topical imidazole derivatives are very effective. Oral ketoconazole or itraconazole are needed for disseminated or chronic candiasis.

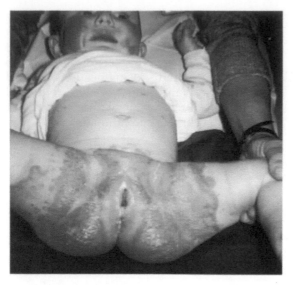

Figure 22.1
Cutaneous candidiasis. There is an extensive involvement of the thighs, lower abdomen, groin and buttocks by *Candida.* At the periphery of the reddish plaques are numerous satellite papules. The surface of the lesions is shiny, probably as a consequence of weeping from the erosions.

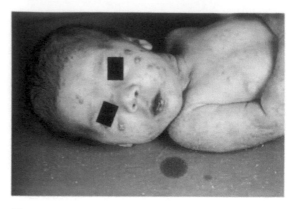

Figure 22.2
Congenital cutaneous candidiasis. Numerous papules and papulopustules are present on the face, trunk and upper extremities. The lesions on the face tend to merge and form nodules with vegetated surfaces.

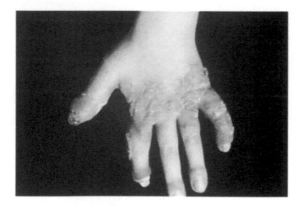

Figure 22.3
Candidal paronychia. These lesions consist of pinkish plaques covered by scales and crusts. Note the involvement of the nail plates as well as the periungueal skin.

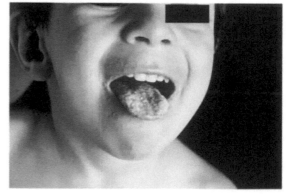

Figure 22.4
Oral candidiasis. White plaques on the tongue are typical of oral candidiasis. Note that the disease also affects the mucocutaneous junctions and the skin.

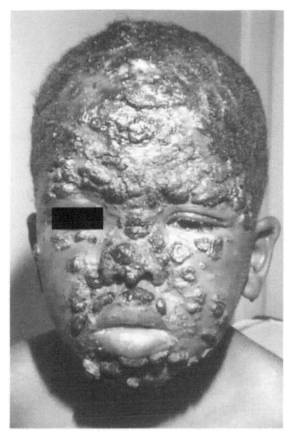

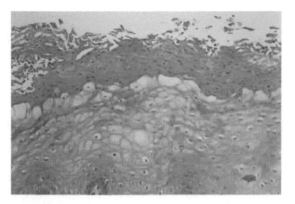

Figure 22.6

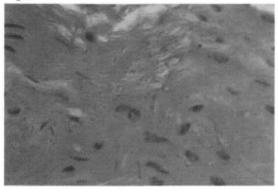

Figure 22.7

Figure 22.5
Chronic mucocutaneous candidiasis. This extensive granulomatous infection (candidal granuloma syndrome) results in markedly hyperkeratotic areas on the face of this immunocompromised child.

Figures 22.6 and 22.7
Candidiasis. Within the markedly thickened parakeratotic cornified layer are numerous pseudohyphae of *Candida albicans.*

23

CAT-SCRATCH DISEASE

Cat-scratch disease produces a primary lesion in the skin and a secondary regional lympadenopathy. It affects children and adults who have been scratched by a cat.

EPIDEMIOLOGY

Cat-scratch disease is mostly a disease of the young and is worldwide in distribution. The disease usually occurs after the age of 3 years, when children begin to play with pets. The skin lesions appear 3–10 days after the scratch of a cat.

CLINICAL FINDINGS

The initial lesion, appearing 3–10 days after a cat scratch at the site of a scratch, is a red papule, 5–10 mm in diameter, which may ulcerate and become covered by a crust (Fig. 23.1). The lesion is usually situated on the limbs or face. Regional lymph node enlargement, without signs of lymphangitis, is noticeable 3–12 weeks after the appearance of the primary lesion and is characterized by red, painful and tender lymph nodes (Fig. 23.2). Nodes suppurate and become confluent in about 20% of patients. Low-grade fever, headache, anorexia, nausea, malaise, myalgia and arthralgia are seen in about a one-third of patients. The primary lesion persists for about 1–2 months. Regional lymphadenopthy usually regresses after a few weeks.

LABORATORY FINDINGS

A positive skin test with Hanger–Rose antigen (induration of more than 5 mm after 72 hours) is indicative of cat-scratch disease.

HISTOPATHOLOGICAL FINDINGS

Confirmation of the diagnosis may be obtained by demonstration of the causative agent with the Warthin–Starry silver stain.

ETIOLOGY AND PATHOGENESIS

The cause of cat-scratch disease is a Gram-negative organism, *Bartonella hanselae*.

MANAGEMENT

Cat-scratch disease subsides without therapy. Incision and drainage of affected lymph nodes should be avoided because fistulas may develop. The efficacy of therapy with tetracyclines and other antimicrobial agents remains controversial.

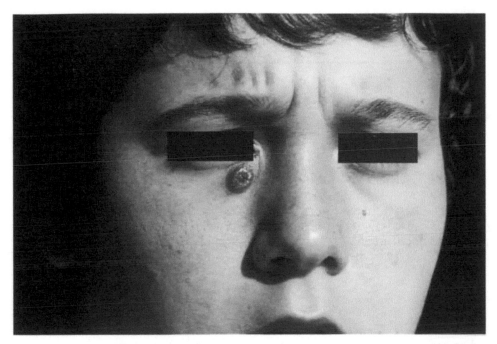

Figure 23.1
Cat-scratch disease. This relatively well-circumscribed, reddish-brown nodule is centrally ulcerated and covered by crusts.

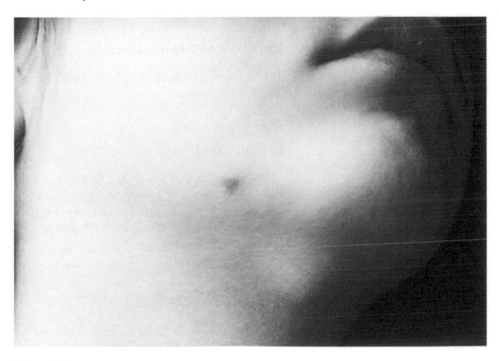

Figure 23.2
Cat-scratch disease. Below and to the left of the small, pink, smooth-surfaced papule is a substantial swelling that represents an enlarged lymph node.

24

CHEILITIS

CHEILITIS GLANDULARIS

Cheilitis glandularis is characterized by a prominent lower lip. It is caused by hyperplasia of the salivary glands and ducts.

EPIDEMIOLOGY

Cheilitis glandularis is an extremely rare disorder observed as early as the first decade of life.

CLINICAL FINDINGS

Cheilitis glandularis consists of painless enlargement and eversion of the lower lip caused by hyperplasia of the salivary glands and ducts. The involved lip has a cobbled surface (Fig. 24.1), and patulous openings of the salivary ducts are visible easily on its surface. Mucus can be extruded from the openings by squeezing the firm lip gently. It has a chronic course.

Complications

Rarely, intense suppuration leads to abscesses, fistulous tracts, ulcers and purulent crusts. This form of the disease has also been called cheilitis glandularis apostematosa. The most serious complication is the development of squamous cell carcinomas.

HISTOPATHOLOGICAL FINDINGS

The salivary glands are enlarged. The salivary ducts within the substance of the glands, the lamina propria and the surface epithelium are widely dilated by abundant acid mucopolysaccharide (mucin). Sometimes, rupture of the distended ducts results in discharge of the mucin into the lamina propria. In response to extravasated mucin, a variably dense patchy infiltrate of inflammatory cells forms. It is suppurative initially; later it is composed mostly of lymphocytes and histiocytes.

ETIOLOGY AND PATHOGENESIS

The cause of cheilitis glandularis is not known.

MANAGEMENT

No treatment for cheilitis glandularis has been successful. Wedge resections of the inner aspect of the lip or vermilionectomy are used to correct cosmetic disfigurement that results from the swollen lip

CHEILITIS GRANULOMATOSA

Cheilitis granulomatosa is characterized by swelling of the lips caused by granulomatous inflammation.

EPIDEMIOLOGY

Cheilitis granulomatosa is an extremely rare disorder. The vast majority of patients are girls.

CLINICAL FEATURES

Cheilitis granulomatosa is characterized by episodes of swelling of the lips that ultimately lead to persistently enlarged lips (Fig 24.2). This sign is one feature of Melkersson–Rosenthal syndrome, which consists of facial swelling, paralysis of a facial nerve and plicate tongue. The swelling is not accompanied by erythema, pruritus or tenderness. The acute episodes last for days only but with each recurrence, the swelling persists longer and becomes progressively more firm. The lips are often everted, which causes the moist surface of mucous membranes to be exposed to air. This results in chapping and fissuring.

HISTOPATHOLOGICAL FINDINGS

The lesions are characterized by granulomas composed of epithelioid histiocytes and surrounded by lymphocytes and plasma cells within the dermis, the subcutaneous fat and skeletal muscle (Figs 24.3 and 24.4).

ETIOLOGY AND PATHOGENESIS

The cause of cheilitis granulomatosa is not known.

MANAGEMENT

There is no satisfactory treatment for cheilitis granulomatosa. Facial swelling may be decreased by corticosteroids injected into the zone of involvement at about monthly intervals. The cosmetic deformity caused by protruding lips may be ameliorated somewhat by wedge resection of the inner margin of the lips. Intralesional injections of corticosteroids should be maintained after surgery to diminish the chances of recurrence.

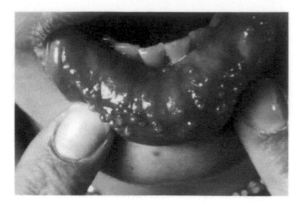

Figure 24.1
Cheilitis glandularis. When the lower lip is folded, as shown here, many glistening translucent papules are revealed. Such papules are full of acid mucopolysaccharides.

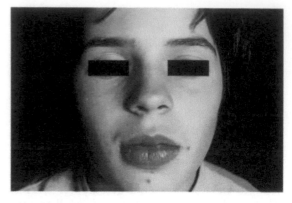

Figure 24.2
Cheilitis granulomatosa. The lower lip of this adolescent is markedly swollen as a consequence of granulomatous involvement of the tissues.

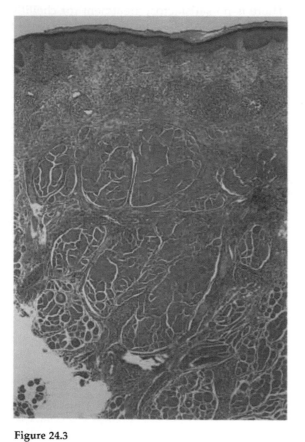

Figure 24.3

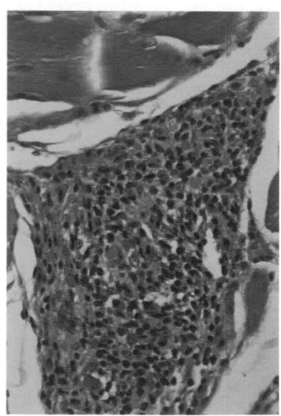

Figure 24.4

Figures 24.3 and 24.4
Cheilitis granulomatosa. Collections of epithelioid histiocytes surrounded by lymphocytes in the lamina propria, submucosa and skeletal muscle of the lip.

25 CONGENITAL MELANOCYTIC NEVI

Congenital melanocytic nevi are proliferations of melanocytes present at birth, or very soon after birth, in the skin and sometimes in the tissues beneath it.

EPIDEMIOLOGY

Congenital melanocytic nevi are present in almost 1% of white newborns.

CLINICAL FINDINGS

Congenital nevi vary considerably in size, shape, color, surface characteristics, and degree of hairiness. Congenital nevi are conventionally subdivided into small (from less than 15 mm up to 50 mm in greatest diameter to) (Fig. 25.1), large (50–200 mm) (Figs 25.2 and 25.3), and giant (greater than 200 mm) (Fig. 25.4).

The color varies from light brown to dark brown or black. Small congenital nevi are usually oval or round; large or giant congenital nevi may assume irregular shapes. The borders may be sharply demarcated or they may merge imperceptibly with surrounding skin.

Congenital nevi may have an uneven 'pebbled cobblestone' and rough surface with or without long coarse and dark hairs. The consistency is usually soft or wormy.

Associations

Large congenital nevi situated in the area of the head and neck may be associated with leptomeningeal melanocytosis and attendant neurological findings, including seizures. Similarly, large congenital nevi in the lumbosacral area may be associated with defects in the underlying spinal column such as meningomyelocele or spina bifida.

Complications

The single most important complication within a congenital nevus is development of malignant melanoma. A giant congenital nevus has a 10–20% chance of having a malignant melanoma develop within it, whereas a small congenital nevus has a less than 1% chance of being the harbinger of a malignant melanoma.

HISTOPATHOLOGICAL FINDINGS

In small congenital nevi, melanocytes are splayed between collagen bundles in the reticular dermis and there is angiocentricity and adnexocentricity of melanocytes (Figs 25.5 and 25.6). Large congenital nevi consist of dense diffuse infiltrate of melanocytes throughout the dermis and often in the subcutaneous fat. Giant congenital nevi may also contain melanocytes below the subcutis; melanocytes may be seen in large blood vessels such as veins in the septa of subcutaneous fat.

ETIOLOGY AND PATHOGENESIS

The cause of congenital nevi is not known, but genetic factors are surely important. They are presumed to occur as a result of a developmental defect in neural crest-derived melanocytes.

MANAGEMENT

Considerable debate continues, without resolution, about the management of both small and large congenital nevi. Many authors contend that all congenital nevi, irrespective of size, should be excised at puberty, when local anesthesia is possible. In giant congenital nevi the risk of melanoma is significant even in the first 3–5 years of life and therefore this type of nevus should be removed as soon as possible. Tissue expanders and tissue cultures using the patient's own normal skin can be used to facilitate removal of very large lesions.

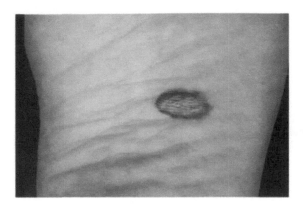

Figure 25.1
Small congenital nevus. This lesion, on the sole, is benign because it is symmetrical in shape, uniform in coloration and relatively well circumscribed.

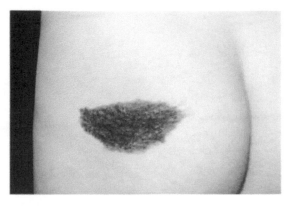

Figure 25.2
Large congenital nevus. This lesion consists of many dark brown papules situated on a tannish patch. Numerous fine hairs cover the nevus.

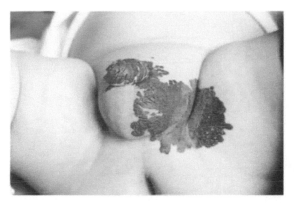

Figure 25.3
Large congenital nevus. This bizarre-shaped, uniformly colored bluish-black plaque has a scalloped and reticulated periphery that, nonetheless, is sharply circumscribed – a sign that it is benign.

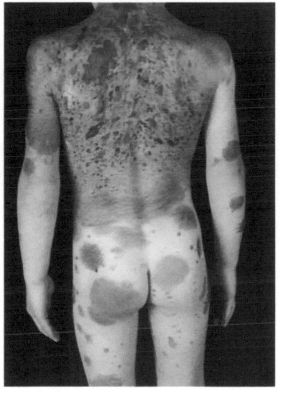

Figure 25.4
Giant congenital nevus. All the widespread pigmented lesions in this boy are congenital nevi. Some are hairy, others are not. Some of the lesions on the shoulders and back are difficult to differentiate clinically from malignant melanomas.

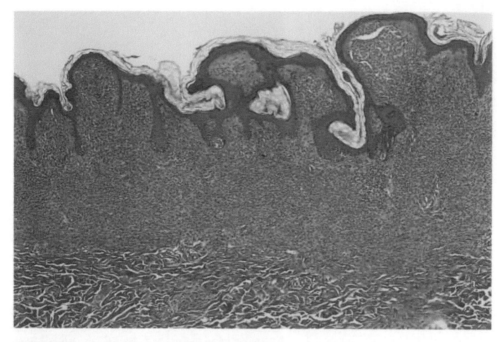

Figure 25.5

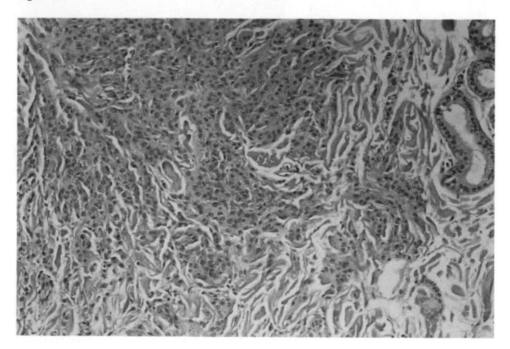

Figure 25.6

Figures 25.5 and 25.6
Small congenital nevus. This nevus is characterized by involvement of the upper half of the dermis and by sparing of the lower half. The melanocytes of the reticular dermis are arranged in two distinct patterns – around blood vessels and between collagen bundles.

Connective tissue nevi are malformations characterized by excessive amounts of either collagen or elastic tissue and sometimes of mucin.

EPIDEMIOLOGY

Connective tissue nevi are rare disorders, although their incidence is probably underestimated.

CLINICAL FINDINGS

Collagenous nevi

Connective tissue nevi that are marked by an excess of collagen are called collagenous nevi or collagenomas. They may be congenital or acquired, solitary or multiple. The lesions consist of asymptomatic yellow–brown or skin-colored patches, papules, nodules or plaques of variable sizes and shapes (Figs 26.1 and 26.2). Their mammillated surfaces have often been compared to that of pigskin. They are usually situated on the trunk or the extremities and persist for life.

Four subtypes of collagenomas have been described:

- isolated collagenoma (Fig. 26.1), which is a patch or plaque in zosteriform distribution that is not associated with other diseases;
- eruptive collagenoma (Fig. 26.2), which presents suddenly with numerous macules that quickly become papules and then nodules;
- familial cutaneous collagenoma, which is typified by numerous, symmetrically distributed nodules and is often associated with extracutaneous abnormalities, particularly cardiac problems;
- Shagreen patch (better termed 'plaque' because its mammillated surface is raised above the surface of surrounding normal skin), which occurs in the lumbosacral area of children with tuberous sclerosis.

Elastic tissue nevi

Connective tissue nevi marked by an excess of elastic tissue are called elastic tissue nevi or elastomas. They, like collagenomas, may be congenital or acquired, solitary or multiple. The commonest forms taken by these hamartomas are:

- dermatofibrosis lenticularis disseminata, which consists of numerous elastic tissue nevi in association with osteopoikilosis (mesenchymal alterations of bone). Taken together, these findings constitute the Buschke–Ollendorff syndrome. The cutaneous lesions are small, asymptomatic papules distributed symmetrically on the lower part of the trunk or the extremities;
- Solitary elastoma, which is a plaque composed of yellowish papules (nevus elasticus of Lewandowsky) or nodules (juvenile elastoma) and is situated principally on the trunk and buttocks; it is seemingly without genetic transmission (Fig. 26.3).

HISTOPATHOLOGICAL FINDINGS

Connective tissue nevi are characterized by alteration in quality and quantity of collagen and elastic tissue in the absence of associated inflammation or neoplasia. Collagenous nevi have thickened collagen bundles, some of which are oriented vertically to the skin surface. The reticular dermis may be thickened (Fig. 26.4). Elastic tissue nevi usually have markedly thickened fibers, either focally or diffusely, within the reticular dermis.

ETIOLOGY AND PATHOGENESIS

The accumulation of collagen and elastin seems to result primarily from overproduction of these substances at a molecular level. A precise molecular defect has yet to be defined.

MANAGEMENT

Collagenous and elastic tissue nevi in themselves are harmless and rarely need to be removed except for cosmetic considerations. The simplest and most effective way to remove them is surgical excision.

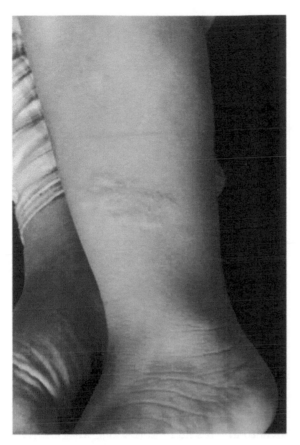

Figure 26.1
Isolated collagenoma. The skin-colored plaque is ill-defined and characterized by a slightly mamillated surface.

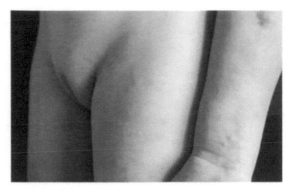

Figure 26.2
Eruptive collagenoma. There are papules and plaques of 'collagenoma' along the left forearm and thigh. The lesions have a smooth surface and are of skin-colored, tan or reddish-brown hues.

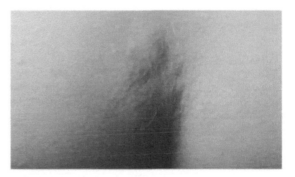

Figure 26.3
Solitary elastoma. Skin colored papules have become confluent to form a slightly elevated plaque.

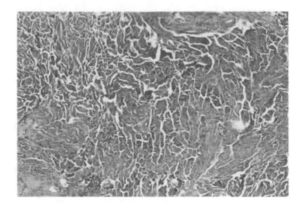

Figure 26.4
Collagenous nevus. Dense collagen bundles arranged mostly horizontally but also vertically to the skin surface thicken the dermis of this mamillated lesion of shagreen plaque.

CONTACT DERMATITIS

Contact dermatitis is an inflammatory reaction. It either occurs within several days of direct contact with an allergen (allergic contact dermatitis) or follows immediately after direct contact with an irritant (irritant contact dermatitis).

EPIDEMIOLOGY

Allergic contact dermatitis occurs in only a small percentage of children who have been exposed to the sensitizing agent. Irritant contact dermatitis is very common in infants.

CLINICAL FINDINGS

Allergic contact dermatitis follows re-exposure to a sensitizing agent and requires several days between first exposure and the development of the dermatitis. In the acute phase the dermatitis consists of well-demarcated plaques of erythema and edema on which vesicles exuding serum and crusts are superimposed (Figs 27.1 and 27.2). In the subacute phase the erythematous plaques show papules and desquamation. The chronic phase consists of plaques of lichenification (thickening of epidermis with enhanced skin lines) and signs of excoriations. All the objective signs are accompanied by itching. The distribution and shape of the lesions depend on the nature of the allergen and often provide clues to its detection. 'Id' reactions (i.e. development of lesions similar to those at the primary site of allergic contact dermatitis, but distant from it) are not uncommon.

Irritant contact dermatitis occurs quickly after first exposure to an irritant. It is charac-terized by well-defined plaques of erythema, vesicles, blisters and erosions (Fig. 27.3). Irritant contact dermatitis usually bypasses the papular stage and, in the subacute stage, crusts and scaling predominate. The common-est example of irritant contact dermatitis in young children is diaper (nappy) dermatitis.

HISTOPATHOLOGICAL FINDINGS

Early lesions of allergic contact dermatitis are characterized by superficial perivascular and interstitial infiltrates composed mostly of lymphocytes (but sometimes of variable numbers of eosinophils), edema of the papillary dermis, and focal spongiosis that may eventually result in spongiotic vesicles (Fig. 27.4).

Fully developed lesions show a somewhat denser infiltrate of similar composition, more marked edema of dermal papillae, psoriasiform hyperplasia, spongiotic vesicles, and scaly crusts composed of parakeratosis and plasma.

Late lesions are marked by features of lichen simplex chronicus, a consequence of vigorous and prolonged rubbing of the persistent pruritic lesions of allergic contact dermatitis. The findings are of compact orthokeratosis, hypergranulosis, irregular psoriasiform hyperplasia and a papillary dermis thickened by coarse collagen bundles that are oriented perpendicular to the skin surface and parallel to the rete ridges.

Irritant contact dermatitis is characterized by superficial perivascular and interstitial infiltrates of lymphocytes and neutrophils, ballooning of epidermal keratinocytes, ballooning vesiculation and necrosis of keratinocytes.

LABORATORY FINDINGS

Patch tests are necessary to prove a sensitization. In children who are younger than 5 years of age, concentration of the agents used in patch tests should be adjusted (usually to one-half of adult concentration).

ETIOLOGY AND PATHOGENESIS

In children, the most frequent causes of allergic contact dermatitis are nickel (in jewellery), dichromates (in shoes), phenylenediamine, balsam of Peru, neomycin, sulfonamides, antihistamine creams, and rubber in shoes. Among cosmetics, agents that most commonly cause allergic contact dermatitis are moisturizing and cleansing agents, antiperspirants, lipsticks and eye make-up, in that order. The commonest allergenic ingredients in cosmetics are fragrances, followed by preservatives (such as Kathon CG or parabens) and emulsifiers. In the first year of life, allergic contact dermatitis is nearly always a consequence of topically applied vioform, neomycin, or penicillin. Allergic contact dermatitis is an example of type IV delayed hypersensitivity.

Irritant contact dermatitis differs from allergic contact dermatitis because it is not immunologically mediated.

MANAGEMENT

The agent responsible for allergic contact dermatitis should be sought vigorously. Irritants are usually easier to recognize than allergens by history and physical examination. Treatment consists of elimination of the causative allergen or irritant. This alone should bring relief, albeit slowly. Prompt improvement can be effected by topical application of corticosteroids. If there is severe oozing and crusting, compresses with plain water or agents such as aluminium hydroxide should be applied before topical corticosteroids are brought in contact with the affected site. Systemic corticosteroids may be indicated in rare circumstance. Antihistamines help to diminish pruritus, but have no other benefits.

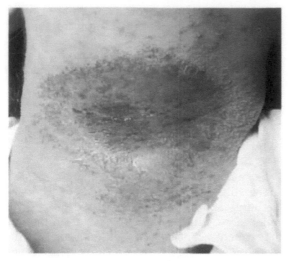

Figure 27.1
Allergic contact dermatitis. Scales, crusted papules and vesicles provide a rim around a weeping erosion. The cause of this dermatitis was topically applied neomycin.

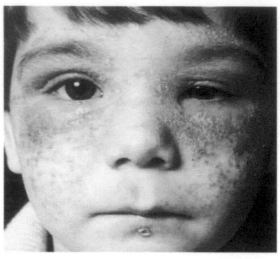

Figure 27.2
Allergic contact dermatitis. In addition to prominent edema of periorbital skin bilaterally, there are papules covered by gray scales and yellow crusts. The dermatitis was a consequence of eyedrops that contained an antibiotic.

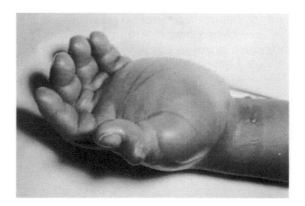

Figure 27.3
Irritant contact dermatitis. The vesicles and bullae were caused by an irritant in this child's mitten. The blisters developed quickly (hours) after the mitten was first worn.

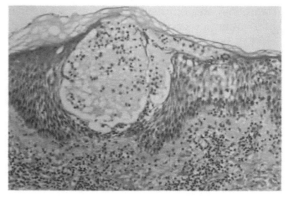

Figure 27.4
Allergic contact dermatitis. This is an early lesion because there is only a single discrete spongiotic vesicle despite the several zones of spongiosis. Furthermore, the cornified layer has a basket-weave configuration devoid of parakeratosis or scaly crusts, a sign of a lesion that is only a few days old.

28

CUTIS LAXA

Cutis laxa is an uncommon disorder of elastic tissue that is characterized by sagging, flaccid, inelastic skin. It may be congenital or acquired.

EPIDEMIOLOGY

Cutis laxa is very rare.

CLINICAL FINDINGS

The skin in cutis laxa hangs in loose folds and gives the impression of being too large for the body. Because the skin is inelastic, it returns slowly to its normal condition after being stretched. The laxity of the skin is particularly evident in the pendulous, drooping folds of the face 'basset hound facies'. Affected children appear far older than their actual years. Lax vocal cords give the voice a hoarse sound. Laxity of joints does not occur usually in cutis laxa.

An inflammatory process, which may be widespread, usually precedes the acquired form of cutis laxa. The eventual laxity may be localized to a discrete zone of the skin (Fig. 28.1) or it may be diffuse.

The congenital form of cutis laxa (Figs 28.2 and 28.3) may be transmitted in autosomal-dominant, autosomal-recessive or, rarely, X-linked fashion. The autosomal-dominant form is the mildest, affects mainly the skin, and may improve without treatment. The autosomal recessive form is more severe and affects organs other than the skin. The X-linked form is thought by some to be related to Ehlers–Danlos syndrome.

COMPLICATIONS

Widespread defects of the elastic tissue in cutis laxa lead to systemic manifestations such as emphysema, bronchiectasis, numerous diverticula of the urinary bladder and the gastrointestinal tract, inguinal, umbilical and diaphragmatic hernias, mitral valve prolapse, aortitis and arterial dilatation.

HISTOPATHOLOGICAL FINDINGS

In the early phase there is a sparse infiltrate of neutrophils aligned along elastic fibers throughout the entire dermis. Later there are neither neutrophils nor elastic fibers (Fig 28.4).

ETIOLOGY AND PATHOGENESIS

It has been shown that cutis laxa starts after exposure to systemically administered drugs, febrile episodes and surgery. How these precipitating events actually induce cutis laxa is not known. It is not known whether the defect in cutis laxa lies in decreased formation of elastin or in increased destruction of it.

MANAGEMENT

Correction of pendulous folds of skin by plastic surgerys offers the only hope for patients with cutis laxa. Even this modality benefits only those in whom the disorder is slight.

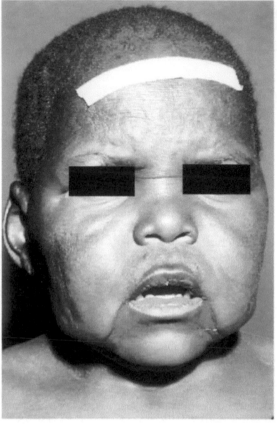

Figure 28.1
Acquired cutis laxa. This condition occurred after Sweet's syndrome in a young black girl. It resulted from loss of elastic tissue following the effects of dense infiltrates of neutrophils in Sweet's syndrome.

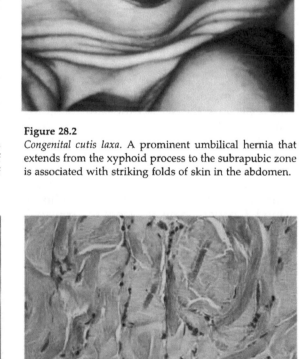

Figure 28.2
Congenital cutis laxa. A prominent umbilical hernia that extends from the xyphoid process to the subrapubic zone is associated with striking folds of skin in the abdomen.

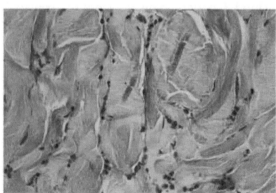

Figure 28.3
Congenital cutis laxa. Pendulous folds of skin on the arm, in the axilla and on the trunk are covered by lanugo hair.

Figure 28.4
Acquired cutis laxa. This is a moderately dense sparse infiltrate composed mostly of neutrophils throughout the entire dermis. The neutrophils are aligned along elastic fibers, and these fibers may eventually be destroyed by them.

29

CUTIS MARMORATA TELANGIECTATICA CONGENITA

Cutis marmorata telangiectatica congenita is a vascular anomaly that is present at birth. It is characterized by a distinctive reticulated pattern that follows the superficial vasculature and tends to fade progressively with time.

EPIDEMIOLOGY

Cutis marmorata telangiectatica congenita is uncommon but not rare.

CLINICAL FINDINGS

The important features of cutis marmorata telangiectatica congenita are livid, reticulated mottling of the skin (Fig 29.1), telangiectasias, phlebectasias and ulcerations with crusts. There may be hints of atrophy but, at times, verrucous or hyperkeratotic lesions may be present. The condition involves circumscribed segments of the skin, usually of a limb, but it may be widespread. The involved areas, in decreasing order of frequency, are the extremities, the trunk, the face and the scalp. The lesions usually fade during the early years of life but clinical improvement is slow, and major lesions can still be seen in adulthood. Cutis marmorata telangiectatica congenita must be differentiated from physiologic cutis marmorata, which is a transient phenomenon in newborns (Fig. 29.2).

Associations

About 50% of children with cutis marmorata telangiectatica congenita have one or more associated abnormalities, among them varicosities, hemiatrophy or hemihypertrophy of a limb, dystrophic teeth, glaucoma, mental retardation, macrocephaly, cerebrovascular malformations and syndactyly

HISTOPATHOLOGICAL FINDINGS

The lesions consist of an increased number of widely dilated venules in the upper part of the reticular dermis (Fig. 29.3).

ETIOLOGY AND PATHOGENESIS

The cause is unknown. Defects during embryonic development and teratogens have been implicated, but nothing has been proven.

MANAGEMENT

A careful search should be undertaken for all associated abnormalities and, if detected, they should be managed promptly and properly. Care of the skin consists only of management of any ulcers that may develop.

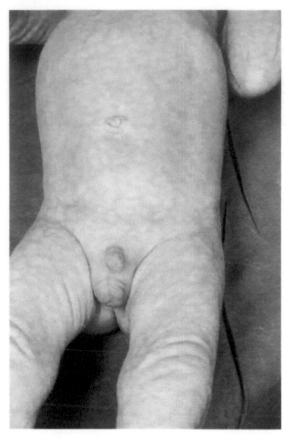

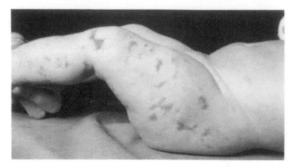

Figure 29.1
Cutis marmorata telangiectatica congenita. Caramel-colored, stellate, atrophic patches are scattered over the extremities. The marble-like quality has been lost as the process has resolved.

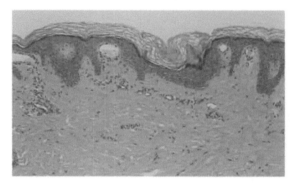

Figure 29.2
Physiologic cutis marmorata. This pattern of 'marbled skin' caused by dilated vessels is a transient phenomenon in newborns and represents a vasomotor reaction to a lowering in the environmental temperature.

Figure 29.3
Cutis marmorata telangiectatica congenita. There is an increased number of widely dilated venules in the upper third of the dermis.

30

DARIER'S DISEASE

Darier's disease is a genodermatosis that is characterized clinically by rough, gray–brown, mostly non-follicular papules that are localized predominantly on the face and the upper part of the trunk. Histopathologically it is characterized by foci of acantholytic and dyskeratotic cells.

EPIDEMIOLOGY

Darier's disease is uncommon but not rare.

CLINICAL FINDINGS

The fundamental lesions of Darier's disease are brownish keratotic papules (Figs 30.1 and 30.2), which may become confluent to form plaques. Sites of predilection are the 'seborrheic areas,' which include the face, the preauricular areas and the ears, the neck, the chest and the midline of the back. Commonly, flat wart-like papules are present on the dorsa of the hands and the feet. Punctate keratoses, either raised or with a central pit, may be seen on the palms and soles. The nails are commonly affected in Darier's disease, and increased brittleness, longitudinal splits and V-shaped notches of the distal part of the nail plate are typical findings. Lesions tend to appear from the age of 5 years through to adolescence. The disease is persistent and long-standing. It is exacerbated during summer and after exposure to ultraviolet light. The oral mucosa in patients with Darier's disease may be affected by white papules clustered in a 'cobblestone' pattern.

Complications

Patients with Darier's disease are susceptible to widespread cutaneous infections by viruses such as herpes simplex, vaccinia and Coxsackie viruses. Less frequently, bacteria or fungi may infect the lesions of Darier's disease.

HISTOPATHOLOGICAL FINDINGS

Darier's disease is characterized by foci of suprabasal clefts, acantholytic dyskeratotic cells in the spinous and granular layers (Figs 30.3 and 30.4) and columns of parakeratotic cells, some of which are acantholytic

ETIOLOGY AND PATHOGENESIS

Darier's disease is inherited as an autosomal-dominant trait. The site of altered gene has been localized in 12q23–24.1

MANAGEMENT

'Keratolytic' ointments and creams that contain all-trans retinoic acid are beneficial. Some children with Darier's disease benefit from oral retinoids, but others do not. Treatment with either 13-cis-retinoic acid or etretinate should be started at a low dose of 0.5 mg/kg per day in two divided doses and increased gradually if needed.

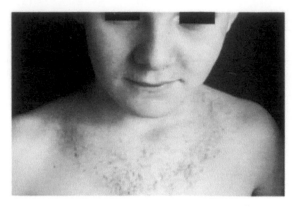

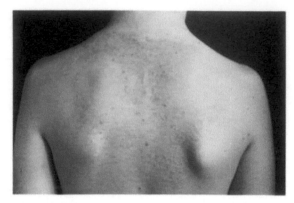

Figure 30.1
Darier's disease. Red–brown keratotic papules are present in semilunar configuration on the upper part of the chest, where they are confined to sites exposed to sunlight.

Figure 30.2
Darier's disease. Red–brown keratotic papules are present in somewhat wedge-shaped distribution on the back.

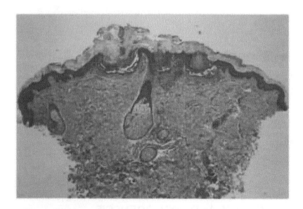

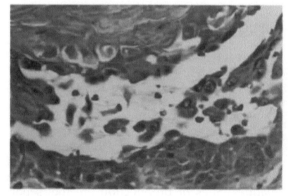

Figure 30.3

Figure 30.4

Figures 30.3 and 30.4
Darier's disease. Several foci of acantholytic dyskeratosis are apparent within the epidermis. Each focus is characterized by a suprabasal cleft, above which acantholytic dyskeratotic cells are present in the spinous, granular and cornified layers. Each focus is topped by column of parakeratosis.

31

DERMATITIS HERPETIFORMIS

Dermatitis herpetiformis is a chronic disorder associated with gluten enteropathy. It is characterized clinically by intensely pruritic papules and vesicles that tend to be grouped in herpetiform fashion. Histopathologically it is characterized by subepidermal vesicles in dermal papillae, in which there are numerous neutrophils.

EPIDEMIOLOGY

The prevalence varies from one person per 10,000 to one person per 80,000, depending on the population studied. In children the peak age of onset is between 3 and 6 years.

CLINICAL FINDINGS

Dermatitis herpetiformis is typified by pink, edematous (urticarial) papules and by vesicles distributed symmetrically over the shoulders, especially the scapulae, the elbows, the back, the sacrum, the buttocks and the knees (Figs 31.1, 31.2, 31.3 and 31.4). Herpetiform grouping of lesions is a helpful, but inconstant, diagnostic feature. Sometimes the only signs are crusted erosions or ulcerations, which are the result of vigorous excoriation, or post-inflammatory hypopigmentation (see Figs 31.1 and 31.4). A child with dermatitis herpetiformis may complain of stinging, burning or itching of the skin, any one of which may herald eruption of fresh papules and vesicles. Ingestion of iodides or overload of gluten dramatically exacerbates the eruption. In the absence of specific therapy, lesions of dermatitis herpetiformis can persist into adulthood.

Associations

A gluten-dependent enteropathy, characterized by patchy atrophy of jejunal villi, occurs in nearly all patients. Immunoglobulin A antibodies binding to the intermyofibril substance of smooth muscle (antiendomysial antibodies) are present in the majority of patients. The incidence of HLA-B8 and DR3 is markedly increased compared with the general population.

LABORATORY FINDINGS

Direct immunofluorescence reveals granular deposits of immunoglobulin A, as well as deposits of complement (C3) and fibrin, at the tips of dermal papillae in the skin around the lesions (Fig. 31.8). Circulating basement membrane zone antibodies are generally not detectable in the serum of patients, although immunocomplexes have been found in 20–40% of patients.

HISTOPATHOLOGICAL FINDINGS

The papules are characterized by collections of neutrophils, neutrophilic nuclear dust, a variable number of eosinophils, microabscesses in dermal papillae (Figs 31.5 and 31.6) and by subepidermal clefts that may contain fibrin. Vesicles are subepidermal and contain mostly neutrophils but also eosinophils (Fig. 31.7).

ETIOLOGY AND PATHOGENESIS

The presence of granular deposits of immunoglobulin A at the dermoepidermal junction and the association of dermatitis herpetiformis with gluten-sensitive enteropathy indicate that a defective mucosal immune response may be pivotal to the development of this disorder in genetically predisposed people. However, the relationship of the gluten-sensitive enteropathy to the skin lesions has been controversial. Following loading of gluten by ingestion, patients develop increased levels of circulating immune complexes to gluten–immunoglobulin A, which are deposited in dermal papillae. Subsequent activation of complement, chemotaxis of neutrophils and release of neutrophilic mediators lead to tissue injury.

MANAGEMENT

In most children, cutaneous and intestinal manifestations of dermatitis herpetiformis may be controlled within 1–6 months of starting a gluten-free diet. Although all types of cutaneous lesions of dermatitis herpetiformis respond dramatically to therapy with dapsone, the accompanying intestinal disorder is unaffected by dapsone. In patients who are unresponsive to diet alone, a combination of gluten restriction and dapsone therapy enables the daily dose of dapsone to be reduced markedly. Patients taking dapsone must have their glucose-6-phosphate dehydrogenase level measured before and during therapy, because dapsone may induce catastrophic hemolysis in patients who are deficient in this enzyme.

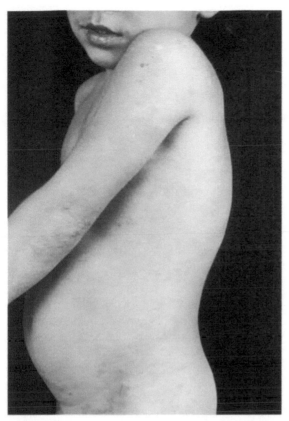

Figure 31.1
Dermatitis herpetiformis. Urticarial papules and crusts are situated near the elbows, and foci of post-inflammatory hypopigmentation are present on the shoulders. Some of the papules have become confluent to form small plaques.

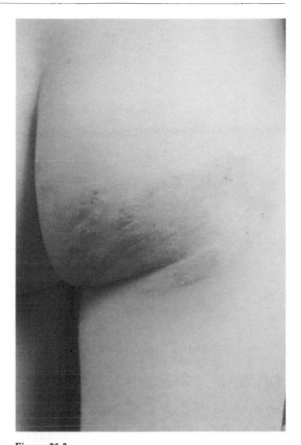

Figure 31.3
Dermatitis herpetiformis. On the buttocks of this child a plaque made up of an edematous papule and vesicles is evident.

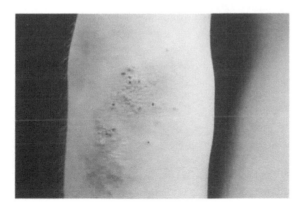

Figure 31.2
Dermatitis herpetiformis. Herpetiform grouping of lesions is a typical diagnostic feature.

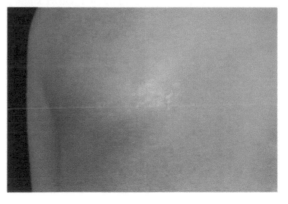

Figure 31.4
Dermatitis herpetiformis. The characteristic distribution of the hypopigmented macule is virtually diagnostic of this disease.

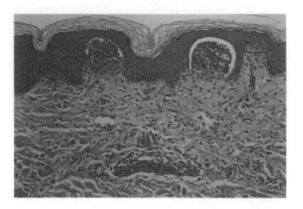

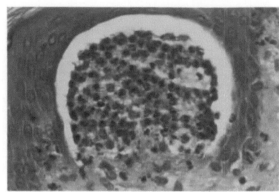

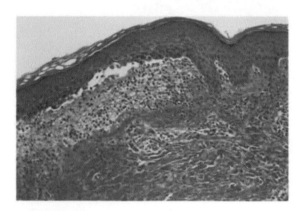

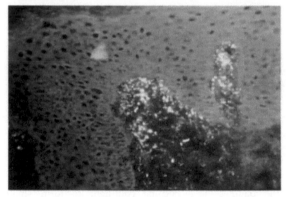

Figure 31.7
Dermatitis herpetiformis. A subepidermal blister contains neutrophils and eosinophils.

Figure 31.8
Dermatitis herpetiformis. Direct immunofluorescence. Most granules of immunoglobulin A are situated near the top of dermal papillae.

32

DERMATOFIBROMA

EPIDEMIOLOGY

Dermatofibroma is the commonest fibro-histiocytic proliferation in adults but it is rare in children.

CLINICAL FINDINGS

Dermatofibromas (Fig. 32.1) are well-defined, usually asymptomatic papules and nodules that range in size from a few millimeters to more than 20 mm, with a mean of about 10 mm. They have a predilection for the extremities, especially the legs. Their color ranges from pink to dark brown and tends to vary from the center of the lesion to the edge. Dermatofibromas, on palpation, can be appreciated to be much deeper lesions than they appear to be on inspection; only a small portion of their mass is elevated above the surface of the skin. Over the course of many years, however, dermatofibromas become progressively flatter and may eventually become depressed below the surface of the surrounding skin.

HISTOPATHOLOGICAL FINDINGS

Dermatofibromas consist of a proliferation of histiocytes and fibrocytes within the dermis, with thickened bundles of collagen at the periphery of the lesion (Fig. 32.2). There is epidermal hyperplasia with hyperpigmentation.

ETIOLOGY AND PATHOGENESIS

In general, dermatofibromas appear within weeks or months after an injury, often a penetrating one.

MANAGEMENT

Dermatofibromas are best left alone. They flatten in time. Surgical excision may be employed for cosmetic purposes. Cryosurgery has been claimed to be effective in some patients.

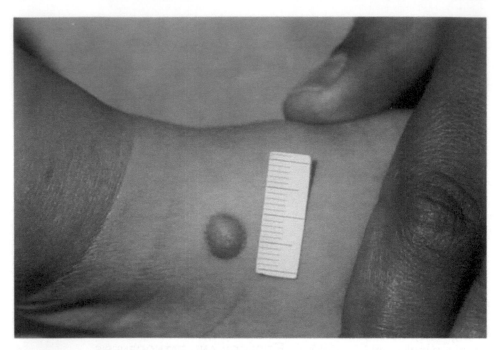

Figure 32.1
Dermatofibroma. This dome-shaped, red–brown, firm nodule appeared a few weeks after a penetrating trauma.

Figure 32.2
Dermatofibroma. Numerous fibrocytes and histiocytes are seen to be associated with coarse bundles of collagen. All the components are arrayed haphazardly.

33 DERMATOFIBROSARCOMA PROTUBERANS

Dermatofibrosarcoma protuberans is a low-grade sarcoma. It is characterized clinically by agminated papules, nodules and, eventually, tumors. Histopathologically, it is characterized by short fascicles of cells with some wavy nuclei in the dermis and subcutis. Its grows slowly and rarely metastasizes.

EPIDEMIOLOGY

Dermatofibrosarcoma protuberans is rare in children.

CLINICAL FINDINGS

A typical lesion of dermatofibrosarcoma protuberans begins as a macule. Within months it becomes a small, raised, nipple-like projection (Fig. 33.1), then a nodule, and sometimes a tumor. Some macules eventually become patches that evolve into plaques (Fig. 33.2) on which nodules and tumors may supervene. The lesions, which are firm, often have an orange, red, violaceous or brown hue. If tumors become very large, they may ulcerate, but this is uncommon. In 1–5% of patients, dermatofibrosarcoma protuberans may be pigmented. Sites of predilection are the upper part of the trunk, the proximal extremities, the head and the neck. Lesions grow slowly for years. Persistence locally after attempts of excision is the rule, but metastases are uncommon.

HISTOPATHOLOGICAL FINDINGS

Dermatofibrosarcoma protuberans is a non-epithelial neoplasm constituted by cells with oval and wavy nuclei arranged in fascicles that interweave within the dermis, subcutaneous fat and often in tissues that underline them (Figs 33.3 and 33.4). Mucin is present in variable quantities.

ETIOLOGY AND PATHOGENESIS

The cause of dermatofibrosarcoma protuberans is not known. Trauma has been claimed to precede the onset in 25% of cases.

MANAGEMENT

Dermatofibrosarcoma protuberans must be excised widely and deeply if cure is to be effected. Persistence (recurrence at a local site) of neoplastic cells after apparently complete excision of dermatofibrosarcoma protuberans is notorious and may pose serious problems in management because the neoplastic cells grow steadily and unremittingly downwards and outwards. Radiotherapy after surgical excision is said to decrease the incidence of local recurrence. Moh's micrographic surgery is claimed to be the treatment of choice.

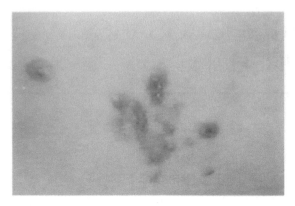

Figure 33.1
Dermatofibrosarcoma protuberans. Orange–brown papules and poorly circumscribed plaques are present on the chest.

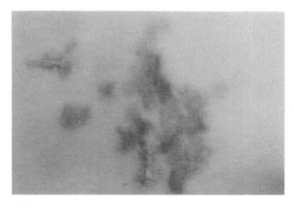

Figure 33.2
Dermatofibrosarcoma protuberans. The orange–brown patches and plaques are relatively early lesions of this low-grade sarcoma.

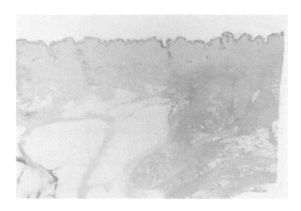

Figure 33.3

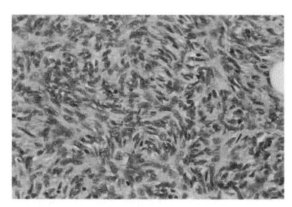

Figure 33.4

Figures 33.3 and 33.4
Dermatofibrosarcoma protuberans. An increased number of oval and spindle-shaped cells arranged in short, interwoven fascicles can be seen throughout the dermis and markedly widened septa in the subcutaneous fat. Nuclei are not atypical, and mitotic figures are few. A neoplasm such as this one may eventually extend into fascia as well into skeletal muscle.

34

DERMATOMYOSITIS

Dermatomyositis is a systemic disease of unknown cause that particularly involves the skin and skeletal muscle.

EPIDEMIOLOGY

Dermatomyositis is uncommon but not rare. It tends to begin in children aged between 5 and 10 years.

CLINICAL FINDINGS

Changes in the skin in most children with dermatomyositis are evident by the time a physician first sees them. A pink to violaceous suffusion of the skin of the eyelids may extend to involve the nasal bridge and the malar areas (Fig. 34.1) and may also include the ears. The color of the eruption has been likened to that of heliotrope, a flower. Discrete scales may partially cover the discoloration. Edema on the eyelids may be prominent (Fig. 34.2), even dramatic, as may be telangiectasia.

Symmetrical, scaly redness is present on the extensors of the extremities, particularly the elbows, knees, medial malleoli and finger and toe joints. Papules and, less often, small plaques (plaques of Gottron) tend to form, particularly on the fingers (Fig. 34.3). Skin that overlies joints may be atrophic and may even ulcerate. The combination of hyperpigmentation and hypopigmentation, atrophy and telangiectases over the extensor surfaces is known as poikilodermatomyositis. Severe cutaneous expression of dermatomyositis may be marked by telangiectases of periungual folds and nail beds.

Calcinosis (Fig. 34.4) is present in 50% of children affected by dermatomyositis. It may appear as small, hard deposits or as large, tumorous deposits, mostly in the subcutis. Calcium may accumulate in intermuscular fascial planes. These foci of calcification may cause great debility.

Malaise and fatigue may precede the onset of symmetrical weakness of proximal muscles that is so characteristic of dermatomyositis.

Involvement of the esophagus, in as many as one-third of patients, results in difficulty in swallowing and a heightened risk of aspiration of food.

With the use of systemic corticosteroids, about 90% of patients with childhood dermatomyosistis survive the disease with little residual disability.

Complications

Severe muscle involvement may lead to life-threatening paralysis of the respiratory muscles. Deposits of calcium are purported to lead to widespread tissue necrosis. Dystrophic calcification may impair the mobility of joints and limbs. Aspiration and hyperventilation may follow involvement of esophageal and chest muscles.

LABORATORY FINDINGS

Diagnosis may be confirmed by muscle enzyme studies, electromyography and muscle biopsy:

- muscle enzyme studies show elevation of creatine phosphokinase, aldolase, lactate

dehydrogenase and aspartate aminotransferase, together with increased urinary
creatinine excretion (> 200 mg per 24
hours);
• electromyography shows a myopathic
pattern;
• muscle biopsy reveals sparse infiltrates,
mostly of lymphocytes, around venules in
the connective tissue that envelops muscle
fascicles, and segmental necrosis within
muscle fibers with loss of cross-striations.

HISTOPATHOLOGICAL FINDINGS

The skin lesions are characterized by thinned
epidermis, vacuolar alteration at the
dermoepidermal junction, a thickened
basement membrane and a sparse, superficial
infiltrate of lymphocytes around superficial
venules and along the dermoepidermal
junction. Mucin can be seen in the reticular
dermis (Figs 34.5 and 34.6).

ETIOLOGY AND PATHOGENESIS

The cause of dermatomyositis is not known.
The characteristic nature of the lesions associated with the typical humoral autoimmune
abnormalities has led to the hypothesis that
the disorder results from a genetically determined aberrant autoimmune response to
myotropic infectious agents such as viruses
and *Toxoplasma gondii*.

MANAGEMENT

Most children with dermatomyositis require
treatment with systemic corticosteroids, such
as prednisone 1–2 mg/kg per day. This treatment prompts regression of inflammatory
lesions in the skin, reduces signs and
symptoms of inflammatory changes in skeletal muscle and returns muscle enzyme levels
to normal. In some children, even high doses
of corticosteroids may not suffice to control
the activity of dermatomyositis. The addition
or substitution of other immunosuppressants,
such as methotrexate, azathioprine or
cyclosporin A, may benefit such children.
Plasmapheresis has been used effectively in
children whose disease is resistant to all kinds
of drug therapy. In all cases, a diet high in
calories and proteins is important because
skeletal muscles become progressively wasted
during the course of the disease.
Physiotherapy is required if mobility is to be
maintained and contractures are to be
prevented.

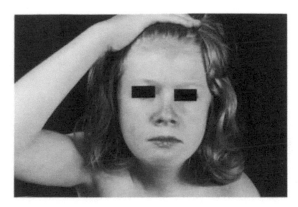

Figure 34.1
Dermatomyositis. In addition to faintly red lesions on the forehead, the eyelids, the malar regions and the nose, this adolescent has discrete scales on the upper and lower lips.

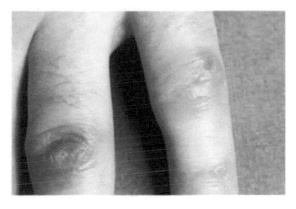

Figure 34.3
Dermatomyositis. The lesions that overlie the joints are known as Gottron's papules. These discrete, slightly violaceous papules are covered by scales.

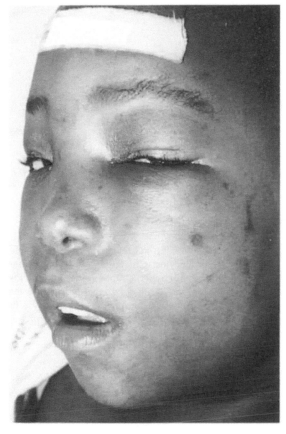

Figure 34.2
Dermatomyositis. The eyelids of this youngster are markedly swollen and have a violaceous hue, a common presentation for dermatomyositis. The discoloration, which appears purple against the black skin, is seen as heliotropic in white skin.

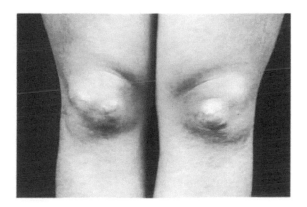

Figure 34.4
Dermatomyositis. In the skin above the knees, deposits of calcium can be seen as white specks. There are also telangiectases and hints of atrophic scars.

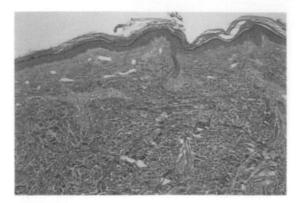

Figure 34.5

Figures 34.5 and 34.6
Dermatomyositis. Note the sparse, superficial perivascular infiltrate of lymphocytes with numerous telangiectases, the focally thinned but hyperkeratotic epidermis with loss of rete ridges, and the focally smudged dermoepidermal junction. These are typical findings of dermatomyositis. Abundant granular basophilic material (mucin) is present between collagen bundles.

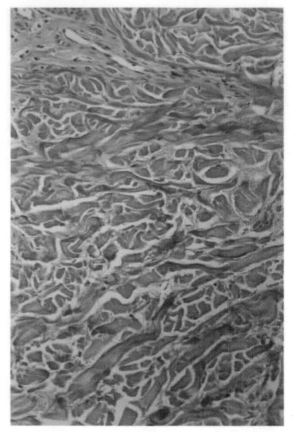

Figure 34.6

35

DERMATOPHYTOSIS

Dermatophytosis refers to cutaneous infection by any of the microscopic fungi. This common infectious process, often referred to by lay persons as tinea or 'ringworm', expresses itself in a variety of clinical and histopathological forms.

EPIDEMIOLOGY

Fungi can colonize the skin of every human being. Dermatophytosis is very common in warm climates, especially where humans and animals live in close proximity.

CLINICAL FINDINGS

Tinea capitis

This infection of the scalp occurs most commonly in children aged between 6 and 10 years of age. It is commoner in black than in whites. The transmission is usually from person to person or from animal to person. Two types of infection may be distinguished: ectothrix and endothrix. These terms indicate the presence of spores outside ('ecto-') a hair shaft or within it ('endo-').

Ectothrix infection is usually caused by *Microsporum* spp. It is characterized by invasion occurring outside hair shafts. Clinically it causes patches of scalp alopecia with scales (Fig. 35.1), the so-called 'gray patch'. Hair shafts break off slightly above scalp.

Endothrix infection, usually caused by *Trichophyton* spp., consists of an invasion of spores within the hair shaft. It may cause black dots tinea capitis, which is characterized by diffuse and poorly circumscribed patches of alopecia caused by the breaking off of hairs near the surface. Each black dot is caused by a fallen hair. It may also present as a kerion, a boggy, tender, purulent, painful mass (Fig. 35.2), from which hairs fall out and can be pulled out without pain.

Favus is an intensely inflammatory tinea capitis caused by *Trichophyton schoenleinii*. It consists of yellow, cup-shaped aggregations of fungi and skin debris (Fig. 35.3). The lesions have an extremely unpleasant, 'mousy' odor and result in cutaneous atrophy and scarring.

Tinea corporis

This infection of glabrous skin may be prompted by *Trichophyton*, *Microsporum* and *Epidermophyton* spp. It is transmitted by contact with infected animals or people or with contaminated soil. Lesions begin around hair follicles as red macules that soon become papular and spread centrifugally to form rings. These rings consist of red, scaly, sharply marginated patches with vesicles and pustules at the margins. There is a progressive peripheral enlargement and a central clearing, which produces a configuration of concentric rings (Fig. 35.4). Lesions may fuse and so assume a polycyclic pattern. Zoophilic lesions are more inflammatory. Pruritus is frequently present.

Tinea faciei

This condition behaves in an identical way to tinea corporis (Fig. 35.5).

Tinea cruris

This infection, usually caused by *Trichophyton* and *Epidermophyton* spp., is mostly seen in postpubertal boys. It begins on the upper and inner part of the thighs and resembles the lesions of tinea corporis, except that maceration is more common and central clearing is less common.

Tinea pedis and tinea manuum

The organisms that most often provoke this dermatosis are *Trichophyton* and *Epidermophyton* spp. Three clinical patterns are recognized:

- a vesicular form consisting of a patch of vesicles or pustules (Fig. 35.6);
- an interdigital form that is characterized by maceration, peeling and fissuring of toe webs;
- a scaly form that involves the entire sole and sides of the feet (moccasin type).

LABORATORY FINDINGS

Dermatophytosis is diagnosed by demonstrating hyphae and spores in scrapings of cornified cells of the skin, the nail plate or hair shafts after treatment with potassium hydroxide. Diagnosis also is achieved by demonstrating fungi on culture media such as Sabouraud's agar or Dermatophyte Test Medium. Wood's lamp examination can be useful for tinea capitis induced by *Microsporum* spp., in which it shows bright green fluorescence.

HISTOPATHOLOGICAL FINDINGS

Hyphae are easily demonstrated in cornified cells of stratum corneum (Fig. 35.7) and in the inner sheath and hair of follicles (Fig. 35.8) in sections stained by hematoxylin and eosin or by periodic acid–Schiff. Nearly every histopathological pattern of inflammatory disease in the skin may be assumed in response to dermatophytic infection.

ETIOLOGY AND PATHOGENESIS

Organisms responsible for the majority of dermatophytic infections, are *Trichophyton rubrum, Trichophyton tonsurans, Trichophyton mentagrophytes, Epidermophyton floccosum* and *Microsporum canis*. Dermatophytes flourish in warm and moist surroundings. For this reason, dermatophytosis is nearly endemic in many tropical countries. Infection by dermatophytes is limited to cornified cells (i.e. stratum corneum, nail plates and hair shafts). Dermatophytes are believed to penetrate cornified cells by virtue of the effects of keratinolytic proteinases, many of which have been isolated. Cellular immunity plays a role in defence against dermatophytes. Incidence of dermatophytosis is increased in patients who have diseases marked by reduced cellular immunity

MANAGEMENT

Topical agents (imidazoles and allylamines) are effective for treatment of dermatophytoses of skin but not of hair. They must be applied twice daily, usually for 2–4 weeks. This treatment should be continued for at least 1 week after clearing of the lesions.

Systemic agents are required for treatment of tinea capitis, onychomycosis, and moccasin type tinea pedis and for extensive infections of glabrous skin. In the pediatric age group, griseofulvin is the drug of choice (20 mg/kg per day), but it is only active against dermatophytes. Itraconazole and terbinafine have been used in children, with excellent results.

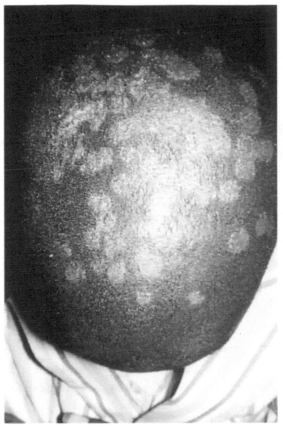

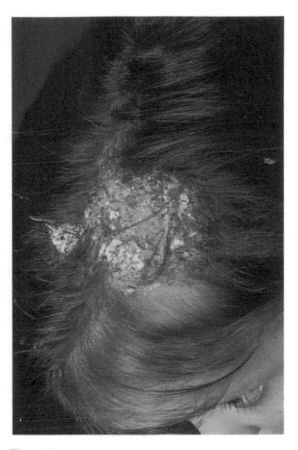

Figure 35.1
Tinea capitis. Numerous grayish and scaly patches and plaques, some of them confluent, cover the scalp of this African youngster. The cause was *Microsporum auduinii*.

Figure 35.2
Tinea capitis. This large, nummular, boggy, very painful tumor with hair loss and multiple pustules and crusts is a typical kerion. Pressure on the lesions causes the discharge of pus.

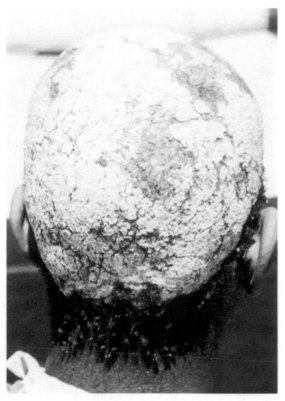

Figure 35.3
Tinea capitis. Chalky, hyperkeratotic and crusted plaques, typical of favus, cover the entire scalp of this South African boy. The zone at the base of the occiput has a honeycomb appearance. Cup-like aggregations of *Trichophyton schoenleinii* near the vertex are known as scutula.

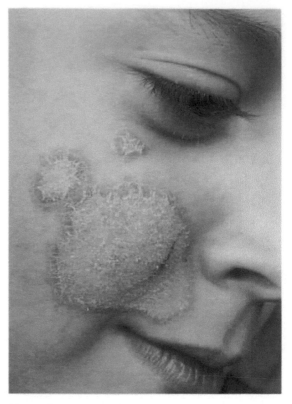

Figure 35.5
Tinea faciei. Borders of this arcuate, annular and serpiginous lesion on the face are constituted of papular vesicles covered by scales.

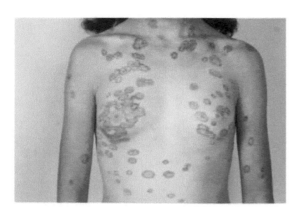

Figure 35.4
Tinea corporis. Numerous reddish, annular, scaly lesions, some of them arrayed in concentric rings, are characteristic.

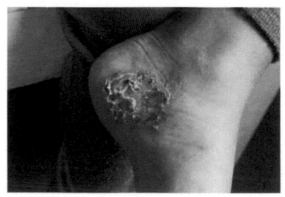

Figure 35.6
Tinea pedis. This well-circumscribed plaque with scalloped borders has some pustules at the periphery as well as a yellow and red crust. The crust has become detached from the centre of the lesion.

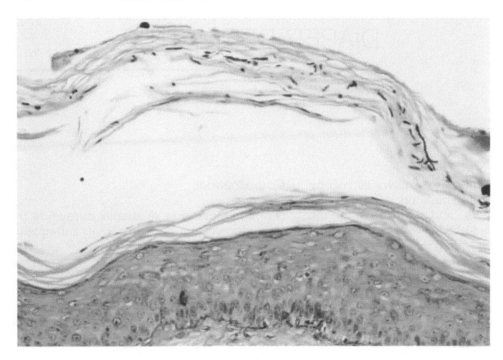

Figure 35.7
Dermatophytosis. The thickened cornified layer is seen teeming with hyphae.

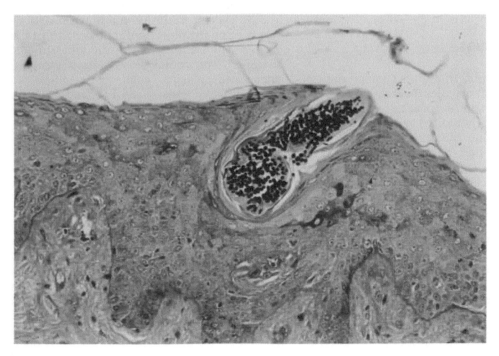

Figure 35.8
Dermatophytosis. The hair shaft and the inner sheath are both filled with fungi.

36

DIAPER DERMATITIS

'Diaper dermatitis,' also known as 'nappy dermatitis,' is an inflammatory condition that occurs in infants and that follows the combined effects of occlusion and irritation in the diaper region.

EPIDEMIOLOGY

This condition was very common in Europe and North America in the 1970s but it is now much rarer owing to improvements in the quality of disposable diapers.

CLINICAL FINDINGS

Clinically, diaper dermatitis is typified at first by shiny, reddish macules that tend to become confluent and form plaques (Fig. 36.1). Lesions are usually limited to convex surfaces of the pubic region, the genitalia, the buttocks, and the upper part of the thighs. At times, discrete, barely elevated, flat-topped, oval papules may accompany the plaques. In long-lasting cases, papules or nodules, which may be isolated or grouped and fully evolved or ulcerated, may be present. These are known as syphiloid dermatitis of Sevestre–Jacquet (Fig. 36.2). In other cases, one or more red–brown nodules and tumors, measuring as much as several centimeters in diameter, arise on convex areas as well as in the crural region. These large, dark nodular and tumorous lesions have been termed granuloma gluteale infantum (Fig. 36.3). Without treatment, diaper dermatitis is likely to persist until the use of diapers stops.

Complications

Secondary infection of diaper dermatitis by staphylococci and *Candida albicans* is frequent.

HISTOPATHOLOGICAL FINDINGS

Fully developed lesions of diaper dermatitis (i.e. granuloma gluteale infantum) are slightly domed and characterized by compact orthokeratosis, marked hypergranulosis, irregular psoriasiform or pseudocarcinomatous hyperplasia, prominent edema of the upper part of the dermis, and a dense, usually patchy infiltrate, made up predominantly of neutrophils, in the upper half of the dermis. The infiltrate is not monomorphous, however, but contains numerous lymphocytes and plasma cells in addition to neutrophils (Figs. 36.4 and 36.5). Karyophagocytosis is common.

ETIOLOGY AND PATHOGENESIS

Many factors are thought to play a causative role in diaper dermatitis. Among them are friction caused by paper or plastic diapers, excessive humidity and maceration, prolonged contact with urine and feces, ammonia produced by the breakdown of urea, secondary bacterial infections, irritation by chemicals contained in diapers or used in cleaning them, and irritation by soap and detergents. However, there is as yet no evidence that links any of these factors conclusively and definitively to the causation of diaper dermatitis.

MANAGEMENT

The frequency of diaper dermatitis correlates directly with the duration of skin contact with feces, and inversely with how often nappies are changed. Therefore, nappies should be changed as often as possible if diaper dermatitis is to be avoided. Tight-fitting diapers also should be avoided and plastic diapers should be shunned entirely. The skin should not be washed with soap but with warm water only. Every effort must be made to keep the skin dry. Non-infectious inflammatory changes may be managed with such time-tested preparations as zinc oxide cream or Lassar's paste. In the Sevestre–Jacquet form of the condition, topical preparations of antibiotics may be used for a few days to decrease likelihood of bacterial infection through erosions. Occlusive agents and potentially irritating agents should not be used.

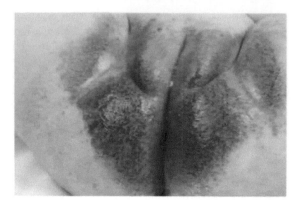

Figure 36.1
Diaper dermatitis. These bright red plaques are eroded, crusted and scaly. Many tiny papules are seen at their periphery.

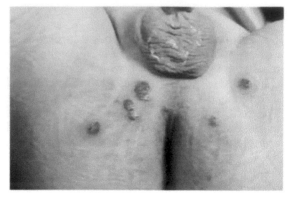

Figure 36.2
Diaper dermatitis. Syphiloid dermatitis of Sevestre–Jacquet. The red–brown papules and nodules covered by scaly crusts resemble lesions of secondary syphilis. The changes are but one manifestation of diaper dermatitis

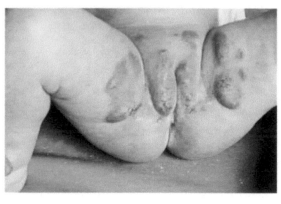

Figure 36.3
Granuloma gluteale infantum. Numerous papules and nodules are situated on top of the plaques. The brown hue indicates that the lesions are long standing. Crusts and scaly crusts cover the erosions and ulcerations.

Figures 36.4 and 36.5
Granuloma gluteale infantum. The lesion is domed because of a dense, brown patchy, lichenoid infiltrate of inflammatory cells. In the upper part of the dermis, blood vessels are dilated. The pallor is evidence of edema. Neutrophils are present within the hyperplastic epidermis. In other foci, lymphocytes and plasma cells predominate.

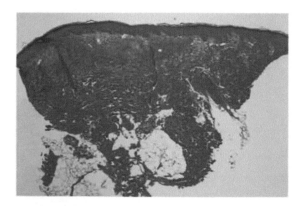

Figure 36.4

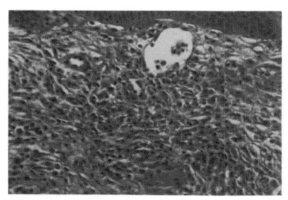

Figure 36.5

37

DYSHIDROTIC DERMATITIS

Dyshidrotic dermatitis, known also as pompholyx and dyshidrosis, is an inflammatory disease in which papules and vesicles are situated mostly on the palms and the soles and along the sides of the fingers and toes.

EPIDEMIOLOGY

Dyshidrotic dermatitis is uncommon before 10 years of age and exceptional before 5 years. From the second decade of life onwards, dyshidrotic dermatitis is among the commoner inflammatory diseases of the skin.

CLINICAL FINDINGS

Tense vesicles, which tend to become coalescent to resemble tapioca, arise along the sides of the fingers. They may ultimately involve an entire palm (or sole) or both (Figs 37.1 and 37.2). If vesicles become confluent, bullae may result. Itching is variable but is often severe. Dyshidrotic dermatitis has an unpredictable course, waxing and waning without apparent cause.

Complications

Extensive vesiculation and secondary infections may cause serious disability by compromising the function of the hands and feet.

HISTOPATHOLOGICAL FINDINGS

Foci of spongiosis and spongiotic vesicles, edema of the papillary dermis, and a superficial, perivascular, predominantly lymphocytic infiltrate are findings in evolving lesions of dyshidrotic dermatitis (Fig. 37.3).

ETIOLOGY AND PATHOGENESIS

The cause of dyshidrotic dermatitis is not known. Despite the name there is no evidence that excessive sweating plays a role. The disease occurs more often in patients with atopic dermatitis. Emotional stress is a possible precipitating factor.

MANAGEMENT

No treatment is consistently effective for dyshidrotic dermatitis, although many have been advocated. Topical corticosteroids are widely used.

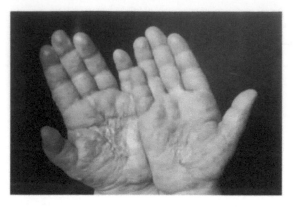

Figure 37.1
Dyshidrotic dermatitis. Nearly the entire volar surface is covered by tiny papules and vesicles, some of which have become confluent and others pustular. Near the wrists the confluence of tiny tense vesicles has eventuated in a multiloculated bulla that looks like tapioca.

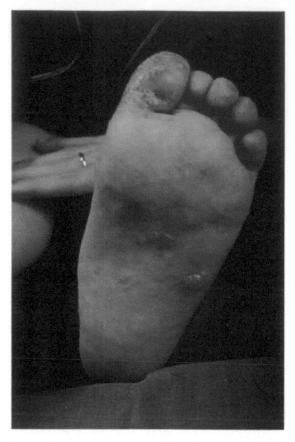

Figure 37.2
Dyshidrotic dermatitis. The toes and the plantar surface of the feet are affected by the inflammatory process at different stages of its evolution, from tiny vesicles to blisters.

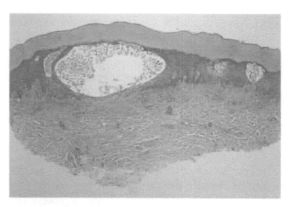

Figure 37.3
Dyshidrotic dermatitis. The lesion on volar skin is characterized by spongiosis and spongiotic vesiculation, psoriasiform hyperplasia and a superficial and mid-dermal (predominantly lymphocytic) infiltrate.

Dyskeratosis congenita (Zinsser–Cole–Engman syndrome) is a rare genetic disorder characterized by a constellation of reticulated hyperpigmentation of the skin, dystrophy of the nails and leukokeratosis on mucous membranes.

EPIDEMIOLOGY

Dyskeratosis congenita is rare. It mainly affects males, and dermatological manifestations generally become evident before puberty.

CLINICAL FINDINGS

Dyskeratosis congenita usually presents itself as slowly progressive skin lesions in the form of reticulate, lacy hyperpigmentation (Fig. 38.1) sometimes accompanied by interspersed zones of hypopigmentation.

Nail dystrophy is found in 98% of patients with dyskeratosis congenita and is expressed as longitudinal grooves in the nails, thinned nails or nearly complete atrophy of the nails.

Leukokeratosis (Fig. 38.2) is present in about 85% of patients and tends to appear on the buccal and lingual mucosa.

Other dermatological manifestations include palmoplantar hyperhidrosis (in 87% of patients), bullae (in 78%), epiphora – a persistent overflow of tears caused by obstruction of the lachrymal ducts and often one of the first symptoms (in 78%), hyperkeratosis of the palms and soles (in 72%), taurodont teeth (in 63%) and aberrations of hair, including alopecia (in 51%).

Hematologic abnormalities occur in more than half of the patients and, as a rule, manifest themselves some time in the second decade of life. Failure of bone marrow to function, with subsequent pancytopenia, is common, as are aplastic anemia, bleeding, and recurrent infections.

Increased susceptibility to neoplasia is characteristic in nearly half of the patients. The neoplasms usually become apparent by the third decade of life. They tend to affect mucous membranes (squamous cell carcinoma in areas of leukoplakia), the pancreas (adenocarcinoma) and the lymph nodes (Hodgkin's disease).

LABORATORY FINDINGS

Anemia is present in about half of patients and is usually the first expression of cytopenia. Neutropenia and thrombocytopenia usually follow shortly, although they may not appear for many years after the onset of anemia. Myeloid and erythroid progenitors in bone marrow are reduced or absent.

HISTOPATHOLOGICAL FINDINGS

The epidermis is thinned focally and is devoid of rete ridges in the thinned foci. Vacuolar alteration is found beneath zones of thinned epidermis. Melanophages and a sparse perivascular infiltrate of lymphocytes are often present in the upper part of the dermis (Figs 38.3 and 38.4). On mucous membranes there may be marked orthokeratosis and parakeratosis, slightly elongated but broadened rete ridges, and variable degrees of nuclear atypia of keratinocytes within the broadened rete ridges.

ETIOLOGY AND PATHOGENESIS

Dyskeratosis congenita is inherited in X-linked fashion, and the responsible gene has been assigned to the Xq 28 locus.

MANAGEMENT

No effective therapy for dyskeratosis congenita is known. Patients with the syndrome should be kept under close observation to detect early signs of bone marrow failure and malignant neoplasms. Topical retinoids may help to decrease leukokeratosis.

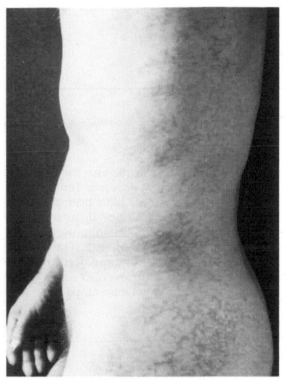

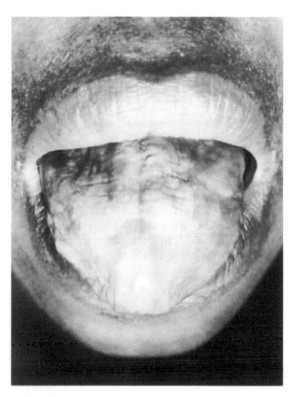

Figure 38.1
Dyskeratosis congenita. Reticulated hyperpigmentation in a patchy distribution covers much of the trunk, the flank and the buttocks of this adolescent.

Figure 38.2
Dyskeratosis congenita. White plaques on the tongue of this black adolescent are a consequence of hyperkertosis. The changes could represent an early stage in the evolution of squamous cell carcinoma.

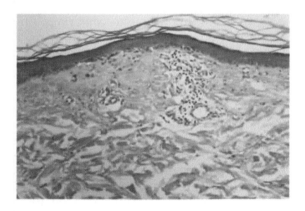

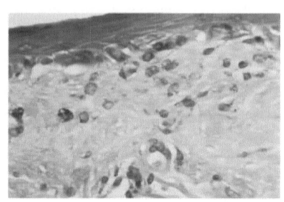

Figure 38.3

Figure 38.4

Figures 38.3 and 38.4
Dyskeratosis congenita. There is a sparse, perivascular, lymphocyte infiltrate beneath a thinned epidermis. The infiltrate obscures the dermoepidermal junction focally, where vacuolar alterations can be seen. Melanophages are present in the upper part of the dermis.

39 EHLERS–DANLOS SYNDROME

Ehlers–Danlos syndrome is not a true syndrome, but a group of at least 10 different disorders characterized by systemic aberration of connective tissue. Hyperelastic or friable skin and hypermobile joints are the findings that most of these disorders have in common.

EPIDEMIOLOGY

Ehlers–Danlos syndrome as a whole is uncommon but not rare.

CLINICAL FINDINGS

The skin in Ehlers–Danlos syndrome is soft, velvety and extremely elastic (Fig. 39.1). In children, once the altered skin has been stretched and released, it returns immediately to its normal position. Increased fragility of the skin in those afflicted by Ehlers–Danlos syndrome causes the skin to split in response to even minor trauma, with resultant formation of atrophic scars of different sizes and shapes (Fig. 39.2). The scars are most commonly situated over bony prominences and extensor surfaces of joints. Healing is slow and sutures repeatedly fail to hold. Areas of trauma also may be sites for development of soft 'molluscoid pseudotumors', which represent abnormal accumulations of collagenous and adipose tissue. The skin bruises easily and hematomas form frequently. Hyperextensibility of joints (Figs 39.3 and 39.4) may result in dislocations, kyphoscoliosis, genu recurvatum and hallux valgus. Hyperextensibility may be so extreme that walking

becomes difficult. Varicose veins may develop in children with the syndrome. Ten forms of Ehlers–Danlos syndrome have been described to date (Table 39.1), and these differ in clinical manifestations, mode of inheritance, and underlying pathological defect. The disease may not become clinically apparent until the child begins to crawl or even to walk. In the absence of visceral involvement, patients may have a normal life span.

ETIOLOGY AND PATHOGENESIS

The causes of Ehlers–Danlos syndrome are described in Table 39.1.

HISTOPATHOLOGICAL FINDINGS

As a rule, conventional microscopy reveals no abnormalities in the skin of patients with Ehlers–Danlos syndrome.

MANAGEMENT

Genetic counselling is crucial to women with types I or IV Ehlers–Danlos syndrome because of the risk of premature rupture of membranes and because of maternal morbidity and mortality. Avoidance of trauma and the use of pressure dressings after trauma are helpful in preventing both cutaneous and joint complications. A surgeon should be highly alert to a diagnosis of Ehlers–Danlos syndrome before performing any operation because of difficulties inherent in the healing of wounds.

Table 39.1 Clinical features, mode of inheritance, and biochemical defect in Ehlers–Danlos syndrome

Type	Main clinical feature	Inheritance	Biochemical defect
I (Gravis)	Hyperextensible, velvety skin; easy bruising; atrophic scars; hypermobile joints; prematurity	Autosomal dominant	Unknown
II (Mitis)	As in type I, but less severe	Autosomal dominant	Unknown
III (Benign hypermobile)	Marked joint hypermobility; skin manifestations almost absent	Autosomal dominant	Unknown
IV (Ecchymotic)	Thin and translucent skin; little joint hypermobility; arterial manifestations; rupture of bowel sometimes	Autosomal dominant or autosomal recessive	Abnormal type III collagen
V (X-linked)	Similar to type II	X-linked	Unknown
VI (Ocular)	Hyperextensible, velvety skin; hypermobile joints; scleral and corneal fragility (recessive)	Autosomal recessive	Lysyl hydroxylase deficiency
VII (Arthrocholasis)	Multiple dislocations; joint hypermobility; soft multiplex skin; scars not abnormal	Autosomal dominant or autosomal recessive	Procollagen conversion abnormality
VIII (Periodontal)	Generalized periodontitis; skin and joint mobility similar to type II	Autosomal dominant	Unknown
IX (Cutis laxa and occipital horn)	Lax, extensible skin; bladder diverticula; inguinal hernias; skeletal abnormalities (recessive)	X-linked	Abnormal copper utilization with deficiency of lysyl oxidase
X (Fibronectin defect)	Similar to type II	Autosomal recessive	Fibronectin defect

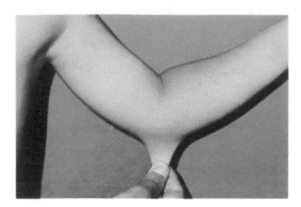

Figure 39.1
Ehlers–Danlos syndrome. Even a gentle tug on the skin elicits dramatic hyperextensibility.

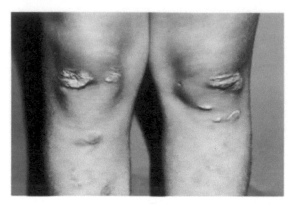

Figure 39.2
Ehlers–Danlos syndrome. There are numerous atrophic scars, like those of anetodermas at sites of previous traumas. Because this condition is characterized by fragility of the skin, subtle trauma may induce scars like these.

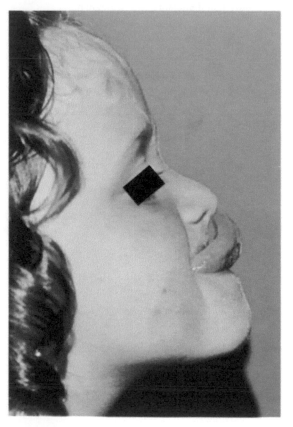

Figure 39.3
Ehlers–Danlos syndrome. Some patients can touch their noses with the tip of their tongues. Note also the atrophic hypopigmented scar on the forehead.

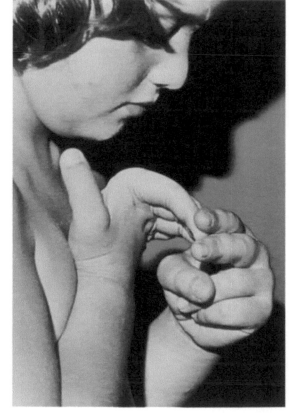

Figure 39.4
Ehlers–Danlos syndrome. This child demonstrates remarkable hyperextensibility of her joints.

ELASTOSIS PERFORANS SERPIGINOSA

Elastosis perforans serpiginosa consists of papules, usually in annular or arcuate configurations. The papules are characterized histopathologically by channels within the surface epithelium; these channels contain altered elastic fibers.

EPIDEMIOLOGY

The disease is uncommon; in about 40% of patients it begins between ages 5 and 10 years.

CLINICAL FINDINGS

The papules of elastosis perforans serpiginosa are asymptomatic, skin-colored to red and keratotic (Fig. 40.1) or crusted. Some of the papules may be umbilicated. Typically, they are 2–5 mm in diameter and are arranged in arcuate (Fig. 40.2), annular and serpiginous patterns. Sites of predilection are the posterolateral aspects of the neck, the arms, the elbows, the knees and the antecubital fossae. Lesions improve without treatment within 5–10 years.

Associations

About 30% of patients with elastosis perforans

serpiginosa also are afflicted by one or more other genodermatoses, such as Ehlers–Danlos syndrome, Marfan's syndrome or pseudoxanthoma elasticum. The disease is especially frequent in people with Down's syndrome.

HISTOPATHOLOGICAL FINDINGS

Elastosis perforans serpiginosa is characterized by an increase in the number of thickened, highly eosinophilic, elastic fibers in the upper part of the dermis and within channels that extend through the surface epithelium, where neutrophils and neutrophilic debris also are lodged (Figs 40.3 and 40.4).

ETIOLOGY AND PATHOGENESIS

Except in the case of lesions induced by penicillamine, the cause of elastosis perforans serpiginosa is not known.

MANAGEMENT

Treatment of elastosis perforans serpiginosa is generally unsatisfactory. Favorable results have been described with liquid nitrogen and stripping with cellophane tape, but only in a few patients.

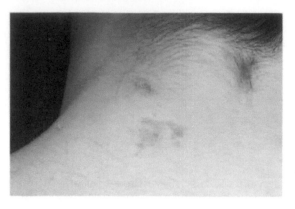

Figure 40.1
Elastosis perforans serpiginosa. Numerous reddish papules with a slight violaceous hue have become confluent to form a small plaque. Scrutiny of the papules reveals a subtle dell within them.

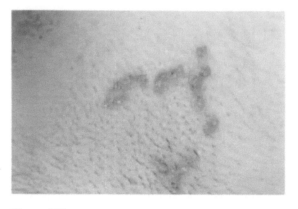

Figure 40.2
Elastosis perforans serpiginosa. The rust-colored keratotic papules situated near the base of the hairline on the posteriolateral neck are arranged in an arcuate pattern rather than a serpiginous pattern.

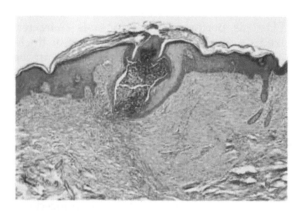

Figure 40.3

Figures 40.3 and 40.4
Elastosis perforans serpiginosa. The epithelial channels shown here are bounded by parakeratosis above and elastic fibers below. Within the channels are numerous neutrophils associated with thick elastic fibers, some of which are stained brightly eosinophilic; others are basophilic.

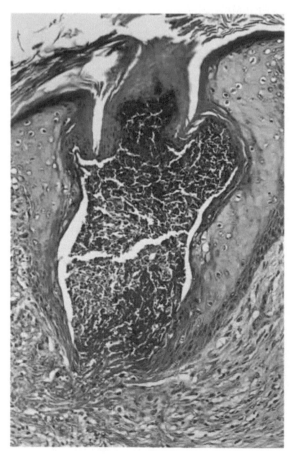

Figure 40.4

Epidermolysis bullosa is a heterogeneous group of hereditary skin diseases characterized by increased fragility of the skin and a tendency to form blisters after minor mechanical trauma. Variants have been classified by electron microscopy as epidermolytic, junctional and dermolytic according to where the plane of separation of blisters occurred.

EPIDEMIOLOGY

Epidermolysis bullosa is considered as a unique entity epidemiologically. It occurs in 1 per 100,000 live births. Dermolytic forms are more frequent than the epidermolytic forms, junctional epidermolysis bullosa being the rarest. National registries have been established in the USA (3000 patients) and Italy (600 patients).

CLINICAL FINDINGS

Epidermolytic epidermolysis bullosa

Three main variants, all inherited as an autosomal-dominant trait, have been described as generalized, localized and herpetiform type.

The generalized (Koebner) type is usually present at birth and consists of blisters that, although widespread, have a predilection for the hands, the feet and the diaper area (Fig. 41.1). Mucosae are rarely involved and the teeth are normal. Dystrophy of the nails occurs in about 20% of patients. Repeated formation of bullae is expected during summer. Some patients improve after puberty.

The localized (Weber–Cockayne) type becomes striking near the end of the 1st year of life when a baby begins to walk. Recurrent bullae develop on the hands and feet (Fig. 41.2). Mucosae are uninvolved, and nails and teeth also are spared. Hyperhidrosis is a complication.

The herpetiform (Dowling–Meara) type causes severe blistering at birth and tends to involve the trunk, face and extremities. Vesicles and bullae are often in a herpetiform pattern. They may house hemorrhagic contents and are surrounded by erythematous borders (Fig 41.3). The lesions resolve rapidly and tend to leave pigmentary abnormalities and milia as sequelae. Mucous membranes are frequently affected. Dystrophy of the nails is common, as is palmoplantar hyperkeratosis. After the age of 7 years, progressive improvement is the rule and life expectancy is usually unaffected.

Junctional epidermolysis bullosa

In the Herlitz type, large bullous and erosive lesions appear at birth on the limbs and the trunk (Fig. 41.6), and because the tendency to re-epithelization is poor (Fig 41.7), healing is often accompanied by the presence of granulation tissue and atrophic scars. Mucous membranes are involved and pharyngeal and laryngeal involvement is common and may lead eventually to a characteristic hoarse voice and asphyxia. The nails are dystrophic. Dental hypoplasia is common, and, as a result, the teeth are malformed and prematurely lost. Severe pulmonary infections lead to a premature death, usually in the 1st year of life. Less severe forms have been noted but life-expectancy is limited to the 2nd decade.

In the non-Herlitz type, bullae recur at sites of trauma on the scalp, face and trunk and leave large atrophic areas as residua (Fig 41.8). Milia are absent. Oral mucosae may be affected during the 1st year of life. The teeth show modifications of enamel, and the nails are absent or dystrophic and thickened. A male pattern alopecia is common in both sexes after puberty. Ophthalmological symptoms are rarely reported. These patients may have a normal life expectancy.

In junctional epidermolysis bullosa with pyloric atresia, widespread bullae and erosions accompanied by severe gastrointestinal symptoms are seen, along with true pyloric atresia. A surgical approach is mandatory. The disease is not always lethal, and some 20% of patients reach adulthood.

Dermolytic epidermolysis bullosa

The dominant (Cockayne–Touraine) type causes a widespread bullous eruption that heals with atrophic, non-mutilating scars in which milia may form, especially on the extensor surfaces of the hands, the elbows (Fig. 41.11), the knees and the feet. On the trunk, in zones seemingly independent of bullae, large, firm, ivory-white, smooth-surfaced papules (albopapuloid lesions) appear. In fact, each of those white papules is a type of hypertrophic scar that develops secondary to subepidermal bullous vesicles. Erosions and scarring of the mucosae are found in 20% of patients, but nails are dystrophic or absent in 80%. The teeth may exhibit modifications of cement and dentine. The course is usually progressive and chronic and associated with considerable morbidity, although generally without life-threatening consequences.

The recessive (Hallopeau–Siemens) type causes widespread bullae that leave scars and milia in their wake. Large ulcerations may be residua of blisters (Fig 41.12). Frequent recurrence of blisters causes cicatricial fusion of the fingers and toes (Fig 41.13) with subsequent contraction. Eventually, the distal parts of the extremities become encased in mitten-like sacs of atrophic skin. Lesions around the mouth and involvement of the oral and esophageal mucosae appear early in the course of the disease and are severe. On occasion, they cause stenosis of these portions of the gastrointestinal tract and scarring. Nails are dystrophic or absent, and the teeth are malformed. The eyes exhibit conjunctival and corneal erosions and scarring with severe impairment of vision. Rarely, bullae, ulcerations and scars affect the inguinal and axillary folds, the neck and the lumbar region. Rarely, there is severe pruritus and the formation of nodular, prurigo-like lesions on the extensor surfaces of the arms and the legs. Severely retarded growth, delayed development, anemia and squamous cell carcinomas that arise in areas of long-standing scars are concurrent findings. The disease is progressive to death at an early age, usually in the 2nd or 3rd decade of life, as a consequence of septic or neoplastic complications.

It must be noted that the relationship 'recessive–severe' and 'dominant–mild' is often false and, in order to avoid mistakes in genetic counselling, only molecular genetic studies should be used together with an examination of the entire family at risk of dermolytic epidermolysis bullosa.

In the variant form, transient epidermolysis of the newborn, the patient experiences bullae at birth that are visible for a short period thereafter. Bullous lesions suddenly disappear within the first 3 months of life. This particular variant seems to be due to some partial release or storage defect of type VII collagen.

HISTOPATHOLOGICAL FINDINGS

Epidermolytic epidermolysis bullosa

Conventional histology is of little use in epidermolysis bullosa (Fig. 41.4). Electron microscopy in epidermolytic epidermolysis bullosa shows that, bullae develop by cytolysis of keratinocytes in the basal layer or just above it. In the Dowling–Meara type, bullae are preceded by aggregation in basal cells of tonofilaments into typical 'clumps', with normal hemidesmosomes (Fig. 41.5). By immunofluorescence, the floor of the bulla is marked by antibodies to type IV collagen, laminin, the antigen of bullous pemphigoid, KF-1 antigen and LH7:2 antigen.

Junctional epidermolysis bullosa

Beneath a subepidermal blister, dermal papillae tend to retain their size and shape. Little or no infiltrate of inflammatory cells can be observed in the blister or in the dermis (Fig. 41.9). Bullae seem to form in the lamina lucida. Common to the various subtypes of junctional epidermolysis bullosa is a decreased number or even the absence of hemidesmosomes, whose anchoring filaments are defective (Fig 41.10). Immunofluorescence has demonstrated antigens of type VII collagen and laminin at the bases of blisters being the antigen of bullous pemphigoid found in the roofs. The monoclonal antibody GB3, which reacts with a normal constituent of the dermoepidermal junction (laminin 5), is absent or markedly reduced in the Herlitz type. Antibodies against collagen type XVII, integrin alpha-6 and integrin beta-4 are used in the diagnosis of the non-Herlitz junctional forms.

Dermolytic epidermolysis bullosa

A subepidermal blister extends down the adnexal epithelial structures. Dermal papillae tend to be preserved in pristine fashion below the blister. A scant infiltrate of inflammatory cells is barely detectable. Fibrosing granulation tissue may occur beneath the blisters. Milia, tiny follicular cysts of the infundibular type (Fig. 41.14), form as a consequence of the blisters. Albopapuloid lesions are slightly dome-shaped and characterized by fibrosis in at least the upper half of the dermis. By electron microscopy, blisters appear to form beneath the basal lamina. Anchoring fibrils appear rudimentary or may be absent. Hemidesmosomes are normal (Fig 41.15). Immunofluorence reveals type IV collagen, laminin and the antigen of bullous pemphigoid in the rooves of the blisters. LH-

7:2 antibody raised against an epitope of type VII collagen is reduced or absent.

ETIOLOGY AND PATHOGENESIS

Epidermolytic epidermolysis bullosa

The epidermolytic forms of epidermolysis bullosa are inherited as an autosomal-dominant trait, even though some pedigree with recessive inheritance has been described. The genes involved in the main forms of epidermolytic epidermolysis bullosa are those of the basal keratins K5 and K14. The clinical severity is related to the relevance of the mutations.

Junctional epidermolysis bullosa

The Herlitz type of junctional epidermolysis bullosa is due to a mutation of one of the three genes that encode for the three proteins that form the laminin 5 protein, which is the most important protein in the hemidesmosomes. These genes are LAMA3, LAMB3 and LAMC2 and are responsible for all the Herlitz phenotypes.

The non-Herlitz type of junctional epidermolysis bullosa is due to genetic defects of the genes that encode for collagen type XVII transmembrane protein and laminin 5 genes.

Junctional epidermolysis bullosa with pyloric atresia is due to a genetic defect of alpha-6 beta-4 integrin. Two different genes are involved – INTGA6 and INTGB4. Molecular biology enables the study of the families at risk for these recessively inherited diseases in order to provide prenatal diagnosis using chorionic villus samples in the 10th or 11th week of gestation.

Dermolytic epidermolysis bullosa

Dermolytic epidermolysis bullosa, inherited as an autosomal-dominant or an autosomal-recessive trait, is a disorder of dermal anchoring fibrils that are formed by the polymerization of type VII collagen. The corresponding gene is mutated. The severity of the disease is linked to the type or position of the mutation. Genetic studies in dermolytic epidermolysis bullosa make prenatal diagnosis possible at an early stage of pregnancy.

MANAGEMENT

No effective treatment is available. Avoidance of trauma is strongly advised at any age and antisepsis of eroded areas daily is mandatory. In particular, pediatricians should help families with regard to nutrition and weaning, in order to avoid mucosal problems and caries. Introduction to school must be encouraged at an early age. In Dowling–Meara epidermolysis bullosa, orthopedic procedures must be undertaken in order to avoid severe sequelae, while low doses of antiserotoninergic drugs, administered systemically, may be beneficial. Surgical procedures on the hands can be useful to relieve contractures but are only temporarily effective. Esophageal dilatation improves deglutition and food intake in patients with severe esophageal stenosis. Enteral feeding, including gastrostomy, may be useful in selected patients. Recent trials with human recombinant erythropoietin has been proposed for severe anemia in affected patients. In general, a multidisciplinary model of care is mandatory in the follow-up of severely affected patients in order to avoid major complications. Transfection studies are in progress in order to obtain gene therapy for these disabling diseases.

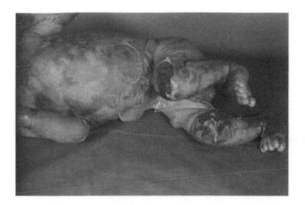

Figure 41.1
Epidermolytic epidermolysis bullosa (generalized type).
Widespread blisters were present since birth in this
newborn.

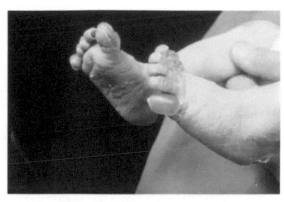

Figure 41.2
Epidermolytic epidermolysis bullosa (localized type). Blisters
in this newborn are localized to the hands and the feet.

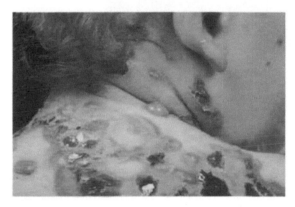

Figure 41.3
Epidermolytic epidermolysis bullosa (herpetiform type). In this
subtype serohemorrhagic bullae in centrifugal arrangement are characteristic and are surrounded by a rim of
erythema.

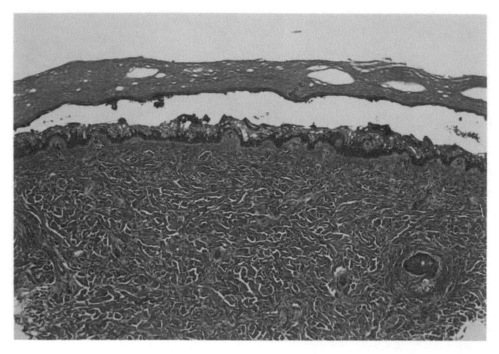

Figure 41.4
Epidermolytic epidermolysis bullosa (localized simple type). The blister forms in the upper portion of the spinous layer. Keratinocytes have abundant pale cytoplasm, which probably reflects intracellular edema.

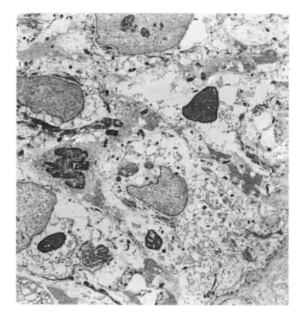

Figure 41.5
Epidermolytic epidermolysis bullosa (herpetiform type). Large cytolytic areas in basal keratinocytes and clumping of tonofilaments are the ultrastructural marker.

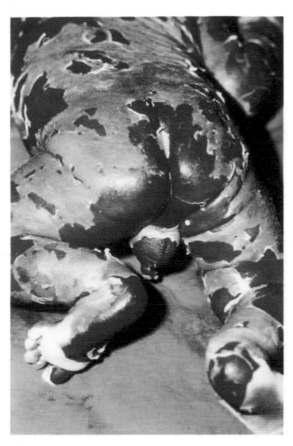

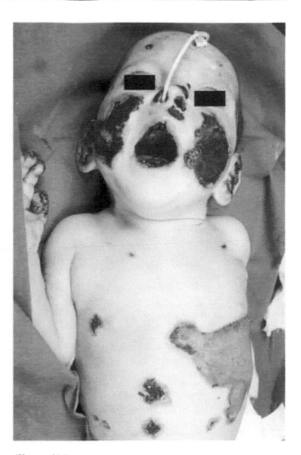

Figure 41.6
Junctional epidermolysis bullosa (Herlitz type). The whole skin of this infant is affected by large bullae that weep when they break, leaving erosions.

Figure 41.7
Junctional epidermolysis bullosa (Herlitz type). Severe recurring erosions are visible on the face and the trunk of this infant.

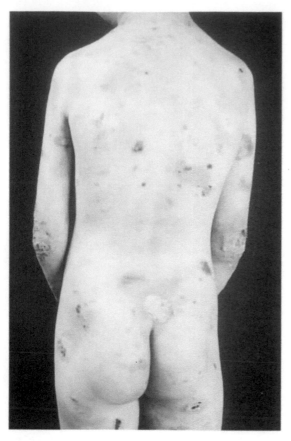

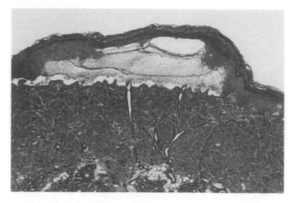

Figure 41.9
Junctional epidermolysis bullosa. A subepidermal blister is
seen to contain fibrin but few inflammatory cells.

Figure 41.8
Junctional epidermolysis bullosa (non-Herlitz type).
Widespread bullous lesions and atrophic scars are
present both on trunk and limbs of this young girl.

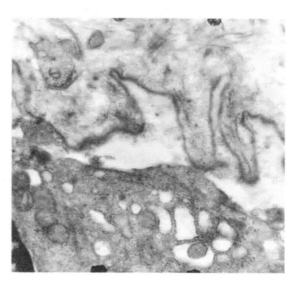

Figure 41.10
Junctional epidermolysis bullosa. By ultrastructure, blisters
are located in the lamina lucida, and hypoplastic or
rudimentary hemidesmosomes are characteristic.

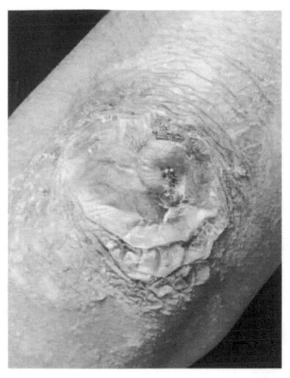

Figure 41.11
Dermolytic epidermolysis bullosa (widespread dominant dystrophic type). The extensive atrophic scars on an elbow are a consequence of recurrent subepidermal blisters at this site.

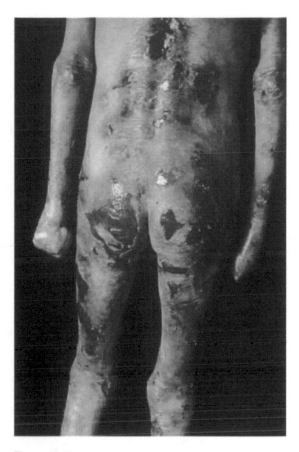

Figure 41.12
Dermolytic epidermolysis bullosa (recessive type). Widespread bullae and large ulcerations leave scars and cicatricial constrictions.

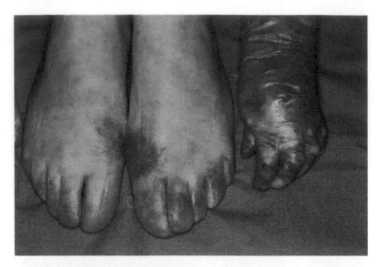

Figure 41.13
Dermolytic epidermolysis bullosa (recessive type). Frequent recurrence of blisters causes cicatricial fusion of the fingers and toes.

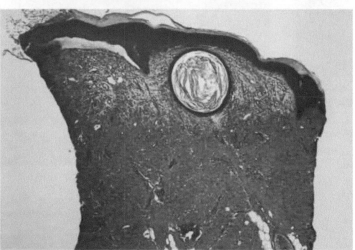

Figure 41.14
Dermolytic epidermolysis bullosa. A broad subepidermal blister extends along a folliculosebaceous unit.

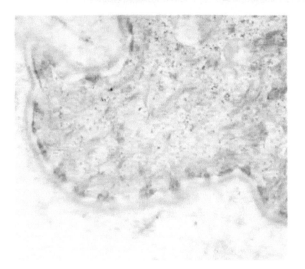

Figure 41.15
Dermolytic epidermolysis bullosa. Ultrastructural examination shows a blister below the lamina densa, with hypoplastic anchoring fibrils and normal hemidesmosomes.

42

EPIDERMOLYTIC HYPERKERATOSIS

Epidermolytic hyperkeratosis (also called bullous congenital icthyosiform erythroderma) is a widespread form of epidermal nevus.

EPIDEMIOLOGY

Epidermolytic hyperkeratosis is rare and is transmitted as an autosomal-dominant trait. However, many cases appear to be sporadic.

CLINICAL FINDINGS

Epidermolytic hyperkeratosis is usually present at birth. The affected newborn is erythrodermic and partially covered by large, flaccid bullae. As the bullae break, they leave residual weeping erosions. Erythroderma alone is seen early in the course and becomes less prominent after infancy, while blisters tend to develop only during the first year of life. After months or years, thick, malodorous gray–brown, verrucous keratotic lesions appear together with deep parallel furrows over virtually the whole skin surface. They are especially prominent on flexural surfaces of the extremities, which assume a rippled appearance (Figs 42.1 and 42.2). The hyperkeratotic lesions persist throughout life.

HISTOPATHOLOGICAL FINDINGS

Epidermolytic hyperkeratosis is characterized by a thickened epidermis in which the normal cohesive organization of spinous and granular cells has been replaced by a markedly vacuolated and feathery appearance, together with clumps of keratohyaline granules. The cornified layer is compactly orthokeratotic (Figs 42.3 and 42.4).

ETIOLOGY AND PATHOGENESIS

The most plausible explanation for epidermolytic hyperkeratosis is mosaicism (i.e. the presence within a single organism of two or more genetically distinct cell lines).

MANAGEMENT

Treatment is unsatisfactory. Oral retinoids may be useful for improving hyperkeratosis, but they may cause an increased tendency to blister.

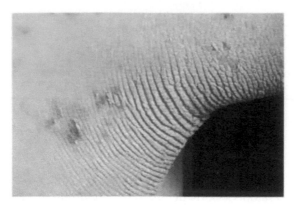

Figure 42.1

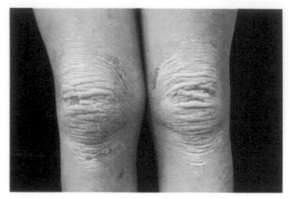

Figure 42.2

Figures 42.1 and 42.2
Epidermolytic hyperkeratosis. Keratotic papules arranged in parallel ridges and deep creases between these keratotic ridges give a rippled appearance to the flexures that is typical of this condition. The few erosions near the axillae presumably represent residua of blisters at that site.

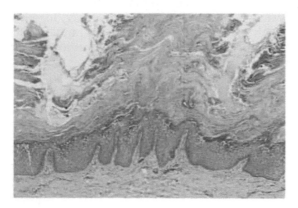

Figure 42.3

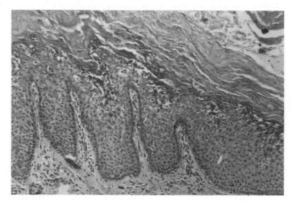

Figure 42.4

Figures 42.3 and 42.4
Epidermolytic hyperkeratosis. The cornified layer is approximately three times the thickness of the viable epidermis. Beneath prominent compact hyperkeratosis, the epidermis is seen to consist of a markedly increased number of kerato-hyaline granules, especially in its upper part, and of a feathery vacuolated appearance of keratinocytes in the spinous and granular zones. That feathery pattern is responsible for the misnomer 'epidermolytic'. In fact, there is no epidermolysis; the epidermal keratinocytes are cohesive.

43

ERYTHEMA ANNULARE CENTRIFUGUM

Erythema annulare centrifugum is an eruption of annular and arcuate red lesions that migrate slowly outwards. It is mainly seen in adults but it has been reported occasionally in children.

CLINICAL FINDINGS

Erythema annulare centrifugum consists of one or more lesions that begin as urticarial papules. The papules enlarge centrifugally to form polycyclic outlines that contain zones either of normal skin or of slightly hyperpigmented skin. The rims of the lesions may be firm, palpable and elevated (deep erythema annulae centrifugum) (Fig. 43.1) or erythematous with delicate scales on the inner position (superficial erythema annulare centrifugum) (Fig. 43.2). Sites of predilection are the trunk and upper limbs, but any part of the integument may be affected. Individual lesions tend to resolve within days or weeks, but new lesions continue to erupt. The condition may last for years. Although itching is present, it is absent in most patients.

HISTOPATHOLOGICAL FINDINGS

The two common types of erythema annulare centrifugum may be classified histopathologically as superficial or deep. The superficial type (Fig. 43.3) shows a superficial perivascular lymphocytic infiltrate, spongiosis in epidermal foci and mounds of parakeratosis. The deep type is characterized by a superficial and deep perivascular infiltrate of lymphocytes, without changes in the epidermis.

ETIOLOGY AND PATHOGENESIS

The causes of erythema annulare centrifugum remain obscure in the large majority of cases. Speculations about the cause in individual cases have included dermatophytes, viruses, infestations and drugs.

MANAGEMENT

Unless an underlying cause is found, no particular treatment has merit for this disease.

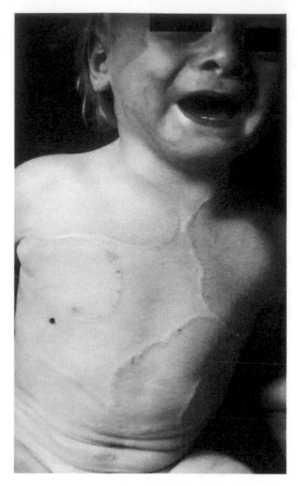

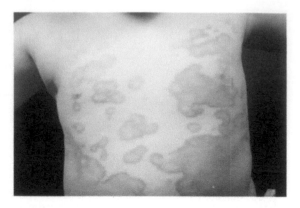

Figure 43.2
Erythema annulare centrifugum (superficial type). Widespread erythematous annular and polycyclic lesions with delicate scaling.

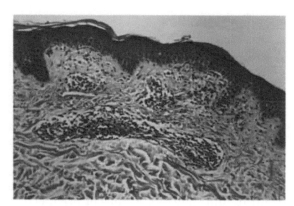

Figure 43.1
Erythema annulare centrifugum (deep type). Arcuate patterns are formed by urticarial lesions on the face and chest of this 4-year-old girl. The borders are sharply demarcated, smooth-surfaced and pink.

Figure 43.3
Erythema annulare centrifugum. Superficial perivascular lymphocytic infiltrate.

44

ERYTHEMA CHRONICUM MIGRANS

Erythema chronicum migrans is a disorder induced by the bite of a deer tick. It represents the principal cutaneous hallmark of Lyme disease.

CLINICAL FINDINGS

Erythema chronicum migrans begins within hours to days after a tick bite. It manifests itself as a red macule or papule that expands centrifugally and clears centrally to become a large annular lesion (Fig. 44.1), sometimes marked by a hemorrhagic punctum at its centre. The borders of the lesions are red, firm and devoid of scales. The thigh, the axilla and the groin are the preferred sites. Although lesions may be asymptomatic, they often itch or burn. The duration of untreated lesions may vary from few weeks to 1 year. In about half of patients, constitutional symptoms (including fever, fatigue, headache, myalgia and arthralgia) may be present.

HISTOPATHOLOGICAL FINDINGS

A superficial and deep perivascular and interstitial lymphohistiocytic infiltrate containing plasma cells is observed (Fig. 44.2). Spirochetes may identified by the Warthin–Starry stain in about 40% of cases.

ETIOLOGY AND PATHOGENESIS

Vectors of transmission of erythema chronicum migrans are ticks of the family Ixodidae, which are widely distributed throughout Europe and the USA. The causative agent, a spirochete named *Borrelia burgdorferi*, has been identified in numerous tissues including skin lesions, of affected patients.

TREATMENT

In children over 8 years of age, tetracycline in the standard oral dose for 10–20 days is recommended, whereas in youger children, oral phenoxynethylpenicillin (50 mg/kg per day) is advised.

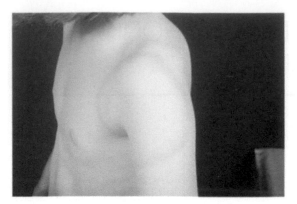

Figure 44.1
Erythema chronicum migrans. An arcuate pink band typical
of a cutaneous manifestation of Lyme disease is seen.

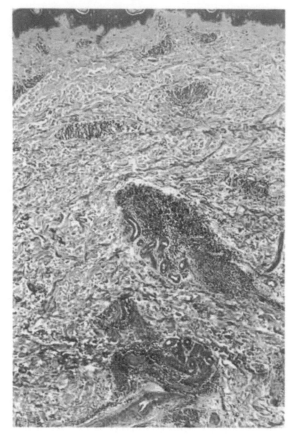

Figure 44.2
Erythema chronicum migrans. Superficial and deep perivascular infiltrate of lymphocytes.

45

ERYTHEMA MULTIFORME

Erythema multiforme is an acute, usually self-limited, often recurrent disease. It is characterized clinically by symmetrically distributed lesions, some of which are often arranged in concentric circles. The lesions favor acral sites and usually affect one or more mucous membranes.

EPIDEMIOLOGY

The incidence of erythema multiforme is not really known, but it may be between 1 in 1000 and 1 in 10,000 of the population. At least 20% of patients with erythema multiforme are children or adolescents.

CLINICAL FINDINGS

Prodromic symptoms such as fever, malaise and headache herald the onset of erythema multiforme in about one-third of cases. These symptoms tend to be commoner in severe forms of the disease. The primary cutaneous lesion is a round, erythematous macule, which becomes papular. The centre of the macular or papular lesion develops a dusky (Figs 45.1 and 45.2) or gray appearance and then blisters. The blister may be either vesicular or bullous (see Fig. 45.2). Often, concentric rings of purpura alternating with rings of edematous erythema form typical 'iris' and 'target' lesions. Cutaneous sites of predilection are the dorsa of the hands, the palms and soles, the forearms, the feet and the face. Lesions on mucous membranes are often present, but not always. Although the mouth (Fig. 45.3) and conjunctiva are the mucous membranes most often affected, any mucosal surface may become involved, including those of the genitalia and gastrointestinal and respiratory tracts.

Erythema multiforme typically runs an uneventful course with no new lesions after about 4 or 5 days. Stevens–Johnson syndrome (see Fig. 45.3) is a severe expression of erythema multiforme with extensive involvement of mucous membranes (e.g. mouth, eyes, genitalia, oropharynx). It is associated with necrotizing tracheobronchitis, meningitis and renal tubular necrosis. The mortality rate for this form of erythema multiforme is more than 5%. So-called toxic epidermal necrolysis begins abruptly with widespread blotchy erythema that has no distinct pattern. Within a few hours, the skin begins to peel in sheets and develops large flaccid bullae. Nikolsky's sign is elicited easily. Involvement of mucous membranes is nearly always severe. Fever and drowsiness are prodromal symptoms. The mortality rate for toxic epidermal neurolysis is about 30%.

HISTOPATHOLOGICAL FINDINGS

Erythema multiforme is an interface dermatitis characterized by lymphocytes around the venules of the superficial plexus and along the dermoepidermal junction, together with ballooning, spongiosis and necrosis of keratinocytes (Figs 45.4 and 45.5).

ETIOLOGY AND PATHOGENESIS

The etiology is unknown. Numerous causative agents seem to be implicated.

Among infective agents herpes simplex virus (for minor episodes of erythema multiforme) and *Mycoplasma pneumoniae* (for severe expressions of the disease) are the most frequent precipitating factors. The commonest drugs triggering the disease are sulfonamides, phenytoin, barbiturates, penicillin and phenylbutazone.

MANAGEMENT

Treatment of an underlying precipiting infection (e.g. with erythromycin for *Mycoplasma pneumoniae* or acyclovir for herpes simplex virus) is mandatary. The role of corticosteroids in the treatment of severe erythema multiforme remains controversial.

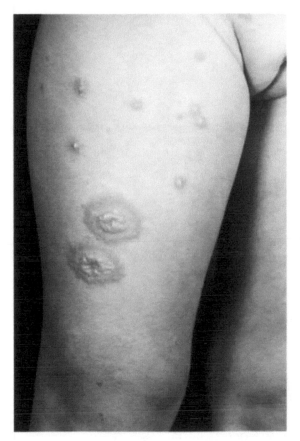

Figure 45.1
Erythema multiforme. The lesions may be papules, vesicles and blisters of different sizes. All three are present here. Concentric rings are characteristic of fully developed lesions.

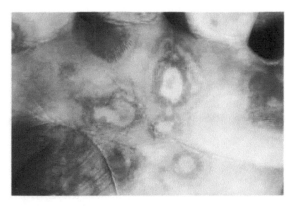

Figure 45.2
Erythema multiforme. The lesions tend to favor the acra, as here, and especially the palms and soles.

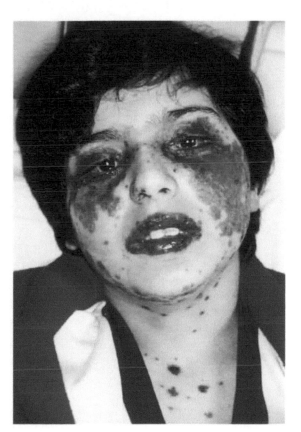

Figure 45.3
Erythema multiforme (Stevens–Johnson syndrome). The hemorrhagic papules and blisters have become confluent on the cheeks and around the eyes. Mucous membranes of the eyes, nose and mouth have been affected by the blistering process.

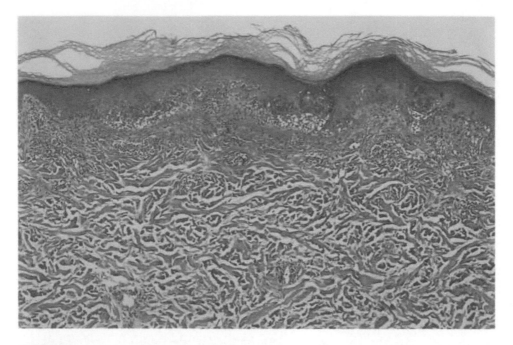

Figure 45.4

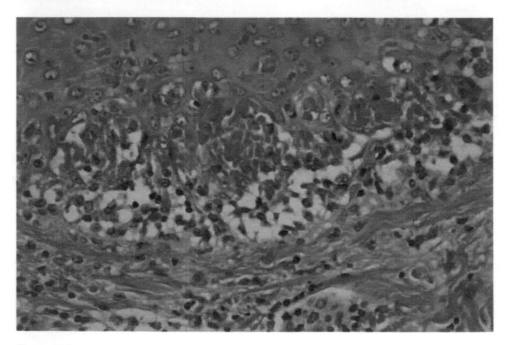

Figure 45.6

Figures 45.4 and 45.5
Erythema multiforme. Lymphocytes are present around vessels of the superficial plexus and along the dermoepidermal junction, where there is also vacuolar alteration. Note the spongiosis and ballooning and the numerous necrotic keratinocytes in the lower part of the epidermis.

ERYTHEMA NODOSUM

Erythema nodosum is a distinctive panniculitis characterized by painful, red patches, plaques and nodules, which have a predilection for the pretibial surfaces.

EPIDEMIOLOGY

Erythema nodosum is rare in the first 2 years of life. The peak incidence of this disease is the peripubertal period. Erythema nodosum is three times more common in females as in males.

CLINICAL FINDINGS

The onset of the lesions of erythema nodosum is often preceded by one or more symptoms and signs (fever, malaise, arthralgia, conjunctivitis or sore throat). Nodules (Figs 46.1 and 46.2) seem to develop rapidly and reach full size within 2 weeks. At first, the bright red, shiny lesions are macules or patches that range in diameter from less than 10 mm to more than 50 mm. These lesions soon become subtly raised, at which time they may be so exquisitely tender that even the weight of linen sheets may be unbearable and so painful that children may refuse to walk. Lesions are firm throughout their course. Their silhouettes tend to be round or oval, but their margins are poorly defined. Typically, only a few lesions are present, but 20 or more may be counted. The pretibial region is most frequently affected, followed by the upper part of the thighs and the buttocks. The lesions are bilateral, but not symmetrical. In most instances, about 10 days after the first lesion has appeared, no new lesions erupt. Within 3–6 weeks, nodules begin to resolve, the redness becomes progressively duller, and the lesions then acquire a purplish cast. As complete resolution nears, lesions take on a yellow–green hue that has prompted the appellation 'erythema contusiformis' because of the resemblance of late lesions of erythema nodosum to a fading bruise. Lesions of erythema nodosum do not suppurate, liquefy or ulcerate. Arthralgias are present in about 50% of patients and affect mainly the ankle joints. Although erythema nodosum is a self-limited disease, recurrences are frequent.

Associations

Erythema nodosum is known to occur in association with sarcoidosis, ulcerative colitis and Crohn's disease, Behçet's disease and erythema multiforme.

HISTOPATHOLOGICAL FINDINGS

In early lesions, scattered neutrophils are seen in slightly widened edematous septa in the subcutaneous fat.

Fully developed lesions are characterized by granulation tissue and granulomatous inflammation in markedly widened septa (Figs 46.3 and 46.4). Lobules affected by foam cells, fat microcysts and membranous fat necrosis appear to be constricted as a result of expansion of the septa.

In late lesions, fibrosing granulomatous inflammation and, eventually, fibrosis in markedly widened septa are observed.

ETIOLOGY AND PATHOGENESIS

Multiple and diverse etiologies have been proposed – tubercolosis, streptococcal infections, chlamydial infections, yersiniosis and histoplasmosis. In the majority of cases, no cause is identified. The precise pathogenesis of erythema nodosum, regardless of cause, also remains obscure.

MANAGEMENT

When the pain is disabling, salicylates and non-steroid anti-inflammatory drugs may be useful. The use of systemic corticosteroids is indicated only in severe cases after an infectious etiology has been excluded.

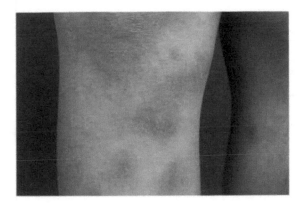

Figure 46.1
Erythema nodosum. The red nodules situated above the anterior tibia represent active evolving lesions of erythema nodosum.

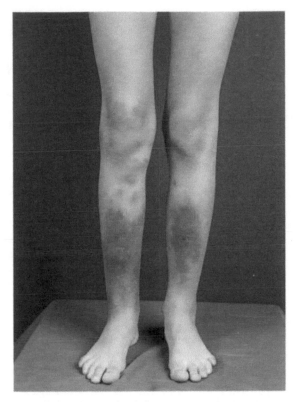

Figure 46.2
Erythema nodosum. The nodules are darkened and have become confluent to form plaques. These findings are expressions of late lesions of erythema nodosum.

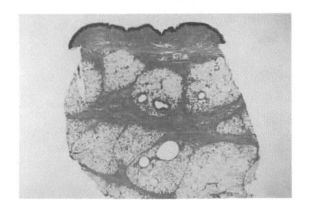

Figure 46.3

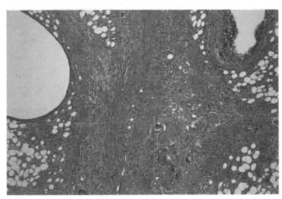

Figure 46.4

Figures 46.3 and 46.4
Erythema nodosum. At scanning magnification (Fig. 46.3), the subcutaneous fat is altered by widened septa that encroach on the fat lobules and constrict them. At higher magnification (Fig. 46.4), a granulomatous inflammation is evident.

47 ERYTHEMA TOXICUM NEONATORUM

Erythema toxicum neonatorum is a self-limited eruption peculiar to newborns. It is so prevalent that it can be considered normal. The condition is marked by widespread tiny pustules that usually occur between the 2nd and 4th days of life, but in many instances the onset may be at birth.

CLINICAL FINDINGS

Lesions usually begin as erythematous 'splotchy' macules (Figs 47.1 and 47.2) that may evolve into edematous papules. Although the lesions may remain macular or papular, many of them progress to tiny pustules. Individual lesions may coalesce, but they resolve without sequelae in a matter of days. The number of lesions ranges from very few to hundreds. Although the palms and soles are spared, the lesions can appear almost anywhere else, especially on the head and neck, the proximal parts of the extremities, the chest and the back.

HISTOPATHOLOGICAL FINDINGS

The lesions consist of collections of neutrophils and eosinophils in follicular infindibula.

ETIOLOGY AND PATHOGENESIS

The etiology and pathogenesis of erythema toxicum neonatorum remain mysterious, despite the commoness of the condition.

MANAGEMENT

No treatment is needed because the lesions are self-limited and disappear nearly as quickly as they develop.

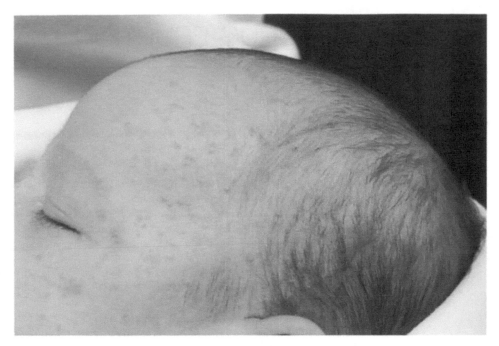

Figure 47.1
Erythema toxicum neonatorum. Discrete papules and papulopustules are scattered over the scalp and cheek of this newborn.

Figure 47.2
Erythema toxicum neonatorum. Macules, papules and tiny pustules are present on the dorsal and ventral surfaces of this newborn.

FIXED DRUG ERUPTION

Fixed drug eruption describes a distinctive cutaneous inflammatory process that is characterized clinically by a recurrence of circumscribed lesions in the same site or sites each time a particular offending drug or chemical is administered.

EPIDEMIOLOGY

The incidence of fixed drug eruption among children has been found to be 1 in 2000. The mean age at the time of onset is 7 years.

CLINICAL FINDINGS

The earliest lesion of a fixed drug eruption is a well-defined, round or oval, red macule. This lesion occurs between 1 and 12 hours after ingestion of a drug in a previously sensitized person. Within a few days, the macule becomes a red–orange–violaceous plaque (Fig. 48.1) whose color closely resembles that of mercurochrome. A bulla may arise on the plaque. An original lesion is often solitary, but recurrent lesions tend to be multiple (Fig. 48.2). Recurrent lesions almost always appear at the exact site or sites of the original eruption. The extremities, the oral cavity, the perioral periorbital and perigenital areas, as well as the genitalia themselves, are the areas most commonly affected. Lesions may be confined to mucous membranes or they may be present on both the mucosae and the skin. Lesions rarely itch or burn. The lesions begin to regress within a few days once the offending drug has been withdrawn. They recur within hours after ingestion of the drug. With repeated attacks, lesions may increase in size and number, and the intensity of pigmentation and the likelihood of its persistence is increased.

HISTOPATHOLOGICAL FINDINGS

In early lesions a superficial and deep perivascular infiltrate that contains neutrophils and eosinophils obscures the dermoepidermal junction.

Fully developed lesions (Figs 48.3 and 48.4) are characterized by intraepidermal vesiculation secondary to vacuolar alteration and also by numerous necrotic keratinocytes within the epidermis and the upper part of epithelial structures of the adnexa.

In late lesions there are numerous melanophages within the papillary dermis.

ETIOLOGY AND PATHOGENESIS

By definition, fixed drug eruption is induced by drugs. Tetracycline and phenolphthalein, sulfonamides and anti-inflammatory agents are the commonest precipitating drugs. The mechanisms of fixed drug eruption are not known.

MANAGEMENT

Identification and elimination of the drug responsible for the eruption is curative. Resolution of lesions may be hastened by the use of oral or topical corticosteroids.

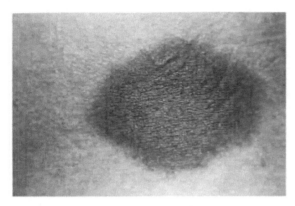

Figure 48.1
Fixed drug eruption. This nummular plaque is characterized by a large central cobalt-blue zone surrounded by a
rim of dusky erythema.

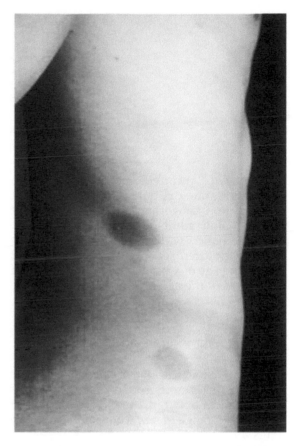

Figure 48.2
Fixed drug eruption. These nummular patches of hyperpigmentation represent post-inflammatory changes.

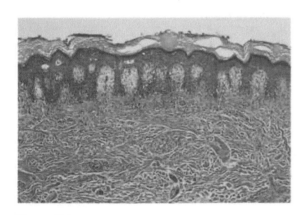

Figure 48.3

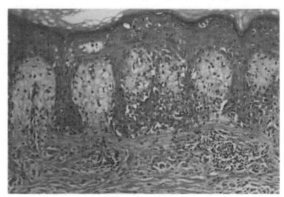

Figure 48.4

Figures 48.3 and 48.4
Fixed drug eruption. This evolving lesion is characterized by a superficial and mid-dermal perivascular mixed cell infiltrate that obscures the dermoepidermal junction. Necrotic keratinocytes are present within the epidermis.

49 GENERALIZED ERUPTIVE HISTIOCYTOSIS

Generalized eruptive histiocytosis is an extremely rare papular, non-lipidic, self healing, non-Langerhans cell histiocytosis. It affects mainly adults. It is characterized by an asymptomatic, widespread eruption. Most cases in children reported to date developed before the age of 4 years. The earliest reported onset was at the age of 3 months.

CLINICAL FINDINGS

The skin lesions consist of an asymptomatic eruption of discrete, round or oval papules that are firm and red–brown or red–blue in color. They range in size from 3 mm to 10 mm (Figs 49.1 and 49.2). These lesions appear in successive crops, may be numerous (from 50 up to 1000) and are distributed on the face, the trunk and the proximal parts of the limbs. They rarely merge into plaques. The oral and genital mucosae are involved only in adults. No visceral lesions have been observed. The patient's general health is good. Permanent remission occurs in months or years.

HISTOPATHOLOGICAL FINDINGS

Conventional microscopy reveals a relatively monomorphous histiocytic infiltrate in the upper and mid-dermis (Figs 49.3 and 49.4). A few lymphocytes may be present. The histiocytes possess a large nucleus and abundant, pale-staining and poorly delimited cytoplasm. These cells are $S100^-$ and $CD1a^-$ and do not contain Langerhans granules.

ETIOLOGY AND PATHOGENESIS

The cause is unknown and the pathogenetic mechanisms are not understood. It has been suggested that generalized eruptive histiocytosis may represent a primitive form of more mature non-X histiocytoses, such as juvenile xanthogranuloma, benign cephalic histiocytosis and multicentric reticulohistiocytosis.

MANAGEMENT

No treatment is necessary because the process tends to resolve completely.

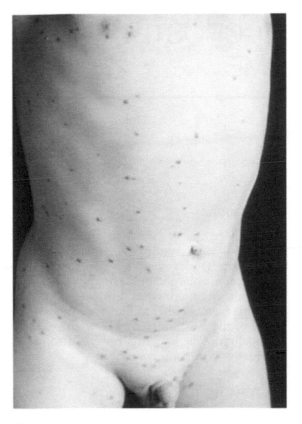

Figure 49.1

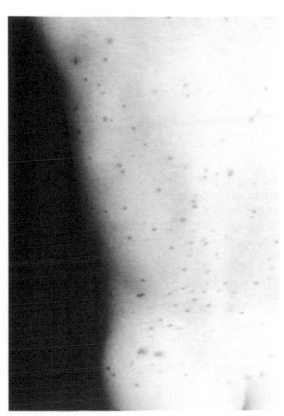

Figure 49.2

Figures 49.1 and 49.2
Generalized eruptive histiocytosis. Numerous discrete, brown macules and smooth-surfaced tan papules are distributed on the chest, the back, the upper thighs, the buttocks and the genital area.

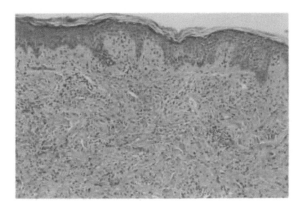

Figure 49.3

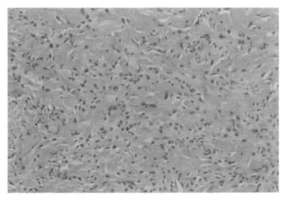

Figure 49.4

Figures 49.3 and 49.4
Generalized eruptive histiocytosis. This papule consists of a dense, diffuse, mixed cell infiltrate composed mostly of histiocytes and lymphocytes.

GIANOTTI–CROSTI SYNDROME

Gianotti–Crosti syndrome refers to a papular or papulovesicular exanthem that is fundamentally spongiotic and is caused by a number of unrelated viruses. Gianotti–Crosti syndrome is typified by an acral distribution and a relatively short, uneventful course.

EPIDEMIOLOGY

As a rule, the eruption occurs in children aged between 2 and 6 years. It is rare in the first year of life and after puberty. Gianotti–Crosti syndrome is common, particularly in the spring and fall. Epidemic hepatitis B virus is a cause of Gianotti–Crosti syndrome in some children, especially in Mediterranean countries and Japan. It now seems, however, that other viruses are more frequently responsible.

CLINICAL FINDINGS

The classical picture of Gianotti–Crosti syndrome is of monomorphic, lentil-sized, papular and papulovesicular lesions distributed symmetrically on the face (Fig. 50.1), the buttocks (Fig. 50.2) and the extensor surface of the limbs (Fig. 50.3). Sometimes the lesions are prominently edematous. They are rarely overtly purpuric. At times, papules may coalesce to form plaques, particularly on the elbows and knees (see Fig. 50.3). The antecubital and popliteal surfaces (see Fig. 50.2) and the trunk (see Fig. 50.3) tend to be spared in Gianotti–Crosti syndrome. Mucous membranes are not affected. In the early eruptive phase, a Koebner phenomenon may be elicited. Itching, when present, is not severe, as evidenced by few excoriations. Lymph nodes, especially in the inguinal and axillary areas, are enlarged, elastic in consistency and freely movable. Skin lesions tend to resolve in a few weeks. The condition does not recur.

Associations

When hepatitis B virus is the cause of Gianotti–Crosti syndrome, acute hepatitis (usually anicteric) is always concurrent. The liver is often enlarged but is not tender. Serum levels of liver enzymes are elevated. The hepatitis begins either at the same time as the onset of the dermatitis, or 1–2 weeks after it. In most patients, hepatitis B virus disappears gradually within a few months.

HISTOPATHOLOGICAL FINDINGS

A superficial and sometimes deep perivascular, predominantly lymphocytic infiltrate is associated with slight edema of the papillary dermis and with foci of spongiosis (Fig. 50.4).

ETIOLOGY AND PATHOGENESIS

Gianotti–Crosti syndrome is an infectious disease caused by various viruses – hepatitis B virus, hepatitis A virus, Epstein–Barr virus, cytomegalovirus, Coxsackievirus, adenovirus, enterovirus, rotavirus and respiratory syncytial virus. In most children, however, no cause is found.

MANAGEMENT

No specific topical treatment is available. Mild corticosteroid creams may be used locally for symptomatic relief, but this is not generally necessary. In the form of the syndrome caused by hepatitis B virus, the hepatitis must be urgently controlled. Family members or children of an affected patient may be carriers of hepatitis B virus.

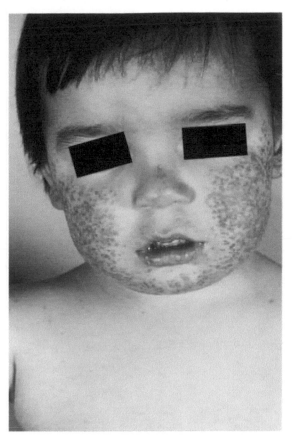

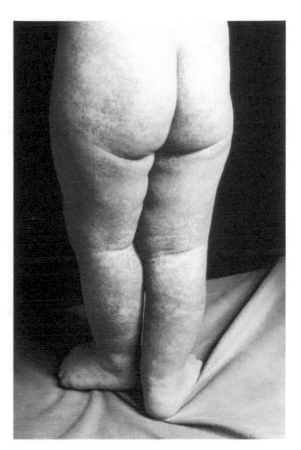

Figure 50.1
Gianotti–Crosti syndrome. There are red–brown, smooth surfaced papules on both cheeks and on the chin. Note that the skin around the nose and mouth is spared.

Figure 50.2
Gianotti–Crosti syndrome. There are countless red–brown, smooth-surfaced papules on the buttocks, the thighs and the legs. The popliteal fossae are mostly spared.

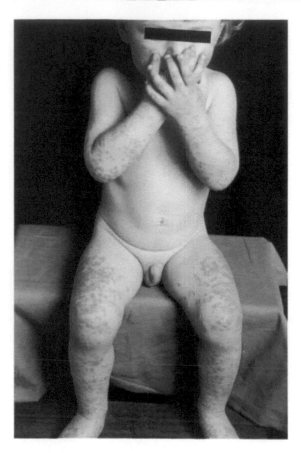

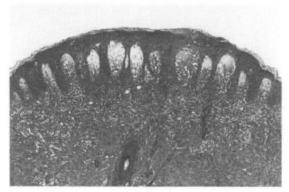

Figure 50.4
Gianotti–Crosti syndrome. This dome-shaped papule is characterized by crust, psoriasiform hyperplasia, focal spongiosis, marked edema of the papillary dermis and a superficial perivascular and interstitial infiltrate of lymphocytes.

Figure 50.3
Gianotti–Crosti syndrome. Extensive involvement of the cheeks and the extremities by red papules. These papules become confluent on the knees. The trunk is spared.

51

GLOMUS TUMOR

Glomus tumors are benign neoplasms. The tumor cells differentiate towards specialized arteriovenous anastomoses (glomus bodies) situated in the deep reticular dermis of acral skin. Clinically, they tend to be blue–red papules; histopathologically, they consist of cells with roundish monomorphous nuclei that encircle small blood vessels. Glomus tumors manifest themselves in two forms – solitary and multiple.

EPIDEMIOLOGY

Glomus tumors are rare in children. Solitary glomus tumors may appear in childhood, but more frequently they arise later in life. Glomangiomas, on the other hand, commonly develop in childhood and are sometimes congenital.

CLINICAL FINDINGS

A solitary glomus tumor usually appears beneath a nail plate as a blue–red, moderately firm painful papule. Rarely is the lesion more than 10 mm in greatest diameter. Tenderness may be felt even in the absence of pressure and may be evoked by a change in temperature. When not subungual, a solitary glomus tumor tends to be positioned elsewhere on the distal part of an extremity (Fig. 51.1). Glomus tumors in multiplicity (sometimes referred to as glomangiomas) range in color from that of the normal skin to reddish blue or dark blue. They often are partly compressible and vary in size from a few millimeters to several centimeters. Glomangiomas can number from very few to several hundred. In some people, glomangiomas are grouped on one part of the skin, especially a limb (localized type), whereas in other people they are scattered over the body (widespread type).

Glomangiomas are not found in subungual regions. Although glomangiomas, unlike solitary glomus tumors, are neither tender nor painful as a rule, individual lesions may become painful even if others are painless. Glomus tumors enlarge slowly and remain stable in size. Evolution of a glomus tumor into a glomangiosarcoma is exceedingly rare.

HISTOPATHOLOGICAL FINDINGS

A solitary glomus tumor (Figs 51.2 and 51.3) is a vascular neoplasm situated in the dermis, usually in a nail bed. The tumor contains distinct lobules, which are composed mostly of cells with remarkably monomorphous, plump oval or round nuclei and scanty cytoplasm (i.e. glomus cells). These lobules surround a small central blood vessel lined by relatively thin endothelial cells. The lobules are separated from one another by fibrous trabecula. Glomangiomas are vascular neoplasms situated in the dermis and sometimes in the subcutaneous fat. They consist of widely dilated, endothelium-lined spaces surrounded by rows of glomus cells.

ETIOLOGY AND PATHOGENESIS

A history of trauma may precede the appearance of the solitary form of the tumor. The familial tendency of glomangioma indicates an autosomal-dominant mode of inheritance.

MANAGEMENT

Complete surgical excision of a glomus tumor is curative.

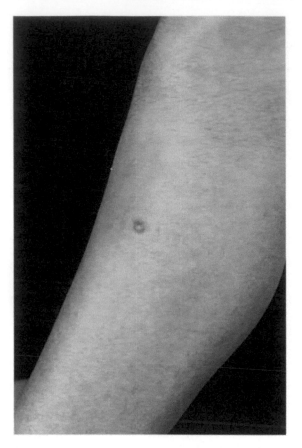

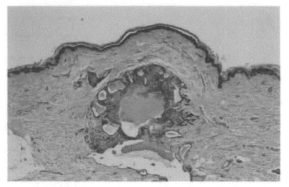

Figure 51.2

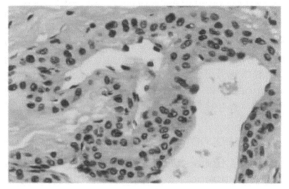

Figure 51.3

Figure 51.1
Glomus tumor. This solitary, smooth-surfaced, pink papule is typical of a glomus tumor.

Figures 51.2 and 51.3
Glomus tumor. This neoplasm is a glomangioma because widely dilated endothelium-lined spaces that contain erythrocytes are lined by rows of large, sometimes oval, relatively monomorphous smooth muscle cells (glomus cells).

52

GRANULOMA ANNULARE

Granuloma annulare is a common inflammatory disease of unknown cause. It is characterized clinically by papules that are often arranged in annular configuration. Histopathologically it is characterized by granulomas, especially in the reticular dermis, which tend to be arrayed in palisades and interstitial fashion.

EPIDEMIOLOGY

Granuloma annulare predominantly affects children and young adults. The subcutaneous form of granuloma annulare occurs almost exclusively in the pediatric age range. More females than males are affected. The localized form of granuloma annulare is common, whereas other forms are relatively uncommon.

CLINICAL FINDINGS

Four types of granuloma annulare (localized, widespread, subcutaneous and perforating) are described. All of these types may appear in children. The most typical expression of granuloma annulare is the localized type; it is characterized by one or more groups of smooth, skin-colored or pink, dome-shaped papules disposed in annular arrangement (Figs 52.1 and 52.2). The rings vary in diameter from 10 to 50 mm. The centre is macular, and the periphery is formed by papules. The lesions favor the distal part of the upper and lower extremities, and they are asymptomatic.

A widespread manifestation of granuloma annulare (Fig. 52.3) is typified by numerous, skin-colored or reddish papules of 1–2 mm in diameter that involve the trunk especially. The tiny papules may be domed entirely or there may be a subtle dell in the center of the dome, the result being an annulus in miniature.

The subcutaneous form of granuloma annulare consists of nodular lesions situated commonly on the legs, the scalp, the periorbital region, the buttocks and the palms. In 25% of those affected, papules of granuloma annulare are confluent.

The perforating type of granuloma annulare (Fig. 52.4) consists of small, skin-colored or reddish, crusted papules. Discharge of pathological material from the dermis is responsible for the crusts that top some of the lesions. Rarely is overt ulceration perceptible. So-called perforating lesions of granuloma annulare are most often situated on the distal parts of extremities and, unlike other variants of granuloma annulare, are reputed to worsen in summer and improve in winter. In the course of months or over a few years, about 70% of lesions heal without therapy and without residual scars.

Associations

A purported association between the widespread form of granuloma annulare and glucose intolerance or overt diabetes mellitus has yet to be substantiated.

HISTOPATHOLOGICAL FINDINGS

Both the localized and widespread forms of granuloma annulare have two basic components – superficial and deep perivascular lymphocytic infiltrates and histiocytes distributed within the reticular dermis in foci and in two patterns, either as palisades around foci of mucin, degenerated collagen, and subtle deposits of fibrin (Figs 52.5 and 52.6), or scattered interstitially among bundles of collagen where mucin tends to be deposited. In all forms of granuloma annulare, histiocytes may be multinucleated or mononuclear. In the perforating form of granuloma annulare, an ulcer is present focally, and beneath it and in continuity with it is a zone of mucin and degenerated collagen, which is partially surrounded by histiocytes. In the subcutaneous form, several discrete foci of histiocytes around zones of mucin, degenerated collagen and fibrin are found within markedly thickened septa of the subcutaneous fat. The septa are also thickened by fibrosis.

ETIOLOGY AND PATHOGENESIS

The cause of granuloma annulare is unknown. Many agents have been implicated, among them trauma and infections. Ultraviolet light doubtlessly plays a role in induction of the widespread tiny papules of granuloma annulare that are confined to sites exposed to sunlight. A role for vasculitis and for cellular immunity has been proposed to explain granuloma annulare, but no unequivocal evidence has been offered to substantiate either hypothesis.

MANAGEMENT

Because the disease in children almost always disappears completely and because no treatment is effective for recurrences, no therapy is necessary. If any treatment is given, it should be one that is harmless (e.g. topically or intralesional corticosteroids).

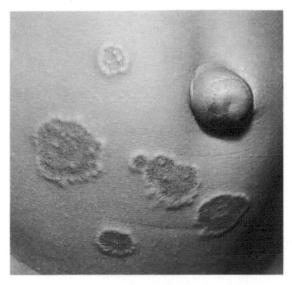

Figure 52.1
Granuloma annulare. These annular lesions are composed of numerous skin-colored papules. The brown contents represent post-inflammatory hyperpigmentation.

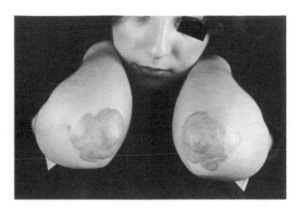

Figure 52.2
Granuloma annulare. There are red–brown, sharply demarcated plaques with discrete papules at the peripheries and within the centers on both elbows.

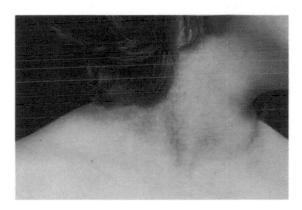

Figure 52.3
Granuloma annulare. This widespread form is manifested by tiny yellow–brown papules, some of which have a subtle annular configuration.

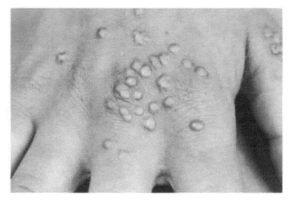

Figure 52.4
Granuloma annulare. Some of the discrete papules have a central dell that gives them an annular appearance. The slight scale on top of some of the papules is an unusual feature for conventional granuloma annulare but is expected for the perforating type.

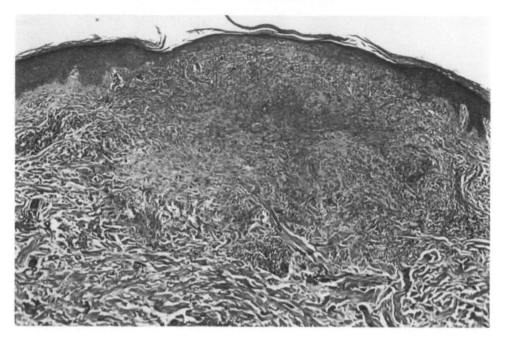

Figure 52.5

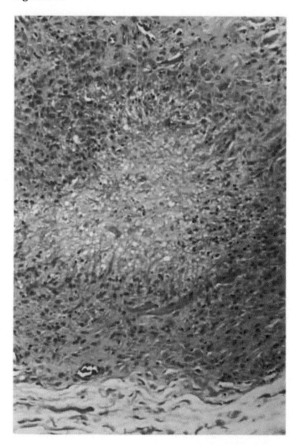

Figures 52.5. and 52.6
Granuloma annulare. Discrete foci of granulomatous inflammation are apparent through the reticular dermis. In each focus, histiocytes are seen to be aligned in a palisade around foci that contain abundant mucin and degenerated collagen.

Figure 52.6

53

HAND-FOOT-AND-MOUTH DISEASE

Hand-foot-and-mouth disease, usually caused by Coxsackievirus, is characterized clinically by an eruption of oblong or oval vesicles rimmed by redness on the distal part of the extremities and on the oral mucosa. Histopathologically it is characterized by intraepidermal vesicles that result from severe ballooning of keratinocytes.

EPIDEMIOLOGY

Hand-foot-and-mouth disease is a common disease that chiefly affects children under 10 years of age. It usually occurs as an epidemic in day care centers and in schools between late spring and autumn.

CLINICAL FINDINGS

Cutaneous findings often are preceded by one or a few days of slight fever, malaise, diarrhea and a mouth that is so sore that the child may refuse to eat or drink. Painful vesicles, surrounded by zones of erythema, appear in the mouth, most frequently in the gingivolabial grooves, and on the tongue, buccal mucosa or hard palate. The blisters break quickly, leaving behind shallow, yellow–gray ulcerations. In about 20% of children affected, submandibular lymphadenopathy is palpable. Two-thirds of patients are affected by typical skin lesions on the fingers (Fig. 53.1), the toes, the sides of the feet (Fig. 53.2) or the palms and the soles. The vesicles are oblong or oval with gray roofs and areolae of erythema. The vesicles tend to be aligned along lines formed by creases. The cutaneous lesions may vary in number from a few to over 50, and they may be asymptomatic or tender. Lesions generally resolve in 7–10 days.

HISTOPATHOLOGICAL FINDINGS

An intraepidermal vesicle marked by reticular alteration formed as a consequence of severe ballooning of keratinocytes, especially in the spinous zone (Fig. 53.3), is the histopathological hallmark of hand-foot-and-mouth disease.

AETIOLOGY AND PATHOGENESIS

Hand-foot-and-mouth disease is typically caused by enteroviruses, most commonly Coxsackievirus A16. The route through which the virus enters the body is the buccal mucosa or the intestinal tract. After infection of regional lymph nodes, the virus spreads to the mucosa and skin via the blood.

MANAGEMENT

Because the eruption and disease run a short course, only supportive care usually is necessary. In some children whose oral mucosae are severely affected, intravenous hydration may be required until intake of liquids by mouth is sufficient.

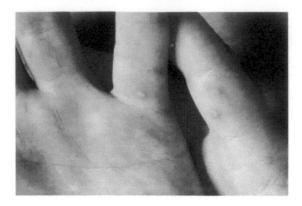

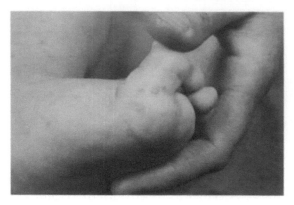

Figure 53.1
Hand-foot-and-mouth disease. There are numerous oblong vesicles surrounded by erythema on the palms. The vesicles have gray surfaces, a sign of necrosis of the epidermis.

Figure 53.2
Hand-foot-and-mouth disease. Oval, round and oblong papulovesicles are present on the medial aspect of the foot. A red rim surrounds some of the vesicles.

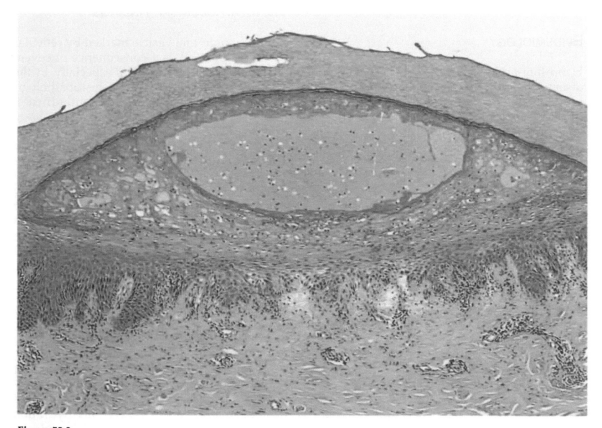

Figure 53.3
Hand-foot-and-mouth disease. There is intraepidermal vesicle within a zone of epidermal necrosis characterized by pink-staining keratinocytes that contrast with the blue-staining keratinocytes found in normal epidermis. Note the keratinocytes and pyknosis in the zone of necrosis.

54

HERPES SIMPLEX

The term herpes simplex refers to a group of infections caused by the human herpes simplex virus. The infections caused by herpes simplex virus type 1 and herpes simplex virus type 2 are conventionally classified as primary and recurrent. The cardinal clinical feature of herpes simplex is clusters of vesicles on top of red bases.

EPIDEMIOLOGY

Herpes simplex is one of the commonest infections of humans. Primary infection type 1 occurs mainly in infants and young children; primary infection type 2 occurs mainly after puberty. Primary infections are frequently asymptomatic or subclinical. Genital primary disease is more commonly symptomatic than oral.

CLINICAL FINDINGS

Primary infections caused by herpes simplex virus may manifest themselves clinically in six main ways:

- herpetic gingivostomatitis which is the most common primary infection caused by herpes simplex virus type 1 in children between the ages of 1 and 5 years. The infection causes high fever, sore throat and malaise. Painful vesicles in the oral cavity tend to become clustered and eventually form erosions on the buccal mucosa, tongue, palate and gingivae. Vesicles may appear on the lips and in the skin surrounding the lips. Profuse salivation,

fetid breath, dysphagia and regional lymphadenopathy are present in some patients. The oral manifestations usually resolve within 2–4 weeks;
- herpetic keratoconjunctivitis, which results from infections by herpes simplex virus type 1 and is usually expressed as severe conjunctivitis together with erythema, edema and vesiculation of the eyelids and periorbital skin (Fig. 54.1). Pain, photophobia and lacrimation are nearly constant symptoms. The cornea may be involved in about 10% of pediatric patients;
- herpes progenitalis, which refers to infection of genital region by herpes simplex virus type 2. Adolescents are most frequently affected. Local symptoms consist of pain and dysuria. Small vesicles, typically grouped, are present in early lesions. They become confluent, rupture and result in ulcers (Fig. 54.2);
- cutaneous inoculation, which is usually due to herpes simplex virus type 1 and most frequently involves the face, the hands and the feet (Fig. 54.3). A cluster of vesicles on an erythematous and edematous base is characteristic. Lesions may be marked by prominent local inflammation and by systemic symptoms, but these are usually less severe than mucous membrane manifestations. The term 'herpetic whitlow' refers to infection by herpes simplex virus of a hand or a finger;
- Kaposi's varicelliform eruption (eczema herpeticum), which appears in patients who suffer from cutaneous diseases such as atopic dermatitis or Darier's disease. About 5–10 days after the infective umbilicated vesicles appear, first in localized form at sites of already diseased skin and then in widespread array. The lesions usually

progress through vesicular, pustular, eroded and crusted stages (Fig. 54.4). Fever, malaise and generalized lymphadenopathy are present;

• neonatal herpes simplex, which results mostly from infection of an infant by herpes simplex virus type 2 during the passage through the birth canal during parturition. The most common skin lesions are vesicles on an erythematous base, which may eventuate in erosion or ulcerations. Skin manifestations may be localized to a particular site such as the head or buttocks or be disseminated.

Recurrent herpetic infections tend to occur as the same site as the primary one. The first indication of impending reactivation of infection is usually a sensation of burning or itching at the locus of the original infection. Vesicles appear and soon erode to heal without scars in 5–10 days. Recurrent infections are much less florid than the primary infection.

LABORATORY FINDINGS

Clinical diagnosis of primary infection by herpes simplex virus may be promptly confirmed by a Tzanck test on a vesicle. Primary herpes simplex viral infection is documented by obtaining serum and demonstrating seroconversion for herpes simplex virus antibodies by immunofluorescence techniques.

HISTOPATHOLOGICAL FINDINGS

Typical features of infection with herpes simplex virus may be found in epidermal and adnexal keratinocytes of lesions, namely, ballooned epithelial cells with steel-gray nuclei that show margination on their nucleoplasm (Figs 54.5 and 54.6). These changes are most marked within the spinous zone. The epithelial cells tend to become multinucleated, and intraepithelial blisters occur as a consequence of acantholysis.

ETIOLOGY AND PATHOGENESIS

Two major antigenic types of herpes simplex virus have been recognized:

• type 1, which is classically associated with facial infections;
• type 2, which mainly involves the genital area.

Primary infection occurs by direct exposure of a non-immune host to the virus, the route being mucocutaneous contact with an infected person. The virus then migrates and establishes a dormant infection within neuronal cells located in regional nerve ganglia. A hallmark of herpes simplex virus infection is its propensity for recurrence. Triggering factors may be events such as stress, exposure to sunlight, trauma or concurrent illness.

MANAGEMENT

Treatment should be started as soon as possible. Systemic acyclovir is the drug of choice and is effective in mucocutaneous infections, eczema herpeticum and neonatal herpes. Application of topical acyclovir is useful in the treatment of recurrent eruptions and in the prevention of corneal ulcers.

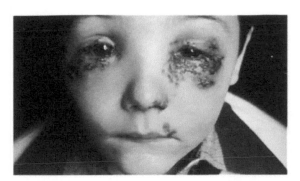

Figure 54.1
Herpes simplex. This is a somewhat unusual presentation of primary herpes simplex because the condition is bilateral, around the eyes. The lesions on the periorbital skin, the nose and the lip are eroded, ulcerated and covered by crusts.

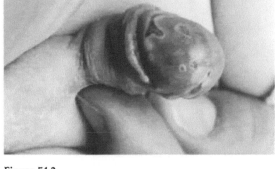

Figure 54.2
Herpes simplex. Primary infection by herpes simplex virus type 2 presents as ulcerated lesions on the glans. Each ulcer is rimmed by a vesicular border, which endows some of them with a donut-like appearance.

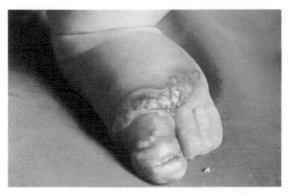

Figure 54.3
Herpes simplex. Primary cutaneous infection characterized by vesiculopustules on dusky-colored skin. Some of the vesiculopustules have become confluent to form a purulent bulla.

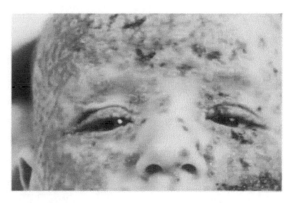

Figure 54.4
Herpes simplex. The diffuse eruption (eczema herpeticum) in this atopic child consists, in part, of umbilicated vesicles, as well as vesicles that have become eroded and crusted.

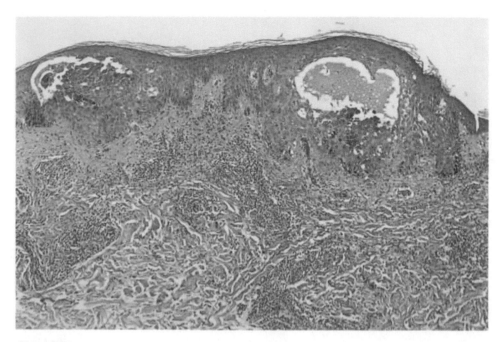

Figure 54.5

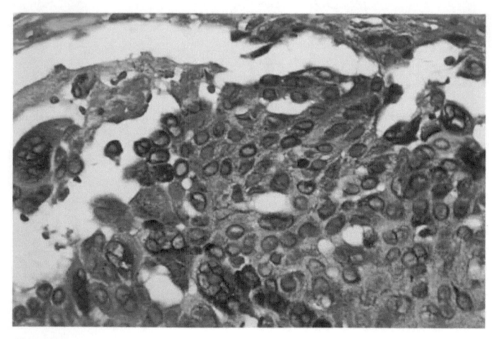

Figure 54.6

Figures 54.5 and 54.6
Herpes simplex. These intraepidermal vesicles contain acantholytic mononuclear and multinucleated epithelial cells. At higher magnification (Fig. 54.6), the nuclei are seen to be steel-gray and the nucleoplasm is exaggerated at its periphery. The cytoplasm is pale and ballooned.

55

HYPERTROPHIC SCARS AND KELOIDS

Hypertrophic scars and keloids are exuberant fibrous repair tissues that follow a cutaneous injury. Hypertrophic scars are fibrosing inflammations that remain localized to the site of injury, whereas keloids extend for a variable distance beyond the site of injury.

EPIDEMIOLOGY

Hypertrophic scars and keloids are unusual before puberty. Boys and girls are equally affected. These lesions are more common in Negroes and in people with darker pigmentation.

CLINICAL FINDINGS

Hypertrophic scars and keloids usually appear within a matter of months after a penetrating injury. They appear as elevated, firm, smooth-surfaced lesions that follow the course taken by the instrument that caused the injury (Figs 55.1 and 55.2). Hypertrophic scars are well circumscribed, whereas keloids often are not. As a rule, hypertrophic scars are linear, whereas keloids may extend in a claw-like fashion. The color may be mildly erythematous in new lesions and paler in older lesions; occasionally older hyperpigmented lesions are seen. The sites of predilection are the ear lobes, the shoulders, the upper part of the back and the chest. Rarely do keloids and hypertrophic scars disappear completely without therapy. They do not become neoplastic. Hypertrophic scars tend to become flatter and softer. Keloids may continue to expand in size for years.

HISTOPATHOLOGICAL FINDINGS

Hypertrophic scars are composed of bundles of fibrillary collagen and fibrocytes aligned parallel to epidermis. Elongated, dilated venules are oriented perpendicular to the surface of the skin.

Keloids are constituted of thick bundles of collagen arranged haphazardly with plump fibrocytes aligned along the bundles (Figs 55.3 and 55.4).

ETIOLOGY AND PATHOGENESIS

The etiology remains unknown, but the accumulated fibrous tissue is associated with increased cellularity, increased metabolic activity of fibroblasts and abnormal proteoglycan content. A familial tendency to form keloids is frequently observed.

MANAGEMENT

In children, hypertrophic scars and small keloids are most commonly treated with pressure or with intralesional injections of corticosteroids. Cryotherapy is said to be a useful therapy occasionally. This treatment may soften the lesions and allow corticosteroids to be injected more easily. X-ray treatment is not recommended in children.

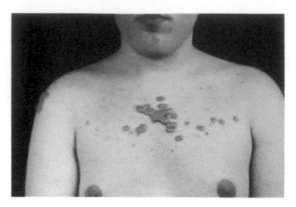

Figure 55.1
Keloids. Numerous pink papules, plaques and nodules are present on the chest of this boy.

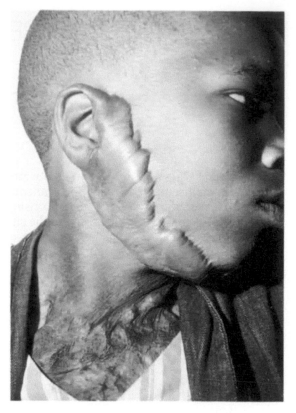

Figure 55.2
Keloids. This extensive plaque on the face is secondary to a burn. Its surface is smooth, and its edges are serrated. On the upper part of the chest there are plaques with post-inflammatory hyperpigmentation.

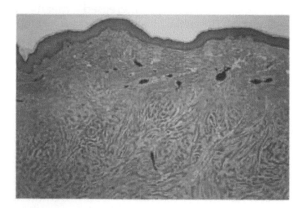

Figurte 55.3

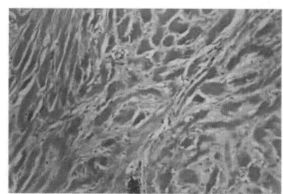

Figure 55.4

Figures 55.3 and 55.4
Keloid. The lesion is constituted of thick bundles of collagen arranged haphazardly, with plump fibrocytes aligned along the bundles.

56

ICHTHYOSIS AND ICHTHYOSIFORM DISORDERS

Ichthyoses are diseases characterized by excessive accumulation of scales on the skin. They consist of a heterogeneous group of hereditary and acquired disorders.

ICHTHYOSIS VULGARIS

Ichthyosis vulgaris (autosomal-dominant ichthyosis) is the commonest and least severe of the ichthyoses. The condition, transmitted as an autosomal-dominant trait, is not present at birth but appears during the 1st year of life.

EPIDEMIOLOGY

Ichthyosis vulgaris is the most frequently encountered form of ichthyosis, with an incidence of about 1 in 300. Both sexes are equally affected.

CLINICAL FINDINGS

The trunk and the extensor surfaces of the limbs are the sites of fine, white scales that may have a 'pasted-on' appearance (Fig 56.1). A mild hyperkeratosis on the forehead and the cheeks can be seen in childhood. Increased palmoplantar skin markings with mild hyperkeratosis are a constant finding, together with sparing of flexures. Follicular hyperkeratosis on the extensor surfaces of limbs is common. Atopy occurs in about one-third of patients. Mild forms can be confused with simple dry skin. Severe cases must be distinguished from mild lamellar ichthyoses.

Clinical improvement is typical in warm and humid climates and during summer. The condition can improve with age. The prognosis is good.

HISTOPATHOLOGICAL FINDINGS

Ichthyosis vulgaris is characterized by laminated orthokeratosis with foci of basket-woven orthokeratosis, a thinned or absent granular layer, a slightly thinned epidermis with diminished undulations between rete ridges and dermal papillae, and plugging of infundibula by orthokeratotic cells (keratosis pilaris) (Fig 56.2). Electron microscopy discloses keratohyaline granules that are typically small and have a crumbly and spongy appearance.

ETIOLOGY AND PATHOGENESIS

Filaggrin, the main protein of keratohyaline granules, is reduced or absent. The rate of epidermal proliferation is normal, but the dissolution of desmosomes in the horny layer seems to be delayed (retention ichthyosis).

MANAGEMENT

Keratolytic agents are helpful. Emollients and ointments should be applied often, preferably after cleansing, in the cold, dry periods of the year. The choice of moisturizers (e.g. urea) is broad, but efficacy should be tested individually.

X-LINKED ICHTHYOSIS (ICHTHYOSIS NIGRICANS)

X-linked ichthyosis (ichthyosis nigricans) is usually a mild form of ichthyosis. It affects males only within the 1st month of life and is characterized by a deficiency of the enzyme steroid sulfatase.

EPIDEMIOLOGY

X-linked ichthyosis has a frequency of between 1 in 2000 and 1 in 6000 births. No racial or ethnic preference has been reported.

CLINICAL FINDINGS

The scales are large (more than 4 mm in diameter), range in color from gray to dark brown (Fig. 56.3) and appear to adhere tightly to the underlying skin. The neck, the trunk and the lower limbs are invariably affected. The disease is most severe on the extensor surfaces, but some degree of flexural involvement is present. The face usually is spared, and the palms, the soles and the nails show no relevant abnormalities. Small comma- or dot-shaped opacities are detectable on the posterior capsule of Descemet's membrane in about 50% of pre-adolescent and adult patients. There is no visual impairment. Cryptorchidism can occur. The association of ichthyosis with mental retardation, seizures and hypogonadism (reported as Rud's syndrome) can also occur. Marked improvement is usually noted during summer. The prognosis is good, even though this condition tends to worsen with age.

LABORATORY FINDINGS

Steroid sulfatase deficiency is detectable in peripheral leukocytes and cultured skin fibroblasts. Increased cholesterol sulfate can be demonstrated in serum, red blood cells and epidermis. Low-density lipoproteins show an increased mobility compared with normal lipoproteins in lipoprotein electrophoresis. Low levels of arylsulfatase C in leukocytes detects female carriers.

HISTOPATHOLOGICAL FINDINGS

X-linked ichthyosis is typified by laminated and compact orthokeratosis that is sometimes associated with tiny foci of basket-woven orthokeratosis. The thickness of the granular zone is increased and the epidermis is slightly hyperplastic. No infiltrate of inflammatory cells is present in the dermis (Fig. 56.4). Keratohyaline granules appear normal on electron microscopy.

ETIOLOGY AND PATHOGENESIS

A steroid sulfatase (arylsulfatase C) deficiency is peculiar to this disorder and produces a retention hyperkeratosis because of a lack of elimination of cholesterol sulfate, which is essential for the cohesion of cells in the horny layer.

MANAGEMENT

Keratolytics are useful. Topical treatment with a cream that contains cholesterol has yielded promising results, especially in younger patients. Aromatic retinoids are rarely necessary.

CONGENITAL ICHTHYOSES

Congenital (lamellar) ichthyoses are a heterogeneous group of severe and generalized diseases of keratinization that are usually inherited as autosomal-recessive traits. They are always apparent at birth. Newborns often have parchment-like sheets that cover the body (collodion baby). Although the heterogeneity of these diseases has been demonstrated, a comprehensive classification is still not available.

EPIDEMIOLOGY

This disorder is extremely rare, with an estimated incidence of about 1 per 300,000 persons.

CLINICAL FINDINGS

Lamellar ichthyosis

The newborn is enveloped in a collodion-like horny layer (Fig. 56.5). Collodion babies are at risk of sepsis and electrolyte imbalances. The increased skin thickness and tautness may lead to abnormal development of the nasal and auricular cartilages. Severe ectropion can lead to permanent corneal opacities. Heat intolerance may result from erythroderma and eccrine duct obstruction. Growth retardation and neurological disturbances can be observed. After the detachment of the collodion envelope, the entire skin appears red and scaly (Fig 56.6). The erythroderma gradually subsides within a few months, or it may persist for life.

The clinical features of the complete form include severe hyperkeratosis with large, adherent scales on the entire body surface (Fig. 56.7); severe ectropion and eclabion may be present together with deformities of ears (Fig. 56.8). In some patients the evolution is more benign, with a less severe, more variable and lighter degree of scaling, and in some babies the clinical presentation is difficult to separate from a dry, atopic skin. These patients are diagnosed only by way of electron microscopy.

Harlequin fetus

Harlequin fetus is the most severe form of the inborn diseases of keratinization. Death occurs *in utero* or shortly after birth because of chest and abdominal constriction. The entire skin is thickened, hyperkeratotic, inelastic and deeply fissured (Fig. 56.9). Ectropion and eclabium are noted. The pinnae may be abnormal or absent. A severe form of ichthyosis congenita develops in those rare instances in which patients have survived beyond the perinatal period.

Autosomal-dominant lamellar ichthyosis

Autosomal-dominant lamellar ichthyosis is a recently described type of congenital ichthyosis with clinical and histopathological features that are similar to those of the recessive forms. Distinctive alterations are demonstrated only in the ultrastructural patterns.

HISTOPATHOLOGICAL FINDINGS

Distinctive features of congenital ichthyoses are hyperkeratosis with corneocytes arranged in laminated and compact fashion, striking hypergranulosis, and epidermal hyperplasia. No infiltrate of inflammatory cells is seen within the dermis (Fig. 56.10). Ultrastructurally, four types of congenital ichthyoses have been characterized:

- type I, with high numbers of lipid vacuoles in the corneocytes but no other specific markers;
- type II, with brick-like, electron-negative crystals in the corneocytes (Fig. 56.11);
- type III, with elongated and laminated membranous structures in the stratum granulosum and the stratum corneum, together with vesicular keratinosome complexes;
- type IV, with elongated membranes associated with prematurity, neonatal respiratory distress, Darier's sign and follicular hyperkeratosis.

In harlequin fetus, compact massive orthokeratosis exceeds the thickness of the remaining epidermis and is also present as plugs within the ostia of adnexal epithelial structures. Autosomal-dominant lamellar ichthyosis shows peculiar alterations, such as a prominent transforming zone between the stratum granulosum and the stratum corneum, which is composed of four to six cell layers.

ETIOLOGY AND PATHOGENESIS

Congenital ichthyoses are usually inherited as autosomal-recessive traits. The mitotic rate is greater than normal and the transit time is reduced (proliferation hyperkeratosis). Several alterations of scale lipids are observed. The gene encoding for transglutaminase 1 has been involved in some pedigrees and two other loci have also been described.

MANAGEMENT

Lubricants and keratolytics are useful. Aromatic retinoids can be used in severe cases. Prenatal diagnosis of congenital ichthyosis can be accomplished by ultrastructural examination of fetal skin biopsies obtained at 22 weeks of gestation, but, except for harlequin fetus, the risk of false-negative results is high. Prenatal diagnosis at an early stage of pregnancy via chorionic villi is available only in families in which the genetic defect has been established

NETHERTON'S SYNDROME

Netherton's syndrome is a distinctive disorder characterized by the triad of ichthyosiform dermatosis, trichorrhexis invaginata (bamboo hair) and atopic diathesis.

EPIDEMIOLOGY

Netherton's syndrome is rare. It affects males and females equally.

CLINICAL FINDINGS

This disorder may be present at birth as collodion baby; more frequently, it appears during the first months of life as transient ichthyosiform erythroderma (Fig. 56.12) or as ichthyosis linearis circumflexa. Collodion baby pattern, once considered a separate entity, is present in most cases, and is characterized by slowly migrating, erythematous and scaling lesions with a serpiginous and polycyclic pattern (Fig. 56.13). A distinctive finding is double-edged desquamation at the periphery of the lesions. The face and scalp are often affected (Fig. 56.14) and may remain diffusely red with fine white scales, even into adulthood. By contrast, the palms, the soles and the nails are usually spared. The hair has a dull general appearance and is sparse, short and dry. The hair defect, trichorrhexis invaginata (bamboo hair), is the distinctive feature of this disorder. It is clearly visible in samples analyzed by optical (Fig. 56.15) and scanning electron microscopy, and consists of an intussusception of the distal hair shaft into the proximal portion; this intussusception has a cup-like shape, forming a node. The disease may improve with age and the hair abnormality may disappear.

Associations

An atopic diathesis with elevation of serum immunoglobulin E levels is present in 30–60% of patients. Eczematous lesions frequently overlap the typical erythematous scaling lesions. Anaphylactoid reactions occur in 25% of patients after ingestion of peanuts, nuts, egg , milk or fish.

LABORATORY FINDINGS

A moderate eosinophilia and an elevated level of serum immunoglobulin E are frequent findings. Urinalysis to study aminoaciduria and an accurate observation of the hair at optical and scanning electron microscopy are necessary.

HISTOPATHOLOGICAL FINDINGS

Netherton's syndrome is a spongiotic dermatitis with focal parakeratosis and a sparse perivascular lymphocytic infiltrate.

ETIOLOGY AND PATHOGENESIS

The disease is inherited as an autosomal-recessive trait. Consanguinity has been noted in about 10% of cases. The formation of the invagination of the affected hair depends on a particular softness of the keratogenous zone of the cortex related to a defect of -SH to -SS group conversion of the proteins contained in cortical keratin structures. The gene SPINK5, encoding a serine protease inhibitor, is mutated.

MANAGEMENT

Lubricants are helpful in improving excessive dryness of the skin. The use of topical corticosteroids must be avoided. The use of aromatic retinoid derivatives is controversial; worsening of an atopic manifestation may occur during this therapy. A trial regimen starting with low-dose retinoid followed by progressive adaptation of the dosage to the course of the disease has been effective.

ERYTHROKERATODERMIA VARIABILIS

Erythrokeratodermia variabilis (Mendes da Costa, genodermatose en cocardes, Degos' disease) is a rare genodermatosis characterized by figurate, sharply demarcated, fluctuating patches of erythema and hyperkeratosis that vary in size, shape and distribution over hours or days.

EPIDEMIOLOGY

Erythrokeratodermia variabilis is rare. About 150 cases have been reported in the world literature. The sex distribution is almost equal.

CLINICAL FINDINGS

Erythrokeratodermia variabilis has two distinct morphological components, erythema and hyperkeratosis, one of which can predominate. Bizarre, figurate, sharply demarcated patches of erythema change in size and location from day to day. Rapidly scaling lamellae develop, particularly at the border of the erythematous lesions (Figs 56.16 and 56.17). Later, fixed, figurate and hyperkeratotic plaques appear on normal skin or, less frequently, on erythematous areas. The distribution of the lesions is often symmetrical. The face, the anterior aspect of the body, the buttocks and the limbs are common sites. The palms and soles may be thickened. Mucous membranes, hairs and nails are not involved. The disease is present at birth in about 30% of patients; in other patients it appears during the first few years of life. The course is chronic.

HISTOPATHOLOGICAL FINDINGS

Histopathologic signs of erythrokeratodermia variabilis are seen at scanning magnification as layers of cornified cells of different character, mammillated epidermal hyperplasia, prominent hypergranulosis and a sparse superficial perivascular lymphocytic infiltrate (Fig. 56.18). At higher magnifications, the layers of orthokeratosis are of two types – compact and basket-woven. Electron microscopy reveals a decreased number of keratinosomes, a finding that is characteristic but not specific.

ETIOLOGY AND PATHOGENESIS

The pattern of inheritance is autosomal-dominant. Close genetic linkage between the locus of erythrokeratodermia variabilis and the Rhesus blood group system has been reported. The epidermal proliferation rate is normal. The significance of the decrease in keratinosomes is unclear. It has been suggested that it may result from a disturbance in the mechanisms of cell-to-cell adhesion. The gene GJB3, which encodes for the connexin CX31, is mutated in this disease.

MANAGEMENT

Lubricants and keratolytic agents may be useful. Patients with erythrokeratodermia variabilis have been treated with several oral retinoids, but acitretin seems to be the derivative of choice.

SYMMETRICAL PROGRESSIVE ERYTHROKERATODERMIA

Symmetrical progressive erythrokeratodermia is an extremely rare genodermatosis characterized by slowly progressive plaques of hyperkeratosis on an erythematous base. The plaques are distributed symmetrically on the head, the extremities and the buttocks.

EPIDEMIOLOGY

The condition is extremely rare. About 30 cases have been reported. The sex distribution is about equal.

CLINICAL FINDINGS

In most cases, onset is during the 1st year of life. Lesions of symmetric progressive erythrokeratodermia consist of sharply demarcated, hyperkeratotic, occasionally hyperpigmented plaques surrounded by a narrow erythematous halo (Fig. 56.19). The onset of erythema may be triggered by exposure to heat, cold or emotional upset. The erythematous lesions may improve with age. These lesions are symmetrical on the limbs (Fig. 56.20) and the buttocks and, less frequently, on the face and the trunk. They enlarge slowly and centrifugally.

HISTOPATHOLOGICAL FINDINGS

Lesions of symmetrical progressive erythrokeratodermia show hyperkeratosis with local areas of parakeratosis, psoriasiform epidermal hyperplasia, and a sparse, lymphohistiocytic infiltrate surrounding the vessels of the superficial plexus. Electron microscopy demonstrates that granular cells contain swollen mitochondria and that corneocytes contain many lipid-like vacuoles.

ETIOLOGY AND PATHOGENESIS

The disease is inherited as an autosomal-dominant trait. The rate of epidermal cell proliferation in the lesion is increased.

MANAGEMENT

Topical treatment consists of ointments and keratolytic agents. Oral retinoids have been used with excellent results. In adolescents, psoralen and ultraviolet-A (PUVA) treatment may be effective.

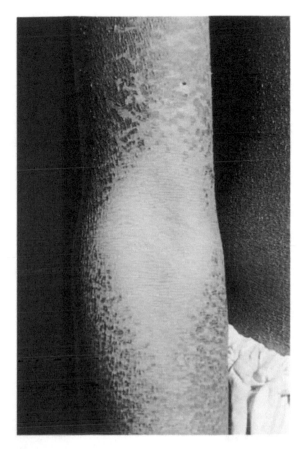

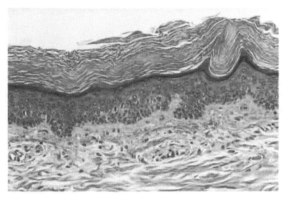

Figure 56.2
Ichthyosis vulgaris. A slightly thinned epidermis, laminated orthokeratosis and hypogranulosis are characteristic features.

Figure 56.1
Ichthyosis vulgaris. Gray, thin scales spare the skin of the antecubital and inguinal region.

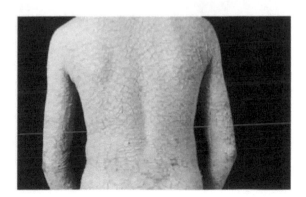

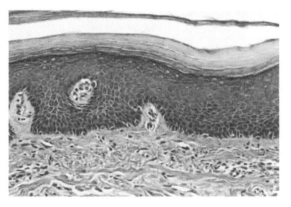

Figure 56.3
X-linked ichthyosis. The widespread, dark, polygonal scales are predominantly large and hyperkeratotic.

Figure 56.4
X-linked ichthyosis. Laminated and compact orthokeratosis, a thickened granular zone and epidermal hyperplasia are characteristic findings.

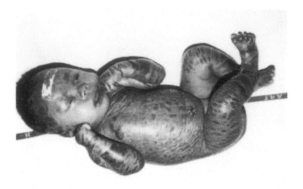

Figure 56.5
Congenital ichthyosis. A typical case of collodion baby in this newborn affected by lamellar ichthyosis.

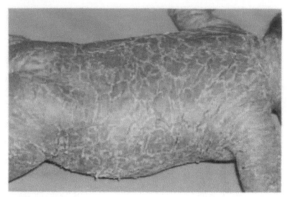

Figure 56.7
Congenital ichthyosis. Erythroderma and large scales are the most prominent feature in this infant.

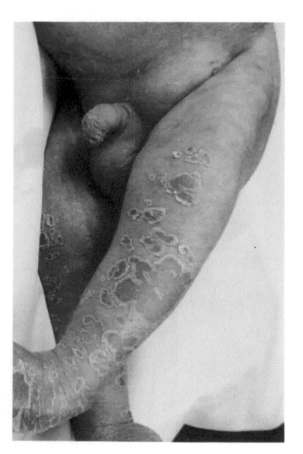

Figure 56.6
Congenital ichthyosis. After a short period, the collodion membrane peels off, leaving large scales.

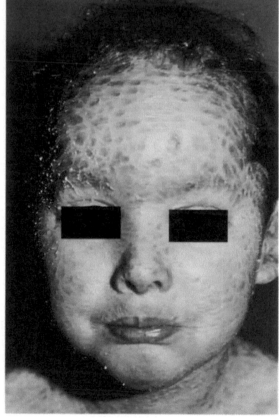

Figure 56.8
Congenital ichthyosis. Ectropion and dark scales can be seen in this young patient affected by lamellar ichthyosis type II.

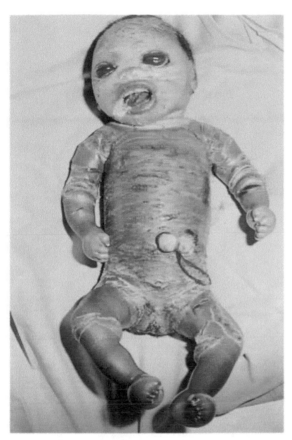

Figure 56.9
Congenital ichthyosis. Harlequin fetus. This fetus is characterized by deep fissures around armor-like plates that give the skin an appearance of an armadillo.

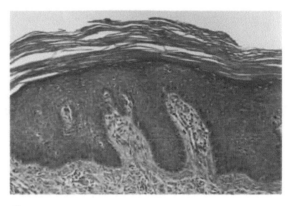

Figure 56.10
Congenital ichthyosis. Orthokeratosis in mostly compact array, a thick granular zone and epithelial hyperplasia are characteristic signs.

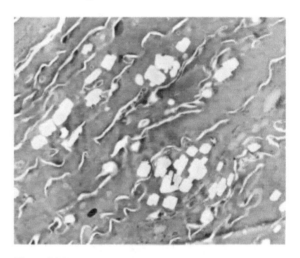

Figure 56.11
Congenital ichthyosis. Ultrastructure reveals groups of rod-shaped, electron-negative crystals in horny cells – pathognomonic markers of lamellar ichthyosis type II.

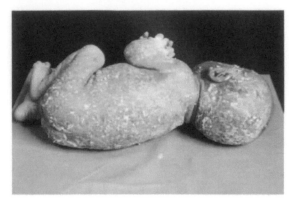

Figure 56.12
Netherton's syndrome. This newborn has widespread erythema covered by scales and scale-crusts. The diagnosis was made because the infant had bamboo hairs.

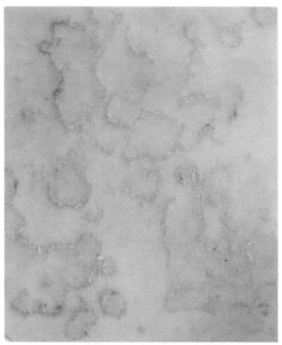

Figure 56.13
Netherton's syndrome. Double-edged desquamation at the periphery of the lesions is a distinctive finding.

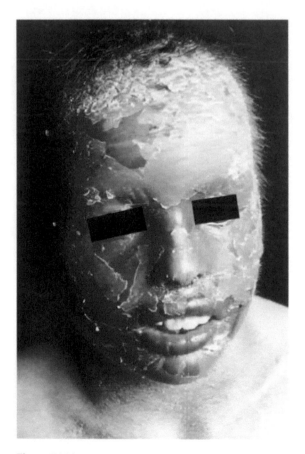

Figure 56.14
Netherton's syndrome. Diffuse erythema and large scales are prominent features. The hairs are short and sparse.

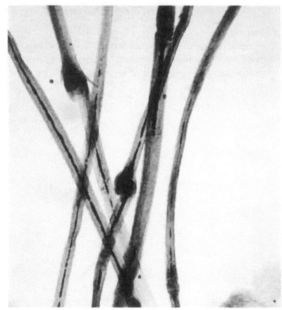

Figure 56.15
Netherton's syndrome. Bamboo joint swelling are typical of trichorrhexis invaginata.

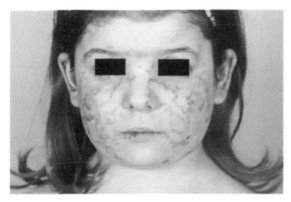

Figure 56.16
Erythrokeratodermia variabilis. Numerous lesions resemble those of gyrate erythema. Reddish papules form arcuate, annular and serpiginous shapes.

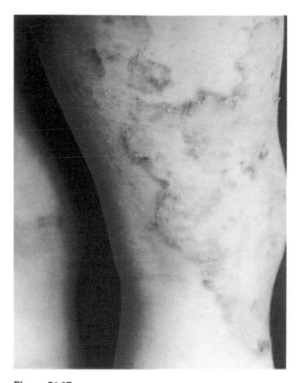

Figure 56.18 (*below*)
Erythrokeratodermia variabilis. A gently mamillated surface covered by orthokeratosis in basket-woven configuration is associated with hypergranulosis and epidermal hyperplasia, which are typical of this condition.

Figure 56.17
Erythrokeratodermia variabilis. The lesions are characterized by scalloped borders along which papules develop, some of which are scaly or crusted.

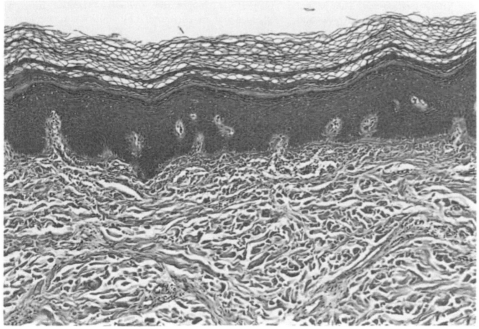

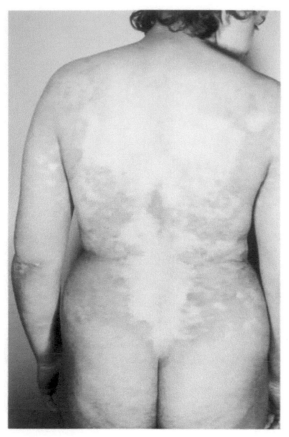

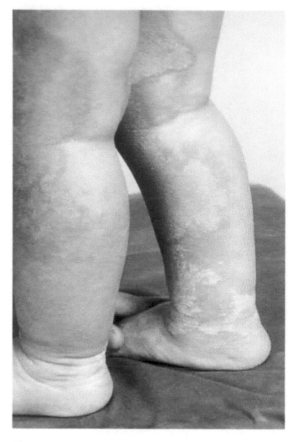

Figure 56.19
Symmetrical progressive erythrokeratodermia. The patient
shows well-demarcated plaques with brownish bases and
whitish scales. The lesions are distributed symmetrically.

Figure 56.20
Symmetrical progressive erythrokeratodermia. Brownish
plaques that are surrounded by white scales characterize
this condition.

Incontinentia pigmenti is a complex, X-linked dominant disease characterized by four overlapping cutaneous stages and numerous neuroectodermal defects.

EPIDEMIOLOGY

Incontinentia pigmenti is rare but it occurs in all races and is usually present at birth. Approximately 95% of affected children are female, suggesting an X-linked mode of inheritance that is lethal in males.

CLINICAL FINDINGS

The first stage begins with erythema from which vesicles and, in time, bullae emerge (erythematous–bullous stage) (Fig. 57.1). Blisters may be present at birth, as may reddish macules and edematous papules. The blisters are at first filled with serum, which in time becomes turbid because of the incursion and disintegration of eosinophils. All of the lesions follow the whorled distribution of Blaschko's lines.

As the vesicular lesions slowly heal, they are replaced in the course of a few weeks by verrucous crusts and keratoses (verrucous stage) (Fig 57.2). The keratotic lesions thicken progressively and affect mainly the limbs, especially the fingers and the toes. Subungual keratoses may be painful.

As the verrucous lesions involute, whorled and linear zones of hyperpigmentation following Blaschko's lines appear (pigmentary stage). These zones occur mainly on the trunk, but the extremities are also often affected (Fig. 57.3). These hyperpigmented lesions represent post-inflammatory changes, even if parents aver that no inflammation occurred at these sites. The pigmented lesions usually fade gradually during late childhood or adolescence.

The fourth stage of incontinentia pigmenti consists of hypopigmented and atrophic skin lesions. These streaks are free of pilosebaceous units and sweat glands. The lack of results from long-term follow-up studies makes it difficult to establish whether hypopigmentation and atrophy represent a chronic evolution of the previous inflammatory or pigmentary stage or an independent feature of incontinentia pigmenti that can arise on previously clinically unaffected skin. Hypochromic and atrophic streaks and macules are distributed in a reticular pattern on the lower limbs or other region of the body, often visible at the legs in the unaware mothers and grandmothers of the child (Fig. 57.4). Although 80% of the vesicular and verrucous lesions come and go in a matter of weeks or months, the pigmented swirls my persist for decades. By puberty, however, they may clear. Hypochromic streaks can represent the only marker for incontinentia pigmenti in adulthood.

In about 80% of patients, associated abnormalities of the hair, the nails, the teeth, the eyes and the nervous system are present. Among these are cicatricial alopecia, nail dystrophy, cone-shaped teeth, anodontia, cataract, strabismus, seizures and mental retardation.

HISTOPATHOLOGICAL FINDINGS

The varied histopathological changes in incontinentia pigmenti parallel the variety of clinical findings. Histopathologically, the course of the disease process can be divided roughly into four stages – vesicular, pseudocarcinomatous, post-inflammatory and atrophic.

In the vesicular stage vesicles of incontinentia pigmenti are spongiotic and filled with eosinophils. Vesicles may be topped by mounds of scaly crusts that contain eosinophils. Beneath the vesicles is a sparse, superficial and deep, perivascular and interstitial infiltrate comprising mostly eosinophils (Fig 57.5).

The pseudocarcinomatous stage is typified by adnexal hyperplasia, especially infundibular, with numerous dyskeratotic cells. The lesion is covered by orthokeratosis and parakeratosis (Fig. 57.6).

Findings in the post-inflammatory stage, unlike those in the vesicular and pseudocarcinomatous stages, are not specific. Only a sprinkling of melanophages in a slightly thickened papillary dermis is noted (Fig. 57.7). Hypochromic lesions show epidermal atrophy and lack of adnexa, without significant melanocytic abnormalities. In the atrophic stage, the papillary dermis is thickened through fibroplasia, dermal papillae are effaced, and the epidermis is nearly devoid of rete ridges.

ETIOLOGY AND PATHOGENESIS

Incontinentia pigmenti is inherited in an X-linked, dominant pattern. The gene has been mapped on the long arm in region Xq 28, close to the factor VIII locus. The mutated gene is 'NEMO' (necrosis factor-kappa B essential modulator–IKKgamma). NEMO is required for the activation of the transcription factor necrosis factor-kappa B and is crucial in many inflammatory, immune and apoptotic pathways. The occurrence of the disease among men with normal karyotype XY may be caused by genetic mosaicism.

MANAGEMENT

No treatment has been helpful consistent in controlling the cutaneous lesions of incontinentia pigmenti. A thorough search of associated malformations is indicated in every affected child, because at least some of these malformations may be surgically correctable.

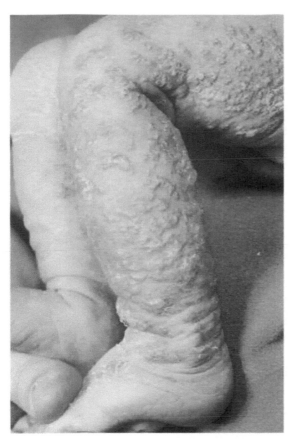

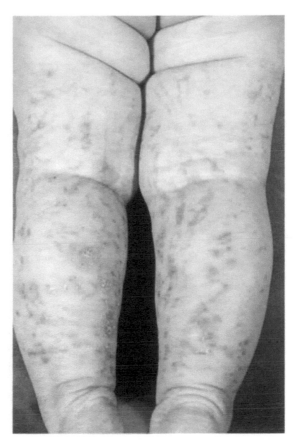

Figure 57.1
Incontinentia   pigmenti   (erythematous–bullous   stage).
Vesicles, pustules, scales and crusts are widespread. Note
that the vesicles are confluent in a reticulated pattern.

Figure 57.2
Incontinentia pigmenti (verrucous stage). Crusts and scale-
crusts are present on top of brownish violaceous papules.
The lesions are arranged in a linear and reticulated
pattern.

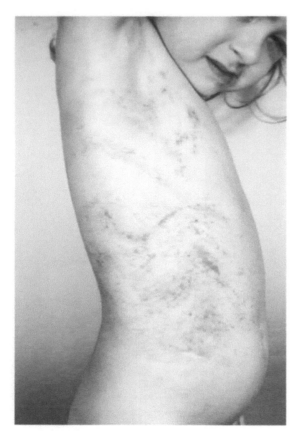

Figure 57.3
Incontinentia pigmenti (pigmentary stage). Whorls of post-inflammatory hyperpigmentation are present where the papules and vesicles formerly were.

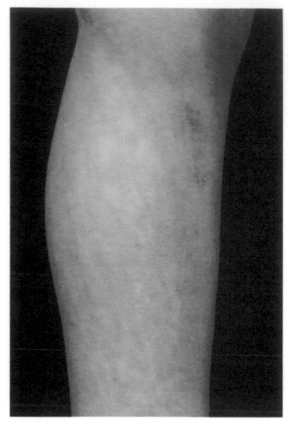

Figure 57.4
Incontinentia pigmenti (hypochromic stage). Whitish and atrophic streaks in the right lower limb show a typical reticulated pattern.

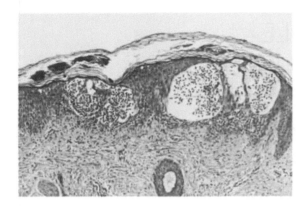

Figure 57.5
Incontinentia pigmenti (vesicular stage). The epidermis is dotted by spongiotic vesicles that are filled with eosinophils.

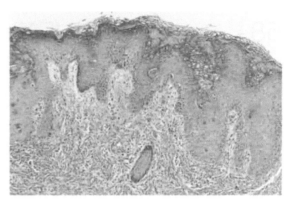

Figure 57.6
Incontinentia pigmenti (verrucous stage). Hyperplasia of the adnexal structures, particularly the infundibula, is associated with innumerable dyskeratotic cells.

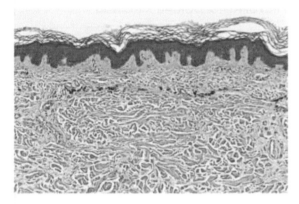

Figure 57.7
Incontinentia pigmenti (pigmentary stage). The numerous melanophages at the base of a thickened papillary dermis indicate an inflammatory process occurring at this site.

58   INFANTILE ACROPUSTULOSIS

Infantile acropustulosis is characterized by crops of eruptive, pruritic vesiculopustules that mainly involve the distal extremities.

EPIDEMIOLOGY

The condition is rare but less unusual in blacks than whites. Males are more frequently affected than females. Onset is generally in the second and third month of life.

CLINICAL FINDINGS

Lesions begin as tiny pink papules that develop rapidly (within 24 hours) into small vesicles or pustules, which are no larger than a few millimeters in diameter. They are extremely pruritic. The hands (Fig. 58.1) and the feet (Fig. 58.2) are the most commonly affected sites; the palmoplantar areas and the sides of the hands and the feet are more often involved than the dorsal surfaces. The scalp (Fig. 58.3), which is occasionally a site of involvement, is regarded by some as a typical location for the condition. The crops of vesiculopustules last for 10–15 days. Recurrent lesions may appear about every 4–5 weeks until the age of 3 years.

Association

Infantile acropustulosis can be associated with atopic dermatitis.

LABORATORY FINDINGS

Laboratory tests reveal a slight leukocytosis and often an eosinophilia. Stained smears of the contents of pustules show mainly neutrophils, although some eosinophils may be present.

HISTOPATHOLOGICAL FINDINGS

The disease is characterized by intraepidermal spongiform pustules arranged horizontally relative to the skin surface (Fig 58.4). In addition to neutrophils, which usually predominate within the pustule, eosinophils may be present in variable number.

ETIOLOGY AND PATHOGENESIS

The cause and mechanism are unknown.

MANAGEMENT

Topical corticosteroids are generally not useful. Antihistamines are effective for controlling the pruritus, but only at high doses. Erythromycin is reputed to give good results. Dapsone (1–2 mg/kg per day) has proved effective in many infants, but its use is not recommended because of possible complications, unless the pruritus is disabling.

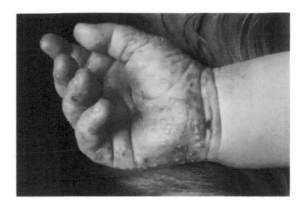

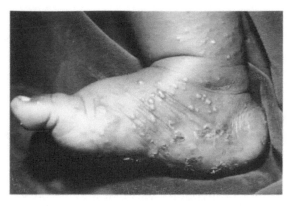

Figure 58.1
Infantile acropustulosis. Discrete pustules and yellow scaly crusts on acral skin are characteristic findings.

Figure 58.2
Infantile acropustulosis. These discrete pustules on the acra are diagnostic. Some of the pustules have resolved with erosions and ulcerations, and others have resolved with scaly crusts.

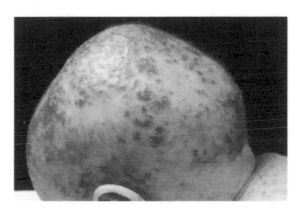

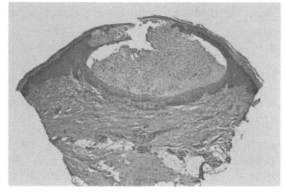

Figure 58.3
Infantile acropustulosis. Numerous rust-brown papules and papulopustules are present on the scalp.

Figure 58.4
Infantile acropustulosis. The tense intraepidermal pustule is situated mostly in the spinous zone, but its roof is formed by the cornified layer.

INFANTILE DIGITAL FIBROMATOSIS

Infantile digital fibromatosis is a benign tumor of myofibroblasts that may be present at birth or appear after the first year of life. It involves the distal phalanx of a finger or a toe.

EPIDEMIOLOGY

Infantile digital fibromatosis is a rare disease.

CLINICAL FINDINGS

Infantile digital fibromatosis, also called 'recurring digital fibroma', is a dome-shaped neoplasm that arises on the distal phalanx of a finger or a toe (Figs. 59.1 and 59.2). Typically, the thumbs and great toes are spared. Lesions may reach a centimeter or more in diameter and, when large, become lobulated or pedunculated. Palpation reveals the lesions to be firm and seemingly adherent to underlying tissues. They range in color from that of skin through pink to red. Their surface is smooth. Spontaneous regression usually occurs in 2–3 years. Recurrences may be expected after surgical excision in 70% of the cases.

HISTOPATHOLOGICAL FINDINGS

Infantile digital fibromatosis is a dome-shaped lesion composed of interweaving fascicles of fibrous tissue that is marked by numerous, plump, oval fibrocytes and coarse, wiry bundles of collagen throughout the dermis and the subcutaneous fat (Figs 59.3 and 59.4). Eosinophilic globules are present within the cytoplasm of fibrocytes.

ETIOLOGY AND PATHOGENESIS

The cause of infantile digital fibromatosis is not known.

MANAGEMENT

Since the lesions of infantile digital fibromatosis tend to involute with time, treatment is not mandatory. When treatment is necessary, complete excision is the treatment of choice.

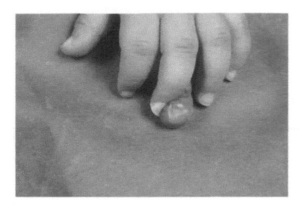

Figure 59.1
Infantile digital fibromatosis. This multilobulated, smooth, shiny, red–brown nodule is confined to a single digit.

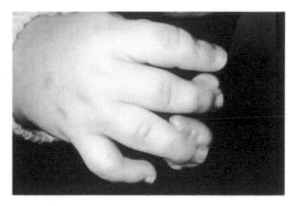

Figure 59.2
Infantile digital fibromatosis. Pink–blue , multilobulated nodules are present on the acral parts of two fingers in this infant.

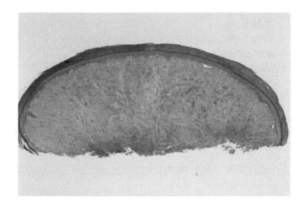

Figure 59.3

Figures 59.3. and 59.4
Infantile digital fibromatosis. This dome-shaped papule is characterized by an increased number of oval or spindle-shaped fibrocytes arranged in fascicles. Collagen, arrayed in thin bundles, is increased markedly.

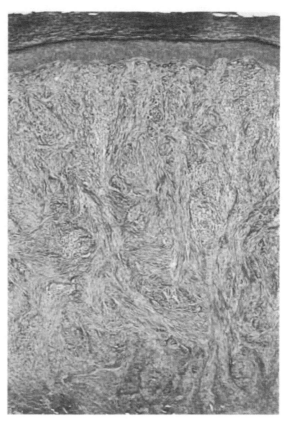

Figure 59.4

60   INFLAMMATORY LINEAR VERRUCOUS EPIDERMAL NEVUS

Inflammatory linear verrucous epidermal nevus (ILVEN) is a unilateral nevus that shows both inflammatory and psoriasiform features.

EPIDEMIOLOGY

The disease is rare. Females are four times as commonly affected as males. The age of onset is early, from birth to 4 years of age, with half of the patients developing the lesions in the first 6 months of life.

CLINICAL FINDINGS

ILVEN consists of discrete, erythematous, scaly, slightly verrucous papules that tend to coalesce and form linear plaques. The lesions are intensely pruritic (Figs 60.1 and 60.2). The lesions are unilateral; most commonly they occur on the left side of the body, especially on the left lower leg. They can be of any length and may involve the nails. Atrophy of the nails may occur. The course of this condition is chronic despite therapy.

HISTOPATHOLOGICAL FINDINGS

The histological appearance is inflammatory and psoriasiform (Fig. 60.3), with the following features:

- moderate acanthosis and papillomatosis;
- thickening of the epidermis;
- elongation of the rete ridges and dermal papillae;
- multiple small areas of spongiosis;
- exocytosis of neutrophils;
- alternating areas of parakeratosis and granulosis;
- perivascular lymphocytic infiltrate in the upper dermis.

ETIOLOGY AND PATHOGENESIS

The most plausible explanation for the existence of ILVEN is mosaicism.

MANAGEMENT

The treatment is unsatisfactory. The wide range of therapeutic trials include topical and intralesional corticosteroids, trichloracetic acid, cryotherapy, laser vaporization and surgical excision.

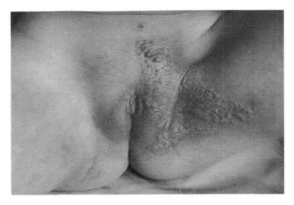

Figure 60.1
Inflammatory linear verrucous epidermal nevus. This pruritic plaque is only slightly elongated but consists of numerous keratotic papules on a reddish base. The hemorrhagic crusts are secondary to vigorous scratching.

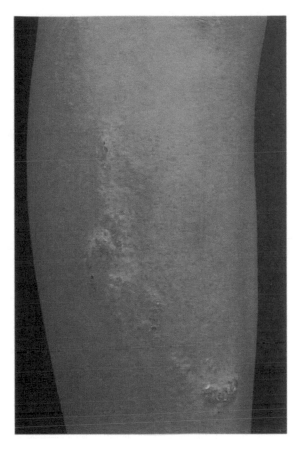

Figure 60.2
Inflammatory linear verrucous epidermal nevus. This lesion on the lower left leg has a somewhat linear configuration and consists of scaly papules whose bases are red–brown.

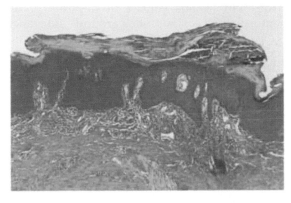

Figure 60.3
Inflammatory linear verrucous epidermal nevus. This lesion is characterized by alternating areas of parakeratosis, thickening of the epidermis, small areas of spongiosis, exocytosis of neutrophils and perivascular lymphocytic infiltrate in the upper dermis.

61 JUVENILE HYALINE FIBROMATOSIS

Juvenile hyaline fibromatosis is a multisystem disorder. It is characterized clinically by skin lesions, gingival hypertrophy, flexor contractures of the joints and osteolytic defects. Histologically it is characterized by deposition of amorphous hyaline material.

EPIDEMIOLOGY

Juvenile hyaline fibromatosis is a very rare disease.

CLINICAL FINDINGS

Juvenile hyaline fibromatosis does not become apparent until a few months after birth. Skin lesions consist of discrete, firm, white papules, pink–violet nodules and subcutaneous nodules of variable consistency (Fig. 61.1). They are found mainly on the scalp, the face, the auricular region, the neck, the limbs, the buttocks and the perineum. Gingival hypertrophy is an expected finding and may be severe. Deforming contractures involve the flexures of joints of the fingers, toes and knees (Fig. 61.2). Osteolytic lesions of terminal phalanges and long bones are often seen on radiological examination. Follow-up reports suggest a reasonable life until at least the second and third decade.

New skin lesions continue to appear but the major problem is represented by the joint contractures, which are disabling and disfiguring.

HISTOPATHOLOGICAL FINDINGS

The skin lesions consist of deposits of an amorphous eosinophilic ground substance (Figs 61.3 and 61.4) that contains chondroid cells. The collagen fibers are thin and decreased in number.

ETIOLOGY AND PATHOGENESIS

Juvenile hyaline fibromatosis is inherited in an autosomal-recessive fashion. It seems to be due to an accumulation of glycosaminoglycans, which influences the macromolecular organization of fibrillar collagen. The probable enzyme deficiency is not known.

MANAGEMENT

Treatment is unsatisfactory. The lesions do not respond to radiotherapy or intralesional corticosteroid injections, and they often recur after excision.

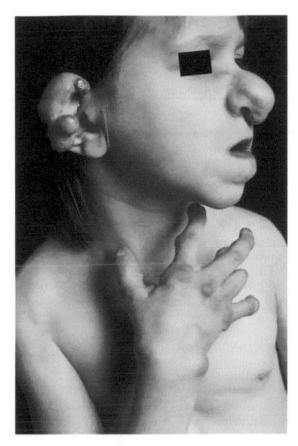

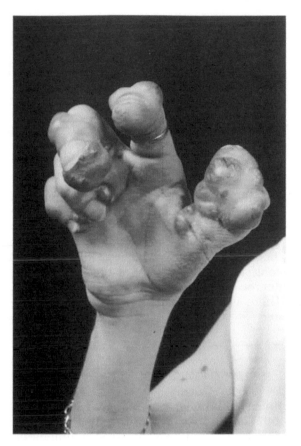

Figure 61.1

Juvenile hyaline fibromatosis. The nose, lips, ears and fingers of this child are disfigured by nodules and tumors, some of which have a brown hue.

Figure 61.2

Juvenile hyaline fibromatosis. The fingers of this patient are markedly distorted by multiple tumors.

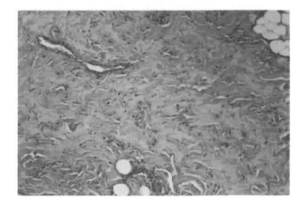

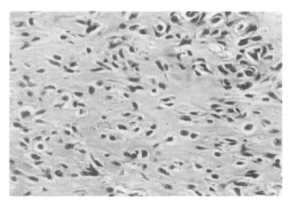

Figure 61.3

Figure 61.4

Figures 61.3 and 61.4

Juvenile hyaline fibromatosis. This lesion is characterized by deposition of amorphous eosinophilic ground substance containing chondroid cells. The collagen fibers are thin and decreased.

JUVENILE XANTHOGRANULOMA

Juvenile xanthogranuloma is a benign, usually self-limited, non-Langerhans cell histiocytosis that is most frequently seen in infants and children. It is characterized by yellowish, asymptomatic nodules located in the skin and other organs. These nodules consist of an infiltrate of histyocytes, and the degree of infiltration progressively increases. There is no accompanying metabolic disorder.

EPIDEMIOLOGY

Juvenile xanthogranuloma is fairly common, although its exact incidence is difficult to determine. Juvenile xanthogranuloma appears within the first 9 months of life in about 75% of cases, with 15–30% of them identified at birth.

CLINICAL FINDINGS

Two clinical variants can be distinguished: a small nodular form and a large nodular form. The small nodular form (Figs 62.1 and 62.2) is characterized by numerous (up to 100) firm, flat to domed, shiny lesions of 2–5 mm diameter. At first, the lesions are reddish brown, but they rapidly assume a yellowish hue. Such lesions remain discrete and are scattered randomly, mainly on the upper part of the body. Mucous membranes are seldom involved.

The large nodular form (Figs 62.3 and 62.4), by contrast, shows single or a few round–oval, translucent, dome-shaped nodules that are 10–20 mm in diameter and pink or yellowish in color; they sometimes exhibit telangiectases on their surface. Occasionally, lesions are exophytic.

Both expressions of juvenile xanthogranuloma usually are asymptomatic, and both may spontaneously resolve in 2–4 years. The term 'giant juvenile xanthogranuloma' has been used to describe lesions larger than 20 mm.

Associations

Several café-au-lait spots and a family history of neurofibromatosis are present in perhaps 20% of people with the small nodular form of juvenile xanthogranuloma. Leukemia manifests in approximately 25% of patients with small nodular juvenile xanthogranulomas. The most common extracutaneous manifestation of the small nodular form of juvenile xanthogranuloma is ocular xanthogranulomas. These lesions are typically unilateral, mostly involve the iris and ciliary body, and may be highly vascular.

The large nodular variant of juvenile xanthogranuloma may be related more often to mucosal lesions. Pulmonary lesions are reported most frequently but bones, pericardium, liver, testes and ovaries may be involved. These lesions are usually asymptomatic and regress spontaneously.

HISTOPATHOLOGICAL FINDINGS

Early lesions of juvenile xanthogranuloma are characterized by a mixed cell infiltrate in which histiocytes, some with foamy cytoplasm, predominate. Fully developed lesions contain more foam cells and Touton giant cells (Figs 62.5 and 62.6). Late-stage lesions show a variable degree of fibroplasia together with a mixed cell infiltrate that houses foam cells.

ETIOLOGY AND PATHOGENESIS

The etiopathogenesis of this condition is unknown. Progressively greater lipidization of histiocytes occurs as the lesions evolve but in the absence of metabolic abnormalities of lipids.

MANAGEMENT

In the absence of associated findings, no treatment is necessary.

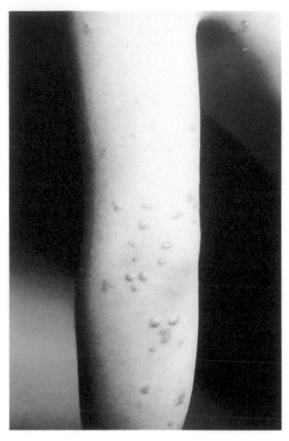

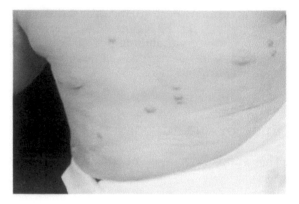

Figure 62.2
Juvenile xanthogranuloma (small nodular form). Many yellowish nodules are evident on the abdomen.

Figure 62.1.
Juvenile xanthogranuloma (small nodular form). This patient shows many discrete, slightly brownish nodules on an upper limb.

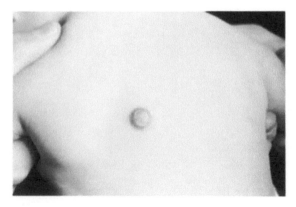

Figure 62.3
Juvenile xanthogranuloma (large nodular form). This solitary brownish nodule is covered by scales.

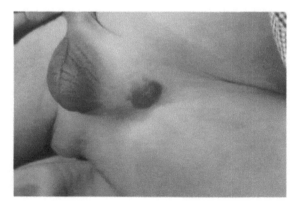

Figure 62.4.
Juvenile xanthogranuloma (large nodular form). A brown nodule is present on the inguinal area.

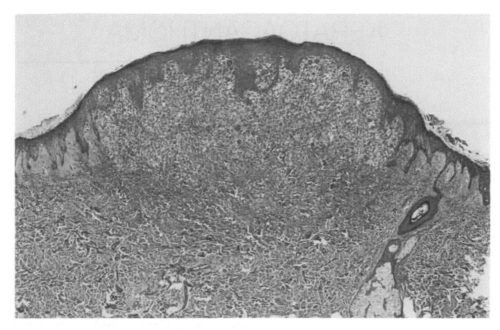

Figure 62.5

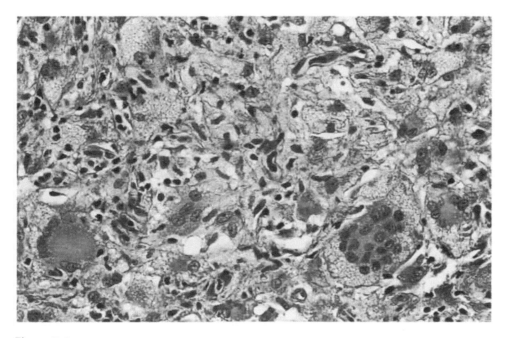

Figure 62.6

Figures 62.5. and 62.6
Juvenile xanthogranuloma (fully developed stage). This dome-shaped nodule is formed mostly by a dense, diffuse infiltrate of foamy macrophages that extends throughout the upper half of the dermis. Touton giant cells, made up of a central amphophilic core surrounded by an annulus of nuclei and encircled by a zone of foamy cytoplasm, are common findings (Fig. 62.6).

63

KERATOACANTHOMA

Keratoacanthoma is a benign, rapidly growing epithelial tumor composed of irregular exoendophytic growth of squamous epithelium that extends into the dermis. It occurs most commonly in a solitary form and more rarely in a multiple form. The multiple form has two variants – multiple, self-healing epitheliomas of Ferguson-Smith and eruptive keratoacanthoma.

EPIDEMIOLOGY

Solitary keratoacanthoma and eruptive keratoacanthoma occur in adulthood and in elderly persons. Multiple, self-healing epitheliomas, in which a familial pattern may be identified, appear in childhood or adolescence.

CLINICAL FINDINGS

Multiple, self-healing familial keratoacanthoma is characterized by the occurrence of numerous self-healing lesions that involve the sun-exposed areas, especially the face and the extremities (Fig. 63.1). Occasionally, the palms and soles are involved. Rarely, tumors are localized and unilateral. Each neoplasm has its beginning in normal skin as a small, firm papule that rapidly assumes the typical dome-shaped, crater-like aspect and size of the solitary keratoacanthoma, but it is set more deeply in the skin. The tumors usually reach full size within 6–8 weeks and disappear in 6 months.

HISTOPATHOLOGICAL FINDINGS

Keratoacanthoma is characterized by a crateriform lesion formed by contiguous, dilated, horn-filled infundibula and by proliferation of aggregations of squamous epithelium at the base of the crater (Fig 63.2).

ETIOLOGY AND PATHOGENESIS

In multiple, self-healing familiar keratoacanthoma, an unknown genetic factor seems to be responsible for most lesions. The genesis and development of this condition is the same as that for solitary keratoacanthoma. The lesion starts with hyperplasia of the infundibulum, with squamous metaplasia of the attached sebaceous glands.

MANAGEMENT

Although spontaneous involution does occur, the shave or curettage of lesions at an early stage may produce good results. In patients with many tumors at various stages of development, the most effective therapy is the administration of oral retinoids.

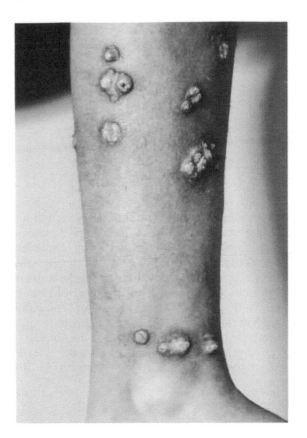

Figure 63.1
Keratoacanthoma. Numerous dome-shaped nodules have central craters plugged by cornified cells. Some of the nodules are discrete, but others tend to merge.

Figure 63.2
Keratoacanthoma. Even an early keratoacanthoma can be recognized as a follicular neoplasm because the crater is formed by dilated infundibula plugged by orthokeratotic cells. At the base of infundibula are prominent proliferations of spinous cells.

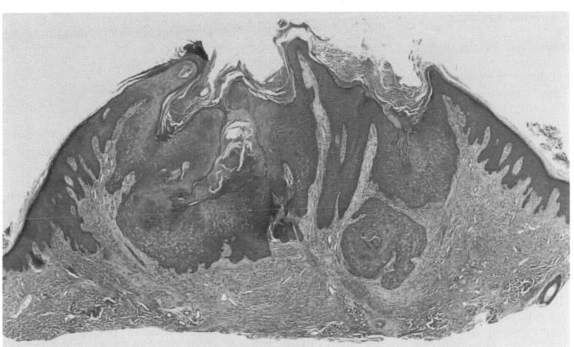

Keratosis pilaris is characterized by small, asymptomatic horny papules distributed mainly on the lateral aspects of the upper parts of limbs, the buttocks and the cheeks.

EPIDEMIOLOGY

Keratosis pilaris is a common disorder that affects about 30% of the population in a more or less evident way. Its occurs mainly in infancy and childhood.

CLINICAL FINDINGS

Keratosis pilaris causes monomorphous, follicular, horny papules that show no tendency to confluence and are localized on the extensor surfaces of limbs, the cheeks and the buttocks (Figs 64.1 and 64.2). These lesions are usually asymptomatic and persistent, tending to improve in summer and to worsen in winter. Typically, the skin in affected areas is rough.

Many clinical variants of keratosis pilaris are known. Among the non-atrophic variants, the most common is keratosis pilaris rubra, in which each lesion is surrounded by more or less evident erythema. Among the variants that leave residual atrophy are keratosis pilaris atrophicans faciei, vermiculate atrophoderma and keratosis pilaris spinulosa decalvans. Keratosis pilaris atrophicans faciei (or ulerythema ophryogenes) involves the upper half of the face, especially the periocular zone, the temporal region and the eyebrows (Fig. 64.3). The skin is erythematous with dissemination of hyperkeratotic micropapules that destroy the follicles. Vermiculate atrophoderma involves the cheeks and the preauricular regions in a symmetrical fashion. The initial erythema is followed by the appearance of follicular hyperkeratosis that leaves tiny atrophic pits. Keratosis follicularis spinulosa decalvans is characterized by diffuse keratosis pilaris associated with a scarring alopecia of the scalp.

Associations

Keratosis pilaris is commonly found in association with atopic dermatitis and ichthyosis vulgaris.

HISTOPATHOLOGICAL FINDINGS

Infundibula are dilated widely by plugs of mostly orthokeratotic cells. These plugs may extend for a short distance above the skin surface, where their tops are conical (Fig. 64.4).

ETIOLOGY AND PATHOGENESIS

Keratosis pilaris is an inherited disease, probably by autosomal-dominant transmission. Keratosis pilaris atrophicans faciei seems to be an autosomal-dominant mutation, with male predominance, even though sporadic cases have been reported. Vermiculate atrophoderma is also an autosomal-dominant disease. Keratosis follicularis spinulosa decalvans seems to have a sex-linked (X chromosome) dominant mode of inheritance. The pathogenesis of keratosis pilaris is still unknown.

MANAGEMENT

Treatment is not usually satisfactory. Emollient creams and mild keratolytic agents have been used with varying degrees of success. The use of systemic retinoids is contraindicated in children, and they are not effective topically.

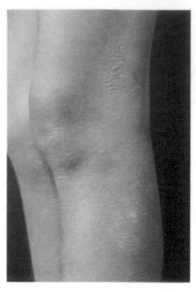

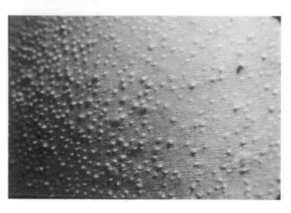

Figure 64.2
Keratosis pilaris. Each of these keratotic papules represents a follicular infundibulum that is dilated and plugged by horny cells.

Figure 64.1
Keratosis pilaris. Keratotic papules are grouped in round patches.

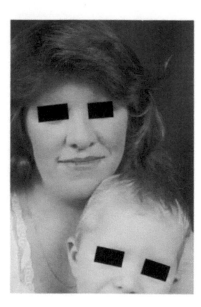

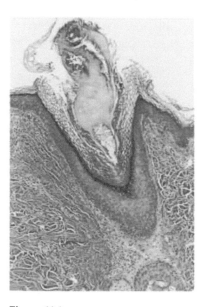

Figure 64.3
Keratosis pilaris atrophicans faciei (ulyerythema ophryogenes). Erythematous skin with keratotic micropapules destroying the follicles affects both mother and son in the periocular area.

Figure 64.4
Keratosis pilaris. Plugs of orthokeratotic cells emanate from the infundibula. These plugs project considerably above the skin surface.

LANGERHANS CELL HISTIOCYTOSIS

Langerhans cell histiocytosis is a disease of unknown cause characterized by the proliferation of a distinct cell type that is S100+ and CD1a+ and contains Langerhans granules in the cytoplasm. Langerhans cell histiocytosis includes four main clinical forms – Letterer–Siwe disease, Hand–Schuller–Christian disease, eosinophilic granuloma and Hashimoto–Pritzker disease.

When the disease involves at least two tissues or organs, the term 'disseminated Langerhans cell histiocytosis' has been proposed.

CLINICAL FINDINGS

Letterer–Siwe disease

Letterer–Siwe disease is the acute, disseminated, multisystem form of Langerhans cell histiocytosis. It begins before 6 months of age in one-third of cases and before 2 years of age in most of the rest. Cutaneous manifestations are very common. They are present in about half of the cases at the onset, whereas they occur in almost all fatal cases and are absent in one-fifth of non-fatal cases. The morphological features of the cutaneous lesions are characteristic. The typical lesions are small translucent papules (1–2 mm in diameter) that are slightly raised, rose–yellow in color (Fig. 65.1) and generally located on the trunk and scalp. The lesions frequently begin to scale and may become crusty. Purpura may appear; it is a poor prognostic sign, especially if petechiae appear on the palms and soles. Cutaneous lesions appear in successive crops. The lesions tend to merge on the scalp, where they have a seborrheic-like appearance, and

on the skin folds. Mucous membrane involvement is rare; when it occurs, it consists of erosions and ulcerations.

Pulmonary involvement may be discerned in more than half of affected children. Bone lesions occur in more than 60% of patients; they tend to be osteolytic and to affect flat bones, cranial bones, and vertebrae. They seem to be more frequent in patients with a favorable prognosis. Teeth may be lost precociously. Marked hepatomegaly, a frequent complication and an unfavorable prognostic sign, is found in two-thirds of patients, particularly those in whom jaundice and other clinical or biological signs of hepatic failure appear. Fewer than one-third of children with splenomegaly survive. Lymphadenopathy is not prominent as a rule, but it has been noted in one-quarter to three-quarters of all cases that end fatally. When thrombocytopenia and severe anemia occur, death is a virtual certainty, especially if splenomegaly coexists and osteolytic lesions are absent. Intercurrent infections are frequent.

Hand–Schuller–Christian disease

Hand–Schuller–Christian disease is the chronic, progressive, multifocal form of Langerhans cell histiocytosis. It begins between the 2nd and 6th years of life in 70% of cases. The disorder is characterized by bone lesions, diabetes insipidus, exophthalmus and mucocutaneous lesions. It is uncommon for all four manifestations to be seen together in the same patient.

Bone lesions are the most frequent manifestations (seen in 80% of cases). They preferentially involve the calvarium, especially in the temporoparietal region, where the infiltrate produces well-delimited osteolytic areas that merge to give a typical 'map' appearance. Bone lesions of the mastoid region may cause otitis media. These lesions are usually painful but not tender.

Diabetes insipidus is present in over 50% of cases, and is easily controlled by vasopressin. It occurs more often in children and in patients with involvement of the skull and the orbit.

Exophthalmus (Fig. 65.2) usually appears later; it is present in 10–30% of cases and may be unilateral or bilateral.

Mucocutaneous lesions are present in about one-third of cases. In the early stage, cutaneous lesions are papular and have the same morphological characteristics as those observed in Letterer–Siwe disease. Mucous membrane lesions are commonly of the noduloulcerative type and involve mainly the gingival tissue and the genital area.

Pulmonary infiltrates are found in less than 20% of cases, whereas hepatomegaly and lymphadenopathy are rare. The initial symptoms of the disease are more frequently diabetes insipidus, chronic otitis media or skin manifestations.

Eosinophilic granuloma

Eosinophilic granuloma is the localized, benign form of Langerhans cell histiocytosis. It is rare during childhoood. Usually, the typical granulomatous lesions affect the bones in the following decreasing order of frequency – the cranial vault, the ribs, the vertebral column, the pelvis, the scapulae and the long bones. The onset is insidious. Mucocutaneous lesions are rare. They are of the noduloulcerative type and preferentially involve the mucous membranes (Fig. 65.3) and the periorificial (perianal, perigenital and perioral) regions.

Hashimoto–Pritzker disease

Hashimoto–Pritzker disease (also called congenital self-healing reticulohistiocytosis) is the benign, self-healing form of Langerhans cell histiocytosis. It is usually present at birth, although it may appear during the first few days of life. Typically, the disease is characterized by the eruption of multiple disseminated, elevated, firm, red–brown nodules, which may be large (Fig. 65.4). These lesions can grow in size and number during the first few weeks of life and then form brown crusts that peel off, occasionally leaving whitish atrophic scars. The absence of mucous membrane lesions is a key feature of Hashimoto–Pritzker disease. Systemic signs are usually absent. Physical and mental development is normal.

In summary, the salient features of Hashimoto–Pritzker disease are:

- multiple or solitary papulonodular lesions;
- sparing of mucous membranes;
- absence of systemic involvement;
- rapid spontaneous regression.

HISTOPATHOLOGICAL FINDINGS

The unifying aspect of the protean clinical symptoms of Langerhans cell histiocytosis lies in its pathological features. The linking histological element of the different lesions is the typical cell of the lesions (Figs 65.5 and 65.6). This cell can be easily identified and differentiated from the non-specific elements of the infiltrate by its size and configuration. It is about four or five times larger than a small lymphocyte, has an irregular, vesiculated, often reniform nucleus, and has abundant, slightly eosinophilic cytoplasm. Three histological patterns are observed in Langerhans cell histiocytosis – proliferative, granulomatous and xanthomatous.

ETIOLOGY AND PATHOGENESIS

The etiopathogenesis of Langerhans cell histiocytosis remains a mystery despite numerous investigative efforts. Viral, immunological and neoplastic pathogenic mechanisms have been considered, but none has been proven.

MANAGEMENT

Treatment strategies depend on whether the disease involves the skin only, bones only, or is multisystem.

Single-system disease of the skin

For disease in children that involves only the skin, observation or topical nitrogen mustard is the treatment of choice.

Single-system disease of bones

Surgery, corticosteroid injections, radiotherapy and monochemotherapy (in multiple bone lesions) are treatments for single-system disease of bones.

Multisystem disease

For multisystem disease, monochemotherapy with vinblastine or etoposide, is the usual treatment. It may be preceded by corticosteroid therapy. Non-responders may be treated with polychemotherapy.

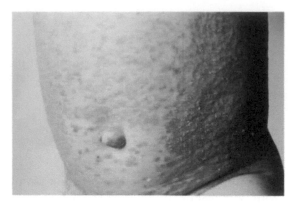

Figure 65.1
Langerhans cell histiocytosis (Letterer–Siwe disease). Brown crusted and scaly papules have become confluent to form plaques. The abdomen is distended by hepatomegaly.

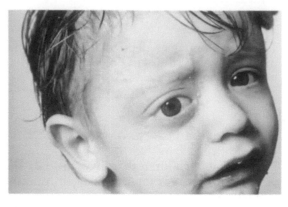

Figure 65.2
Langerhans cell histiocytosis (Hand–Schuller–Christian disease). Tan papules, some covered by scales, are grouped around the eyes and in the region of the temples. Exophthalmos of the right eye is evident.

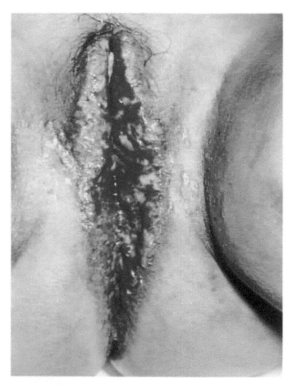

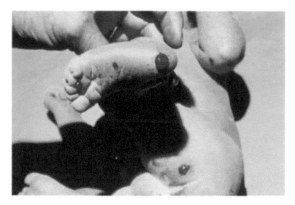

Figure 65.4
Langerhans cell histiocytosis (Hashimoto–Pritzker disease). Multiple disseminated, elevated, firm red–brown nodules, which were present from birth, can be seen.

Figure 65.3
Langerhans cell histiocytosis (eosinophilic granuloma). The vulva in this adolescent is markedly distended by pink papules that have coalesced to form plaques. The plaques are ulcerated and covered by blood and purulent material. Between the vulva and the inguinal folds are many skin-colored papules.

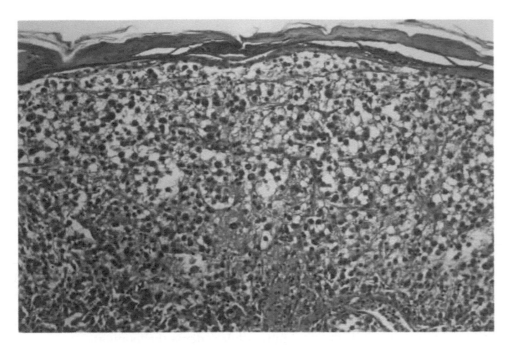

Figure 65.5

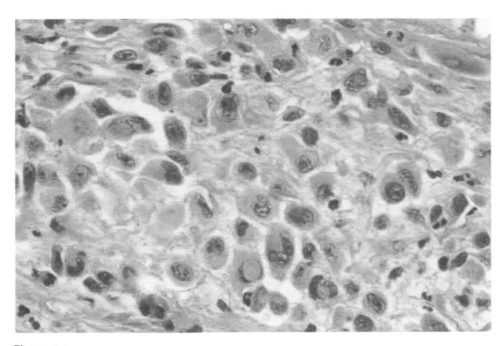

Figure 65.6

Figures 65.5 and 65.6

Langerhans cell histiocytosis. The papule shown here is characterized by an eroded, thinned epidermis covered by crust, beneath which is a dense, diffuse infiltrate of distinctive cells throughout the papillary dermis. These cells (Fig. 65.6) are characterized by bean-shaped nuclei and abundant eosinophilic cytoplasm.

66

LARVA MIGRANS

Larva migrans (or creeping eruption) is a broad term that describes the serpiginous, self-healing eruption caused by the accidental penetration of the skin by infective larvae of hookworms from various animals.

EPIDEMIOLOGY

Larva migrans is found most often in tropical and subtropical areas, especially coastal regions.

CLINICAL FINDINGS

Immediately after larvae penetrate the skin, the patient may experience a mild tingling sensation at the site of entry. The larvae can then lie quiet for weeks or months, or they may immediately begin to creep, with the production of single or multiple, pruritic, erythematous, raised tracks (Figs 66.1 and 66.2). The tracks are formed by papules and vesicles that contain serous fluid. These tunnel-like lesions may give rise to erosions. The leading portion of the track contains the larva, which advances at a rate of a few millimeters each day. The common entry sites are the feet, the hands, the buttocks, the calves, the arms and the thighs. The disease is self-healing in a few months, because humans are a 'dead-end' host.

LABORATORY FINDINGS

Eosinophilia has been observed.

HISTOLOGICAL FINDINGS

The histopathological findings are virtually indistinguishable from those caused by insect bites. There is a superficial and deep, perivascular and interstitial, mixed cell infiltrate made-up mostly of lymphocytes and eosinophils (Fig. 66.3). The papillary dermis is often edematous and the epidermis may house intercellular edema (spongiosis) and intracellular edema (ballooning).

ETIOLOGY AND PATHOGENESIS

The commonest causative agent is *Ancylostoma braziliensis*. Transmission is commoner in hot and rainy seasons because these conditions are appropriate for the development of the egg to the filiform larva stage. Warm sandy beaches contaminated with feces of dogs and cats represent a favorable condition for infection. The soil larvae may penetrate the skin through rhagades and hair follicles.

MANAGEMENT

Larva migrans usually does not require treatment because the worm dies spontaneously. However, this process may take several weeks to months, during which time the patient must endure both intensive pruritus and the discomforting sensation of a worm crawling through the skin. In children only topical treatment such as local freezing with liquid nitrogen, ethylcloride or dry ice under local anesthesia is recommended.

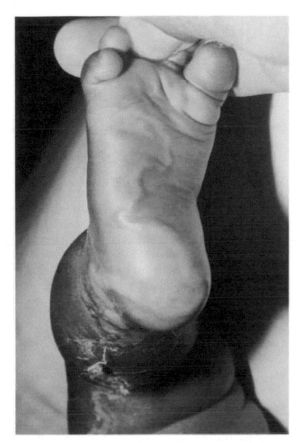

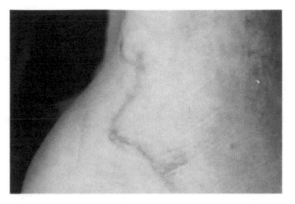

Figure 66.2
Larva migrans. An irregularly shaped, somewhat arcuate track formed by papules and vesicles is visible on the side of the foot.

Figure 66.1
Larva migrans. This serpiginous track winds its way along the entire leg of this child.

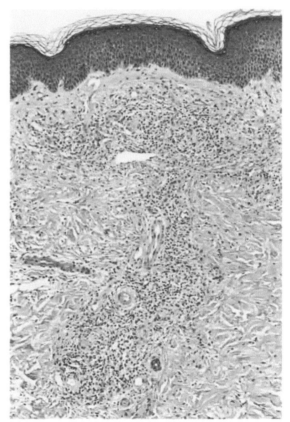

Figure 66.3
Larva migrans. Superficial and deep perivascular and interstitial mixed cell infiltrate of lymphocytes as well as eosinophils scattered among collagen bundles are a non-specific histopathologic finding.

67

LEISHMANIASIS

Cutaneous leishmaniasis (also known as oriental sore or Old World cutaneous leishmaniasis) is a granulomatous disease of the skin caused by *Leishmania tropica* complex (*Leishmania tropica* and *Leishmania major*) and *Leishmania aethiopica*, which are endemic in warm climates.

CLINICAL FINDINGS

The three clinical expressions of cutaneous leishmaniasis are acute, chronic and recidivans. Acute cutaneous leishmaniasis is more common in children. It begins as a single, asymptomatic, pink or red papule, 3–5 mm in diameter, at the site of a sandfly bite. Within 4–12 weeks, the papule evolves to a firm, inflamed, smooth, painful nodule (Fig. 67.1). The nodule enlarges progressively and eventually ulcerates and becomes crusted (Fig. 67.2). After removal, the crusts are soon replaced. After 5–12 months, the noduloulcerative lesions begin to regress from the center and, in time, resolve completely, leaving atrophic, irregular, disfiguring scars. Multiple lesions occasionally occur as the result of several bites by the sandfly that carries the protozoa. Superinfections occur in about 10% of patients, but their course is shorter and the lesions are smaller. The disease appears on the exposed areas of the body, especially the face and the arms.

The chronic form of leishmaniasis occurs only in elderly people, does not ulcerate and lasts for several years.

The recidivans form is rare and consists of new lesions that develop around scars at previously healed sites.

HISTOPATHOLOGICAL FINDINGS

Papules and nodules of acute leishmaniasis are characterized by dense, nodular and diffuse infiltrates composed mostly of histiocytes, neutrophils, and plasma cells. In the cytoplasm of the histiocytes reside numerous organisms of *Leishmania tropica* that appear as tiny blue dots in sections stained by hematoxylin and eosin (Figs 67.3 and 67.4). Such lesions may be eroded or ulcerated and covered by crusts.

ETIOLOGY AND PATHOGENESIS

Leishmania are protozoa of the family Trypanosomatidae. The parasite life cycle includes two forms, an extracellular, flagellated form (promastigote) in the vector and an intracellular non-flagellated form (amastigote) in infected mammals. Cutaneous leishmaniasis is caused by *L. tropica*, *L. major*, and *L. aethiopica*. These organisms are found only in cutaneous locations and do not tend to involve viscera. The most common vectors of the disease are *Phlebotomus papatasii* and *Phlebotomus sergenti*. The transmission occurs by the bite of an infected female sandfly that acquired its infection during a human blood meal 4–7 days previously. The commonest zoonotic reservoirs are gerbils and dogs. The incubation period varies from a few weeks to several months.

MANAGEMENT

The treatment of choice in children seems to be intralesional injection of methylglucamine antimoniate after local anesthesia. The lesions resolve promptly.

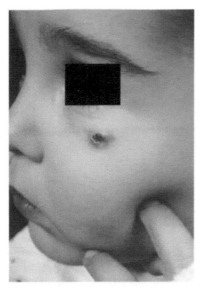

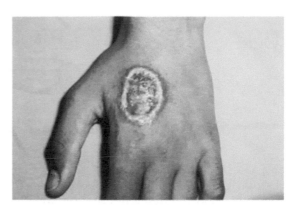

Figure 67.2
Acute cutaneous leishmaniasis. A large crater-like noduloul-cerative lesion with a characteristic sloping edge.

Figure 67.1
Acute cutaneous leishmaniasis. A dark adherent crust is evident at the center of a firm nodule.

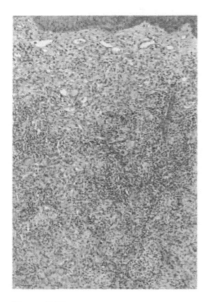

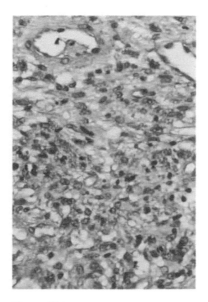

Figure 67.3   **Figure 67.4**

Figures 67.3 and 67.4
Acute cutaneous leishmaniasis. This patchy but diffuse infiltrate, made up mostly of mononuclear cells, harbors macrophages that contain organisms of Leishmaniasis. They are seen as tiny basophilic dots within the cytoplasm of the affected cells. Lymphocytes and numerous plasma cells are present together with macrophages.

68   LEIOMYOMA

Leiomyomas are benign neoplasms that are uncommon in children. They are composed of smooth muscle fibers. Three main types have been recognized, reflecting their different origins or differentiations:

- follicular leiomyoma, which arises from the arrector muscles of hair follicles;
- dartoic leiomyoma, which derives from the dartos muscle or the mamillary muscle of the nipple;
- angioleiomyoma, which originates from the smooth muscles of the blood vessels.

CLINICAL FINDINGS

Follicular leiomyoma appears as firm, red or dark brown nodules that vary in size from a few millimeters to 20 mm. The nodules are mainly situated on the trunk, the extremities and the head (Fig. 68.1). The number of the lesions may vary from few to several hundred. Adjacent tumors may coalesce to form plaques (Fig. 68.2). Single lesions have been observed. The characteristic feature of these tumors is paroxysmal pain induced by trauma, mild pressure or exposure to cold. This is the most frequent variety in children.

Dartoic leiomyoma is a solitary, deeply situated, non-painful nodule. Angioleiomyoma is a solitary, subcutaneous, well-circumscribed, asymptomatic nodule found on the extremities. After an initial period of growth, leiomyomas tend to become stationary. Pain, once established, tends to become progressively more severe.

HISTOPATHOLOGICAL FINDINGS

Leiomyomas have a silhouette of a benign neoplasm made up of myocytes (i.e. cells with elongated nuclei with blunt ends and vacuolated cytoplasm) (Figs 68.3 and 68.4).

MANAGEMENT

The tumors are typically benign, but since they are sometimes painful and also because malignant degeneration has been reported, surgical excision is recommended. Unfortunately, the tumor usually recurs.

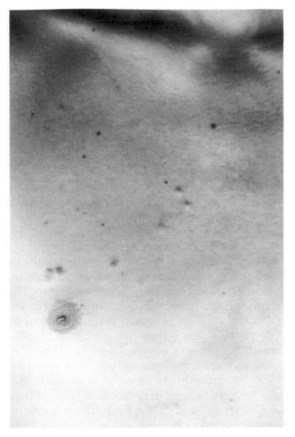

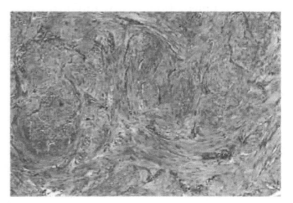

Figure 68.2
Leiomyomas. This cluster of reddish-brown papules and nodules is characteristic of cutaneous leiomyomas. The scar represents the site of a previous biopsy.

Figure 68.1
Leiomyomas. This patient has numerous dull pink and slightly brownish papules and small nodules.

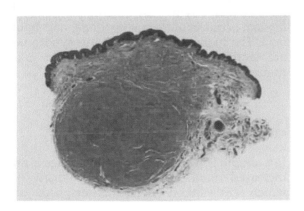

Figure 68.3

Figure 68.4

Figures 68.3 and 68.4
Leiomyoma. This lesion is well circumscribed and consists of fascicles of smooth muscle cells interweaved throughout the dermis.

LENTIGINES

Lentigines are small, dark brown, oval or circular macules that result from an increase in the number of melanocytes at the dermoepidermal junction without formation of nests.

EPIDEMIOLOGY

Lentigines are never present in newborns. They arise most commonly in childhood. They are present only in whites. Both sexes are equally affected.

CLINICAL FINDINGS

Lentigo simplex (or juvenile lentigo) is a macular or slightly raised area of brown or brown–black pigmentation, 1–5 mm in diameter. The pigmentation is fairly uniform, except at the margins where it merges with normal skin. The surface is smooth or slightly scaled (Fig. 69.1). Lentigines may be found on any area of the skin, mucous membrane, and conjunctivae.

Associations

Lentigines may be a distinctive sign of several syndromes. Peutz–Jeghers syndrome (periorificial lentiginosis) is an autosomal-dominant disorder characterized by pigmented spots in the buccal mucosa, the gums, the hard palate and the lips (especially the lower lips) (Fig. 69.1). On the face, the lentigines are concen-trated around the nose and the perioral region. The hands and feet may be affected. The pigmentary changes are present at birth or may develop early in childhood; they are associated with gastrointestinal polyps.

The LEOPARD syndrome or the multiple lentigine syndrome is an autosomal-dominant disorder with protean manifestation. The term LEOPARD is an elaborate acronym designed to help in remembering the various symptoms (lentigines, electrocardiographic abnormalities, ocular hypertelorism, pulmonary stenosis, abnormalities of genitalia, retardation of growth, deafness). Lentigines are always present and may be congenital, or they may appear soon after birth. They grow in number until puberty and are often scattered over the entire body. Cardiac problems are present in 79% of patients and may be detected as conduction disorders.

The LAMB syndrome is an extremely rare cardiocutaneous condition characterized (in a labored acronym) by lentigines, atrial myxoma, mucocutaneous myxoma, and blue nevi. The pigmented lesions of this syndrome are lentigines of the face and vulva and numerous blue nevi.

HISTOPATHOLOGICAL FINDINGS

In a simple lentigo, the dominant change is an increased number of melanocytes, many of which are notably dendritic, disposed as solitary units at the dermoepidermal junction (Fig. 69.2). The epidermis may or may not be thickened. Melanophages may be present in the upper part of the dermis. Simple lentigo is simply an incipient junctional nevus.

ETIOLOGY AND PATHOGENESIS

The cause is unknown.

MANAGEMENT

No treatment is necessary. If the patient requests it, surgical excision should be performed.

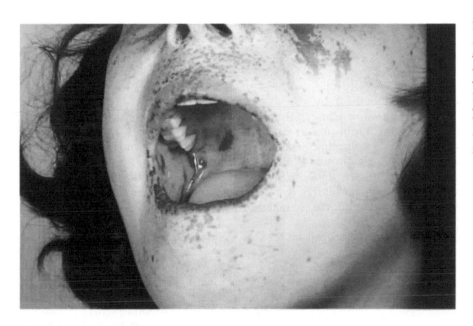

Figure 69.1
Lentigines (Peutz–Jeghers syndrome). Some brown and black macules are discrete and others form patches as a confluence of several elements. The lesions involve the face, the lips and the oral mucosa.

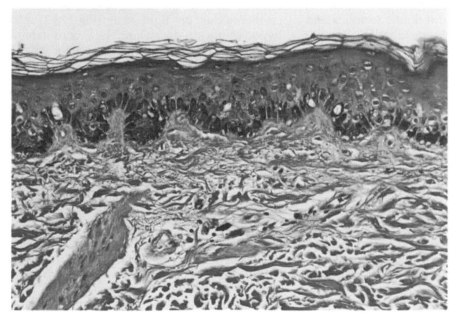

Figure 69.2
Simple lentigo. Epidermal hyperpigmentation in the lower portion of the epidermis together with an increased number of melanocytes arranged as solitary units at the dermoepidermal junction are characteristic of simple lentigo.

Leprosy (or Hansen's disease) is a chronic, systemic, communicable disease caused by *Mycobacterium leprae*. It shows different clinical pictures according to the immune response of the patient. The Redley–Jopling classification recognizes two polar forms (lepromatous leprosy and tuberculoid leprosy, marked respectively by low and high resistance to *M. leprae*), an indeterminate form (characteristic in the early stage of the disease) and an intermediate form (borderline leprosy).

EPIDEMIOLOGY

Leprosy is endemic in central and southern Africa, Asia, Central and South America and Oceania. There are about 12 milion people worldwide with leprosy. Onset of the disease during childhood is rare. The peak age of onset in children is 10–14 years.

CLINICAL FINDINGS

Prodromal manifestations

The onset of leprosy is insidious, with nonspecific symptoms and signs that may last for years. These symptoms and signs include asthenia, loss of weight, fever, headache, arthralgia, myalgia, lymphadenopathy and disorders of sensitivity, such as paresthesia and neuralgia. The only sign that can lead one to suspect the disease is chronic rhinitis with epistaxis.

Indeterminate leprosy

Indeterminate leprosy is characterized by one or a few hypopigmented or erythematous macules, of variable size and with ill-defined borders, on the face, the limbs or the trunk (Fig. 70.1). A sensory deficit may or may not be present, and peripheral nerves are not usually thickened.

Tuberculoid leprosy

Tuberculoid leprosy is the most common form in children. The cutaneous picture is marked by a low number of asymmetrical macular lesions, mostly on the trunk, that appear erythematous on light skin (Fig. 70.2) and hypochromic on dark skin. The lesions extend centrifugally and apparently resolve in the center, eventually acquiring figurated aspects. The borders are clear-cut and elevated. Irrespective of their morphology, the cutaneous lesions of tuberculoid leprosy are anhidrotic, alopecic and anesthetic. The involvement of the peripheral nervous system may precede or follow the skin manifestations and is characterized by sensory, motor, vasomotor and trophic changes. The peripheral nerves, especially the nerves of the head, neck and limbs, are thickened; on palpation, they show hard cylindric or monoliform (rosary grain) tumefactions.

The early sensory disorders are paresthesia, hypoesthesia and neuralgia. Subsequently, heat, pain, and touch anesthesia sets in, both at the sites of skin lesions and in apparently uninvolved areas, such as the cubital border of feet. The motor disorders (peripheral muscular paralysis leading to atrophy, contractures and deformities) appear at a more advanced stage.

The course of untreated leprosy in children is unpredictable, depending on the immunological responses of the individual child. Indeterminate leprosy may subside spontaneously (as occurs in nearly 75% of case); it may remain indeterminate for an indefinite time; or it may progress to lepromatous, tuberculoid or borderline leprosy. Tuberculoid leprosy may last for years and then heal after several periods of worsening and remission. Permanent neurological impairment, however, is common. Lepromatous leprosy may lead to death because of cachexia or intercurrent disease. Borderline leprosy may have its own clinical course as such or evolve to tuberculoid or lepromatous leprosy. The Mitsuda reaction in patients with tuberculoid leprosy is positive.

Lepromatous leprosy

Seen only occasionally in children, lepromatous leprosy involves the skin, the mucous membranes, the viscera and the peripheral nervous system. On the skin, lepromatous leprosy manifests itself as macules, papules, plaques and nodules, which occasionally ulcerate and are then known as lepromas (Fig. 70.3). The lesions are bilateral, symmetrical, clustered or coalescing, roundish or oval. They are of variable size, yellowish or copper red to brown in color, and hard. They arise most commonly on the face (the auricles, the forehead, the nose, the cheeks, the lips and the chin), so patients often show facies leonina. Additional signs include alopecia of the outer one-third of the eyebrows and partial alopecia of hair, eyelashes and beard. Less often, lepromas appear on extensor surfaces of hands and feet. Lepromas may subside, with restitutio ad integrum, or leave brownish pigmentation or hypochromic scars surrounded by a pigmented halo (lepromatous morphea); again, they may undergo deep ulceration and necrosis with involvement of muscles, carti-

lage and bones, leading to extremely severe deformities and mutilations (mutilating leprosy). In lepromatous leprosy, involvement of the eyes may include formation of synechiae, conjunctivitis with ectropion, iritis and iridocyclitis, episcleritis, keratitis, lagophthalmos, chorioretinitis, glaucoma. A common feature is chronic rhinitis with epistaxis, which may cause perforation of the septum and destruction of cartilage. Twenty per cent of patients develop lepromas (often ulcerated) on the oral cavity and in the larynx. In lepromatous leprosy, the Mitsuda reaction is negative.

Borderline leprosy

Borderline leprosy displays clinical, histopathological, immunological and bacteriological features that are intermediate between tuberculoid and lepromatous leprosy. The skin lesions of borderline leprosy (Fig. 70.4) in children correspond to those seen in adults. In borderline tuberculoid leprosy, the healing in the center of plaques is absent or incomplete and the distribution of lesions remains asymmetrical. Sensation within the lesions is diminished but not lost. In borderline lepromatous leprosy, the lesions (nodules and plaques) are numerous and may show a symmetrical distribution.

HISTOPATHOLOGICAL FINDINGS

Indeterminate leprosy

Indeterminate leprosy, as the name implies, cannot be diagnosed as leprosy from histopathological findings alone. The lesion consists of a superficial, perivascular, predominantly lymphocytic infiltrate that may be joined by either foamy or epithelioid histiocytes. As a rule, lepra bacilli cannot be identified in lesions of indeterminate leprosy even if special staining is used. A clue to the diagnosis, however, is the inclination for the lymphocytic infiltrates to be present in and around dermal nerve fascicles.

Lepromatous leprosy

Lepromatous leprosy (Figs 70.5 and 70.6) resembles a xanthoma, formed as it is by histiocytes that have abundant foamy cytoplasm as a consequence of lipid that resides in the walls of myriad lepra bacilli contained within them. The foam cells in lepromatous leprosy form nodules that may be present in the upper half of the dermis or throughout the dermis and even in the subcutaneous fat. The cast of many of the foam cells is bluish gray, a clue to the mycobacterial character of the xanthomatous infiltrate. Ziehl–Nielsen stain and Fite stain reveal innumerable acid-fast bacilli in virtually every foam cell (see Fig. 70.6).

Tuberculoid leprosy

Tuberculoid leprosy, as its name denotes, is characterized by tuberculoid granulomatous infiltrates (Fig. 70.7) within the dermis and sometimes the hypodermis. Histiocytes in tuberculoid leprosy are epithelioid rather than foamy. They form clusters of various sizes and shapes, which, in turn, are surrounded by lymphocytes and plasma cells in variable numbers. The mantle of lymphocytes may be sparse or dense. A characteristic finding is the tendency of the histiocytes to be present around and within dermal nerves. Fite stain does not reveal any acid-fast organisms in tuberculoid leprosy.

Borderline leprosy

Borderline leprosy shows features of both lepromatous and tuberculoid leprosy (Fig. 70.8). Foam cells and epithelioid cells are present and foam cells can be shown to house acid-fast organisms when Fite stain is applied.

ETIOLOGY AND PATHOGENESIS

M. leprae is a straight rod about 3.0 μm by 0.5 μm in diameter. It is alcohol- and acid-resistant. Human to human transmission is the norm. *M. leprae* is eliminated through nasal secretions, saliva and exudates of ulcerated cutaneous lesions. The incubation period is extremely variable, ranging from a few months to about 40 years, with a mean of 2–5 years.

MANAGEMENT

The treatment of leprosy in children is similar to that in adults. Management is presently based on the use of three drugs, dapsone, rifampicin (rifampin), and clofazimine. Dapsone is a bacteriostatic sulfonamide and is the drug of choice. In children, the dose is 2 mg/kg/day; it is usually given with other drugs to avoid resistance. Rifampicin is a bactericidal agent given in the conventional dosage of 10 mg/kg/day. Clofazimine shows bacteriostatic activity and has good anti-inflammatory properties. The standard dosage is 50 mg/day. The treatment regimen with these three drugs should be continued for at least 2 years. Thalidomide and corticosteroids are used in severe leprosy reactions.

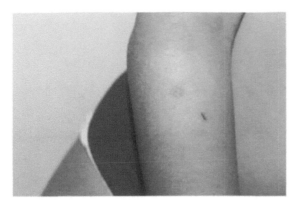

Figure 70.1
Indeterminate leprosy. Slightly hypopigmented macules with well defined borders.

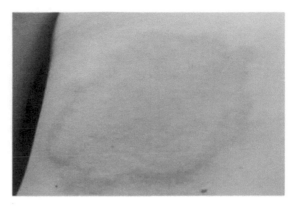

Figure 70.2
Tuberculoid leprosy. A large patch with central healing and a papular, erythematous edge.

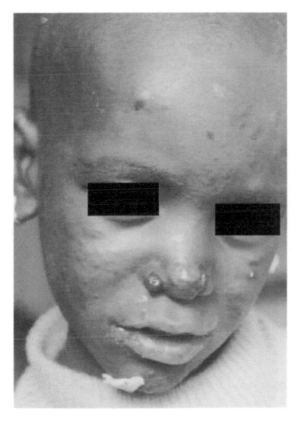

Figure 70.3
Lepromatous leprosy. The nodular eruption is widespread, but the face is the site of predilection. Few lesions on the limbs are ulcerated.

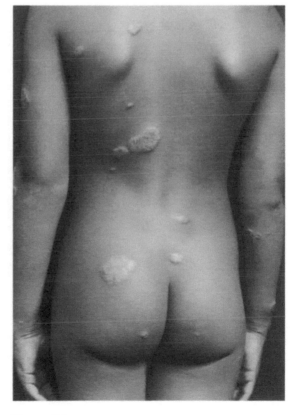

Figure 70.4
Borderline leprosy. Numerous plaques with clear-cut and elevated borders are distributed asymmetrically. The center of the plaques does not tend to heal.

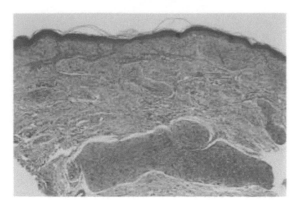

Figure 70.5

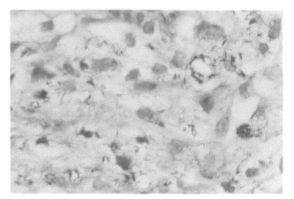

Figure 70.6

Figures 70.5 and 70.6
Lepromatous leprosy. The diagnosis of lepromatous leprosy is suggested by the appearance of elongated, snub-nosed aggregations consisting of pale histiocytes aligned along established vascular plexus. At higher magnification (Fig. 70.6), Ziehl–Nielsen stain reveals numerous acid-fast organisms within histiocytes.

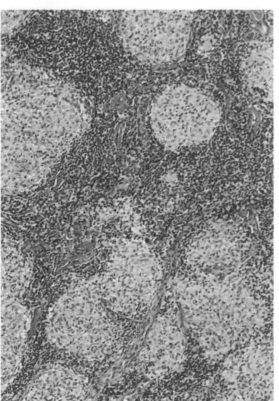

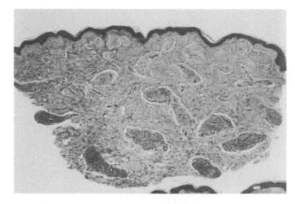

Figure 70.8
Borderline leprosy. This is borderline leprosy because the granulomas consists of both foamy and epithelioid histiocytes with a moderately dense infiltrate of lymphocytes around some of them.

Figure 70.7
Tuberculoid leprosy. The infiltrate consists mostly of epithelioid histiocytes that form nests. Dense lymphocytic infiltrates surround these aggregations.

71

LICHEN AUREUS

Lichen aureus is a rare asymptomatic dermatosis of unknown origin, now classified into the group of pigmented purpuric dermatoses. The eruption consists of roundish or irregular, erythematous, purpuric papules, coalescent in patches, and mostly distributed on the limbs.

CLINICAL FINDINGS

Lesions of lichen aureus begin as red–purple, flat-topped papules of 1–3 mm in diameter. They are sometimes surmounted by fine, adherent scales. With time, the papules join to form plaques, and their color changes to shades of green–yellow, rust, bronze and even dark brown (Fig. 71.1). Failure of lesions at all stages to blanch on diascopy is characteristic. Plaques of lichen aureus are generally solitary, oval, well-circumscribed and small, usually not exceeding 30–50 mm in diameter. Rarely, plaques up to 200 mm in diameter may be seen, as may linear or multiple lesions. Lichen aureus is typically unilateral. Sites of predilection include the lower part of the leg, the thighs, the trunk and the upper extremities, in that order. Pruritus may be noted in early lesions, although most papules are asymptomatic. The lesions tend to regress in months or years.

HISTOPATHOLOGICAL FINDINGS

An infiltrate composed mostly of lymphocytes is present around the vessels of the superficial plexus and in band-like array in a thickened papillary dermis. Usually, the dermoepidermal junction is not obscured by the infiltrate. In early lesions, erythrocytes are extravasated in the papillary dermis (Fig. 71.2). Later, extravasated erythrocytes are few, but siderophages may be numerous throughout the thickened papillary dermis.

ETIOLOGY AND PATHOGENESIS

The etiology of the dermatosis is unknown. The postulated pathogenesis of lichen aureus is a capillaritis triggered by an infective focus that may sensitize the capillaries.

MANAGEMENT

Lichen aureus is unresponsive to topical or systemic treatment, but the disease is not disturbing and there is a slow tendency to spontaneous healing.

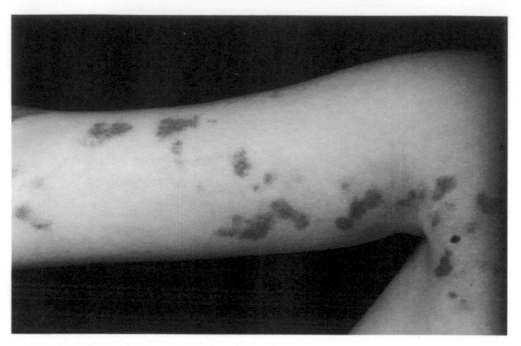

Figure 71.1
Lichen aureus. Asymptomatic, irregularly shaped rusty patches with a zosteriform pattern are seen here.

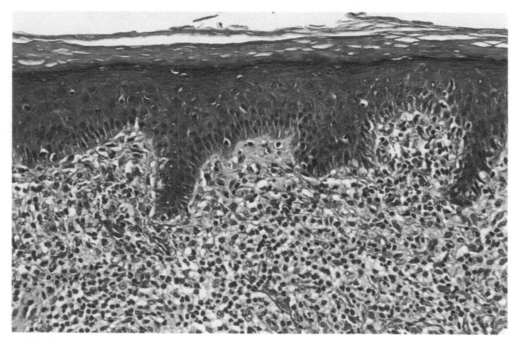

Figure 71.2
Lichen aureus. Lichen aureus is distinguished from other lichenoid dermatitides by the presence of numerous extravasal erythrocytes or siderophages (or both) within the lichenoid infiltrates of lymphocytes, as is evident in this section.

72

LICHEN NITIDUS

Lichen nitidus is an uncommon, chronic, self-healing eruption that is characterized by small, skin-colored papules, especially on the extremities, the abdomen and the penis.

CLINICAL FINDINGS

The fundamental lesion is a tiny translucent papule that is flat-topped and glossy. Although larger lesions may be polygonal (by filling the polygonal areas bounded by pre-existing skin markings), most papules of lichen nitidus are perfectly round, small enough to fit comfortably within skin markings, and strikingly uniform in size and shape (Figs 72.1 and 72.2). They vary in color from alabaster to yellow to pink, but most are skin-colored. The papules are exquisitely well demarcated, and may be arranged discretely in linear array, as a result of a Koebner response, or in agminated groups. Areas of predilection include the flexor surfaces of the ankles, wrists and forearms; the extensor areas of fingers, elbows and knees; the lower abdomen; and the genitalia. The palms and soles may also be involved. The lesions are generally asymptomatic; pruritus, when present, is mild. Lichen nitidus lasts from a few months to a few years, although 70% of patients experience complete resolution within 1 year of onset.

HISTOPATHOLOGICAL FINDINGS

Fully formed lesions display discrete granulomatous balls in widened dermal papillae beneath thinned suprapapillary plates (Fig. 72.3). These plates may harbor slight spongiosis and are often surmounted by slight focal parakeratosis or scaly crusts. The rete ridges partly embrace the granulomas.

ETIOLOGY AND PATHOGENESIS

The monomorphic aspect of the papules and the granuloma-like structure that characterize lichen nitidus have set this disease apart; its etiology is still unknown.

MANAGEMENT

Treatment is not required. When pruritus is present, local corticosteroids can be useful; rarely, systemic corticosteroids are needed, but they are not always effective.

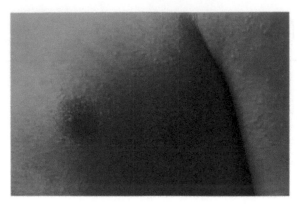

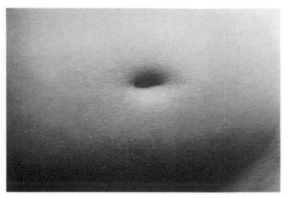

Figure 72.1
Lichen nitidus. Most papules are perfectly round and sharply demarcated. These lesions tend to be arranged in groups, but they are not confluent.

Figure 72.2
Lichen nitidus. Most of these innumerable, tiny, whitish papules are discrete, but some are arranged in a linear fashion as an expression of the Koebner phenomenon.

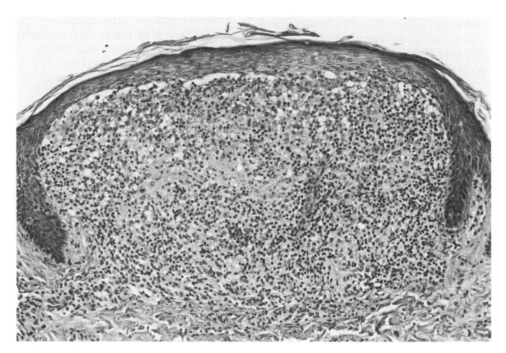

Figure 72.3
Lichen nitidus. A ball of epithelioid histiocytes, which is peppered by lymphocytes, fills the widened dermal papilla. The infiltrate obscures the dermoepidermal junction, where vacuolar alterations have resulted in a subepidermal cleft.

73

LICHEN PLANUS

Lichen planus is a self-limited, pruritic eruption characterized by flat violaceous papules that involve especially the extremities and the mucous membranes. The disease is rare in childhood, but not exceptional.

CLINICAL FINDINGS

The classic lesions of lichen planus in children, as in adults, are small, shiny, flat-topped, polygonal, violaceous papules (Fig. 73.1). Thin scales may be seen on top of some lesions. Wickham's striae (a network of fine whitish lines) can be observed on papules when they are confluent in plaques (Fig. 73.2). Lesions in friction areas may rapidly become subtly hyperkeratotic. The Koebner phenomenon may be easily induced (see Fig. 73.1). Upper and lower limbs are common sites of involvement in children, although the trunk, the neck and, in a few cases, the face can be involved. Lesions of lichen planus on the buccal mucosa (Fig. 73.3) and genital mucosa seem to be less common in children than in adults. The reticular variety is the most frequent type of oral lesion. Involvement of nails is, in the authors' experience, not as rare as described and may even precede the cutaneous lesions. Itching varies in severity and may be absent altogether. Although the classic form of lichen planus is the commonest in infancy, all other variants (annular, linear, hypertrophic and bullous forms) are sometimes seen. Lichen planus is chronic but it has some tendency to remission and exacerbations. In most cases, spontaneous healing occurs in a few years.

HISTOPATHOLOGICAL FINDINGS

The papules of lichen planus, in their fully developed expression, have distinctive changes – compact orthokeratosis, wedge-shaped hypergranulosis, jagged epidermal hyperplasia and a lichenoid infiltrate of lymphocytes that fills a thickened papillary dermis and obscures the dermoepidermal junction in company with vacuolar alteration and necrotic keratinocytes; these keratinocytes are known variously as Civatte bodies, colloid bodies and hyaline bodies (Fig. 73.4).

ETIOLOGY AND PATHOGENESIS

The etiopathogenesis of lichen planus is unknown. Emotional stress can precipitate an eruption. Drugs may induce lichen planus-like manifestation. A viral origin cannot be excluded.

MANAGEMENT

Treatment is mainly symptomatic, with topical corticosteroids and systemic antihistamines administered for mild forms of the disease. Topical coal tar or ointments with a small percentage of salicylic acid may be used for hyperkeratotic forms. In children, systemic corticosteroids can be given for widespread, disturbing forms of lichen planus. Psoralen and ultraviolet-A treatment is not recommended for children.

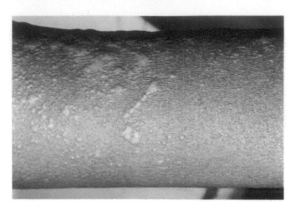

Figure 73.1
Lichen planus. The flat-topped, reddish papules are both discrete and linear. The latter is a consequence of scratching and is the expression of the Koebner phenomenon.

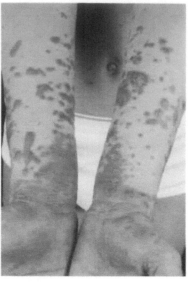

Figure 73.2
Lichen planus. Numerous papules have formed plaques as a consequence of confluence. Some of the lesions are characteristic of lichen planus because they are polygonal, slightly violaceous and scaly. Wickham's striae in a reticulated pattern are evident.

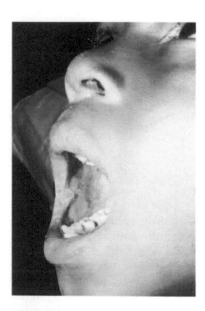

Figure 73.3
Lichen planus. Lesions are present on the lips and the buccal mucosa. The whitish, lacy, reticulated pattern is typical of lichen planus.

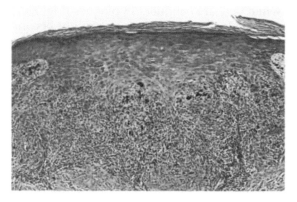

Figure 73.4
Lichen planus. This tiny papule exhibits compact orthokeratosis, wedge-shaped hypergranulosis, jagged epidermal hyperplasia and a superficial perivascular lymphocytic infiltrate that is band-like in a thickened papillary dermis and obscures the dermoepidermal junction.

74

LICHEN SCLEROSUS ET ATROPHICUS

Lichen sclerosus et atrophicus is a distinctive chronic disorder of the skin and mucous membranes that is characterized by atrophy in the anogenital area and white papular lesions on the rest of the skin.

EPIDEMIOLOGY

Most cases (85%) in children occur before the age of 7 years. Ninety percent of patients are female.

CLINICAL FINDINGS

Extragenital lesions are mother-of-pearl or ivory in appearance, irregular or polygonal, flat-topped and firm papules (Fig. 74.1). Their surface typically shows follicular hyperkeratosis with plugging and delling. The papules may coalesce to form plaques. They are asymptomatic. The sites of predilection are the upper parts of the trunk, the neck and the upper extremities. Anogenital lesions in girls occur in a figure-of-eight pattern on the vulva and perianal area (Figs 74.2 and 74.3). Follicular plugging and delling are usually absent. Bullous, erosive, hemorrhagic, rhagadiform and hyperplastic forms have been described. Patients frequently complain of soreness, itching and dysuria. In boys, the lesions appear as a balanitis xerotica obliterans and cause phimosis. Approximately two-thirds of anogenital lesions involute before or at the time of puberty without atrophy. In the remaining one-third of cases, the condition persists with atrophy of the labia minora and the clitoris in girls, and with phimosis in boys.

HISTOPATHOLOGICAL FINDINGS

A fully developed lesion of lichen sclerosus et atrophicus is marked by compact orthokeratosis, a thinned epidermis, sclerosis, telangiectases in a thickened papillary dermis, and a superficial, perivascular lymphocytic infiltrate. The infiltrate, which is considerably compressed beneath the epidermis, is actually present around venules of the superficial plexus (Fig. 74.4). Fully formed lesions are often accompanied by widely dilated infundibula and upper portions of eccrine ducts, both of which are plugged by orthokeratotic cells. When those structures rupture, granulomatous inflammation results. Infrequently, blisters form beneath the epidermis and the subepidermal blister may house numerous erythrocytes.

ETIOLOGY AND PATHOGENESIS

The cause of lichen sclerosus et atrophicus is unknown. The predominance in females and the frequent spontaneous pubertal involution suggest that low levels of ovarian hormones may be a pathogenic factor.

MANAGEMENT

There is no specific treatment. In anogenital lichen sclerosus et atrophicus, topical application of corticosteroids may be useful for controlling itching. Topical progesterone or estrogen provide an alternative approach in prepubertal girls. Circumcision is often necessary for balanitis xerotica obliterans.

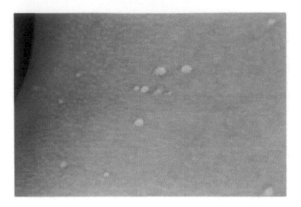

Figure 74.1
Lichen sclerosus et atrophicus. These macules and papules are typical findings. The white zones are the consequence of sclerosis in the upper portion of the dermis and loss of melanin from epidermis. Note the dells in the center of some lesions. They represent dilated ostia of epithelial adnexal structures plugged by cornified cells.

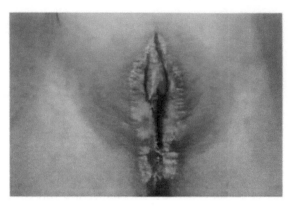

Figure 74.2
Lichen sclerosus et atrophicus. White papules have become confluent to form plaques around the vulva and the anus.

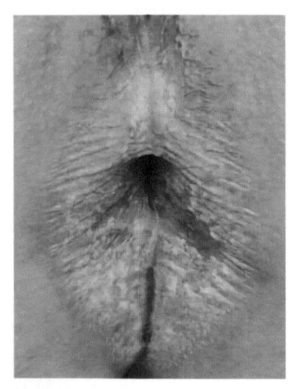

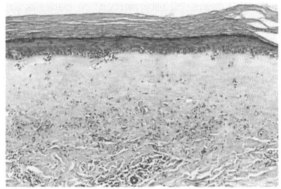

Figure 74.4
Lichen sclerosus et atrophicus. This lesion is characterized by a superficial perivascular, interstitial, predominantly lymphocytic infiltrate; a papillary dermis that is thickened by sclerosis and is pale-staining; a thinned epidermis devoid of the usual undulations between rete ridges and dermal papillae; and compact orthokeratosis.

Figure 74.3
Lichen sclerosus et atrophicus. The process primarily involves the perianal region with whitish plaques that are hyperkeratotic. The accentuation of the skin markings is a consequence of superimposed lichen simplex chronicus.

75 LICHEN SIMPLEX CHRONICUS AND PRURIGO NODULARIS

Both lichen simplex chronicus and prurigo nodularis are common skin lesions that result from persistent and prolonged rubbing.

CLINICAL FINDINGS

Lichen simplex chronicus results from long-standing rubbing across a relatively broad front of skin. As a consequence of this action, lichenified plaques form. 'Lichenification' means 'thickening', and the plaques are characterized by slight induration, accentuation of skin markings, hyperpigmentation and, sometimes, slight scaling.

In contrast, the papules and nodules of prurigo nodularis (Fig. 75.1) result from massage of a discrete point in the skin, usually by the ball of the finger. Resultant papules and nodules have all the features of lichen simplex chronicus but in a domed configuration. These lesions arise chiefly on the extremities. A picker's nodule is simply a lesion of prurigo nodularis that is eroded and crusted as a consequence of lively scratching. Only cessation of rubbing leads to regression of lesions.

HISTOPATHOLOGICAL FINDINGS

Lichen simplex chronicus may be characterized either by compact orthokeratosis and hypergranulosis in the context of folliculosebaceous units or by compact orthokeratosis, hypergranulosis and coarse bundles of collagen arrayed in vertical streaks in a thickened papillary dermis (Fig. 75.2). Prurigo nodularis demonstrates the same features of lichen simplex chronicus but in dome-shaped lesions.

ETIOLOGY AND PATHOGENESIS

Lichen simplex chronicus and nodular prurigo are the result of rubbing and scratching

MANAGEMENT

The treatment of these disorders consists of relieving the itch with corticosteroid creams, injection of corticosteroids and oral antihistamines.

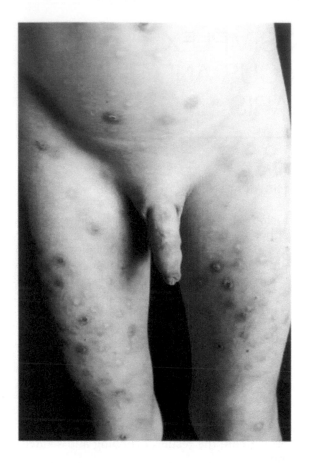

Figure 75.1
Prungo nodularis. The dome-shaped, hyperpigmented, smooth nodules are lesions of prurigo nodularis. The ulcerated and crusted lesions are picker's nodules.

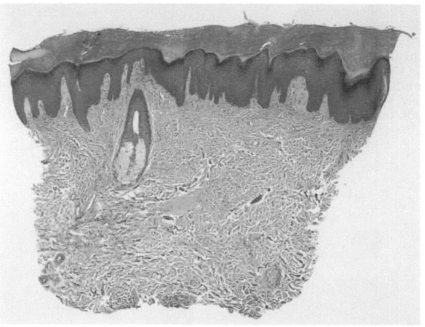

Figure 75.2
Lichen simplex chronicus. Even at scanning magnification; this lesion can be identified as lichen simplex chronicus because the cornified layer vaguely resembles a palm or sole and yet a folliculosebaceous unit is present in the section. The epidermal changes of compact orthokeratosis, hypergranulosis and irregular psoriasiform hyperplasia are a consequence of vigorous rubbing.

76

LICHEN STRIATUS

Lichen striatus is a self-limited eruption that consists of grouped papules in linear array that usually form a band on one side of the body.

EPIDEMIOLOGY

Lichen striatus is the commonest childhood acquired, self-limited linear eruption that follows Blaschko's lines. The age of onset is between 4 months and 15 years. The mean age at diagnosis varies from 3 to 5 years.

CLINICAL FINDINGS

The fundamental lesion of lichen striatus is a round papule that varies in color from pearly white to dark red (Figs 76.1, 76.2 and 76.3). The surface may be smooth or slightly verrucous. Papules appear suddenly and are clustered in bands along Blaschko's lines (Figs 76.1, 76.2 and 76.3). These bands vary in width from a few millimeters (Fig. 76.1) to 50 mm (Fig. 76.2), but generally lesions form a single, unilateral band. In some cases, the band is short, merely a few centimeters in length, but in others, it may stretch from the vertebral column along an entire limb to the tip of one or two digits, even extending to the nails and causing onychodystrophy. In patients with more than one band, the lesions may appear on one half of the body in segmental distribution. The lesions are predominantly distributed on the limbs in two-thirds of cases and on the trunk in the remaining one-third. Lichen striatus is not usually accompanied by any subjective symptoms. Lesions last a few months (the mean duration is 10 months) and then disappear spontaneously, leaving hypochromic sequelae in 50% of cases.

HISTOPATHOLOGICAL FINDINGS

Fully developed lesions of lichen striatus are characterized by focal parakeratosis, focal spongiosis, necrotic keratinocytes and a superficial and deep perivascular infiltrate of lymphocytes and histiocytes that are focally band-like in the papillary dermis and that obscure the dermo-epidermal junction (Figs 76.4 and 76.5). The epidermis may be psoriasiform and the lichenoid infiltrate may be dense.

ETIOLOGY AND PATHOGENESIS

The etiology and pathogenesis of the disease are still unknown. It has been suggested that the transient cutaneous band of lichen striatus might be induced by a somatic mutation that involves skin cells. Keratinocytes may be the target cells derived from a modified clone spread according to Blaschko's lines.

MANAGEMENT

Treatment is not required.

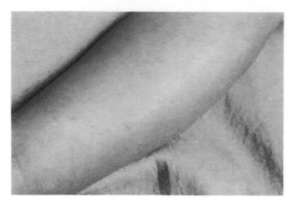

Figure 76.1
Lichen striatus. Pink, slightly hyperkeratotic papules are in a somewhat linear arrangement.

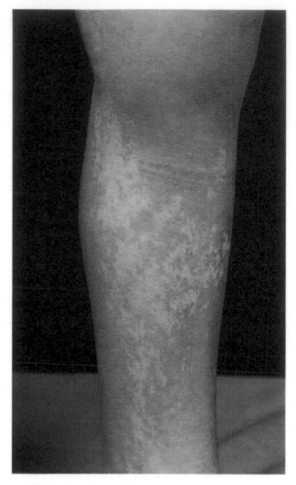

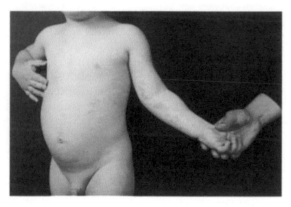

Figure 76.3
Lichen striatus. This 3-year-old boy has red papules in a somewhat linear array on the left upper limb and the left half of the trunk. Hypochromic post-inflammatory sequelae are visible on the trunk.

Figure 76.2
Lichen striatus. This irregular band of whitish, slightly scaling papules is more than 50 mm in width. Individual papules are evident at the periphery of the band.

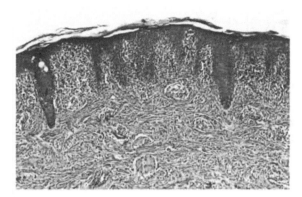

Figure 76.4

Figures 76.4 and 76.5
Lichen striatus. This lesion is typified by a superficial and deep perivascular and periadnexal lymphocytic infiltrate, as well as by patchy lymphocytic infiltrate in the upper part of the dermis that obscures the dermoepidermal junction. The infiltrate is present within the epidermis, together with spongiosis and necrotic keratinocytes. Parakeratosis is also found.

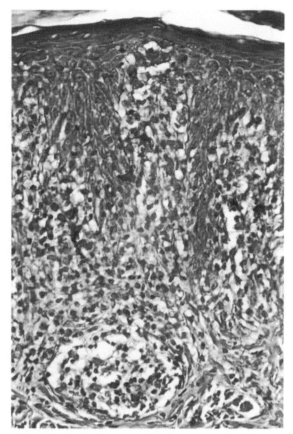

Figure 76.5

77

LIPOATROPHY

Lipoatrophy is characterized by the absence of subcutaneous tissue. Three types of lipoatrophy are recognized – localized lipoatrophy, partial lipoatrophy and total lipoatrophy.

EPIDEMIOLOGY

Lipoatrophy is a rare condition.

Localized lipoatrophy

Localized lipoatrophy consists of discrete loss of subcutaneous fat in a well-circumscribed area of the body (Fig. 77.1). The best known types of localized lipoatrophy are annular lipoatrophy, lipoatrophy of the ankles, and lipodystrophia centrifugalis abdominalis infantilis.

Annular lipoatrophy is characterized by a circular, depressed band, 10 mm wide and 5–20 mm deep, that encircles an upper limb. The lesion usually is unilateral and is accompanied by distal edema. Pain with muscle weakness may be associated features.

Lipoatrophy of the ankles manifests itself as a symmetrical, asymptomatic, depressed band, about 100 mm wide, preceded by a non-inflammatory swelling of the subcutaneous tissue.

Lipodystrophia centrifugalis abdominalis infantilis is characterized by a well-demarcated, depressed area of subcutaneous atrophy with evident blood vessels surrounded by a raised, slightly scaly and erythematous border. The lesion gradually enlarges centrifugally to involve the abdomen and neighboring regions. This form of localized lipoatrophy usually appears before the age of 3 years and tends to remit after puberty.

Partial lipoatrophy

Partial lipoatrophy is characterized by partial, usually symmetrical, slowly progressive loss of subcutaneous fat in different parts of the body. It appears after a febrile illness. The cephalothoracic variety (or Barraquer–Simons syndrome) involves the face, the neck, the shoulders, the upper extremities and the trunk. Lipoatrophy of the Dunnigan type affects the trunk and the limbs. Lipoatrophy of the Köbberling type is restricted to the extremities (Fig. 77.2).

Total lipoatrophy

Total lipoatrophy (or Seip–Lawrence syndrome) is characterized by complete loss of subcutaneous fat over the cutis tegument. The onset, usually before the age of 2 years, is insidious and without inflammation in the areas of fat loss. Typically, the face (Fig. 77.3) is the first part of the body affected, and the patient's aspect is characteristic – the zygomatic bones are prominent, the temples are hollowed and the cheeks are sunken. The skin is easily picked up into folds, but its elasticity is normal. Other prominent skin manifestations are diffuse hyperpigmentation, hypertrichosis and acanthosis nigricans. Insulin-resistant diabetes, hypertrophy of the external genitalia and hyperhydrosis are frequent associations.

HISTOPATHOLOGICAL FINDINGS

Lipoatrophy is a predominantly lobular, rather than septal, panniculitis. A dense, diffuse infiltrate of mononuclear cells, especially histiocytes but also lymphocytes and even some plasma cells, is distributed throughout the lobules (Fig. 77.4). In time, foam cells (histiocytes replete with lipid) appear as a consequence of adipocytic necrosis.

ETIOLOGY AND PATHOGENESIS

The etiopathogenesis of the localized form is unclear. It has been suggested that these disorders may result from an abnormal vulnerability of the fatty tissue to pressure or repeated trauma. Partial lipoatrophy seems to be an expression of an autoimmune disorder. Total lipoatrophy is transmitted as an autosomal-recessive trait.

MANAGEMENT

All the suggested treatments are disappointing.

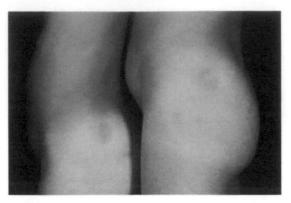

Figure 77.1
Localized lipoatrophy. These lesions, present at birth in siblings, are examples of the localized form of lipoatrophy, in which the gullies are a consequence of loss of subcutaneous fat.

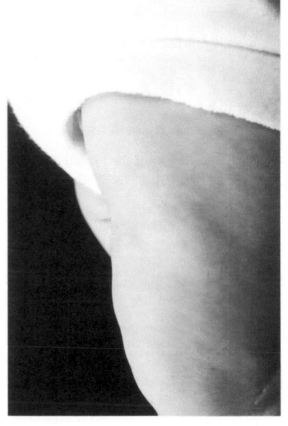

Figure 77.2
Partial lipoatrophy. This slowly progressive depression of the skin appeared on the anterior aspect of the right thigh during the 2nd month of life.

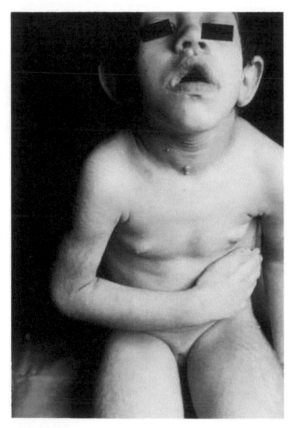

Figure 77.3
Total lipoatrophy (Seip–Lawrence syndrome). Note the characteristic loss of subcutaneous fat beneath the entire skin. Acanthosis nigricans and hypertrichosis are associated conditions.

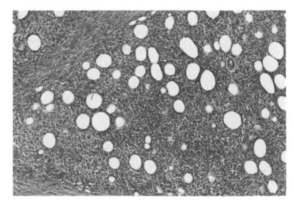

Figure 77.4
Lipoatrophy. This predominantly lobular panniculitis is marked by patchy infiltrates of mononuclear cells, histiocytes chief among them.

LINEAR IMMUNOGLOBULIN A DERMATOSIS OF CHILDHOOD

Linear immunoglobulin A (IgA) dermatosis of childhood is a benign vesiculobullous eruption with a typical annular pattern that involves mainly the pelvic and perioral regions. There are linear deposits of IgA in the basement membrane zone.

EPIDEMIOLOGY

Linear IgA dermatosis of childhood is rare.

CLINICAL FINDINGS

The disorder is marked by the appearance, on apparently healthy or erythematous skin, of tense bullae up to 10 mm in diameter, filled with clear or hemorrhagic fluid. Eruption of new bullae around healing lesions leads to typical rosette and jewel-like patterns (Figs 78.1 and 78.2). Pruritus is often present. Sites of predilection are the perioral region (see Fig. 78.1), the lower part of the trunk (Fig. 78.2), the inner thighs and the genitalia (Fig. 78.3), but the disease may be generalized from the onset. Mucous membranes may be involved, most frequently the ocular and oral mucosae. Spontaneous remission occurs in most patients before puberty.

LABORATORY FINDINGS

Direct immunofluorescence reveals linear IgA at the dermoepidermal junction in all patients. In about 60% of patients, indirect immunofluorescence reveals circulating IgA antibodies against the basement membrane zone.

HISTOPATHOLOGICAL FINDINGS

The earliest changes in papules of linear IgA dermatosis are noted around vessels of the superficial plexus and at the tips of dermal papillae. A sparse infiltrate of lymphocytes encircles venules of the superficial plexus, and a sprinkling of neutrophils arranged as solitary units is positioned in the uppermost portion of the dermis along the course of undulations of rete ridges and dermal papillae. In time, the number of neutrophils attracted to the tips of dermal papillae increases, often accompanied by 'dust' of neutrophilic nuclei (karyorrhexis) (Fig. 78.4). When vesicles form, biopsy reveals subepidermal blisters, within which are neutrophils (Fig. 78.5).

ETIOLOGY AND PATHOGENESIS

Because HLA B8 is considered a marker for hyperimmune responders, increased levels in linear IgA dermatosis (as in dermatitis herpetiformis) may explain the increased incidence of anti-basement membrane zone and other autoantibodies. The source of the autoantibodies that is responsible for the disease is unknown. It has been demonstrated that the majority of the IgA that forms the deposits is IgA_1. This finding may suggest an extraintestinal origin for the antibodies, which is in agreement with the absence of gluten-sensitive enteropathy in patients with linear IgA dermatosis.

MANAGEMENT

A gluten-free diet is ineffective, but both dapsone and sulfapyridine have been used successfully. The appropriate starting dose of dapsone is 2–3 mg/kg per day until the eruption is controlled; the dose is then gradually reduced to a minimum maintenance dose of 0.5–1 mg/kg per day. Dapsone is less effective in treating this disease than it is in managing dermatitis herpetiformis. Patients may respond also to sulfapyridine (60–200 mg/kg per day) with a maximum daily dose of 3 g. Prednisolone is added at a dose of 0.2–1 mg/kg per day when dapsone or sulfapyridine alone fails to give good results. Linear IgA dermatosis responds well to combined treatment with dapsone and systemic corticosteroids.

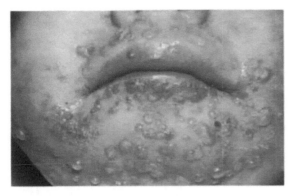

Figure 78.1

Linear immunoglobulin A dermatosis of childhood. The peri-oral region is a site of predilection. Many tense vesicles have ruptured and are weeping, resulting in serous crusts.

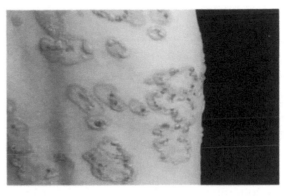

Figure 78.2

Linear immunoglobulin A dermatosis of childhood. Tense vesicles are present in arcuate and annular configurations that resemble rosettes. At the base of the vesicles, the skin is but slightly inflamed.

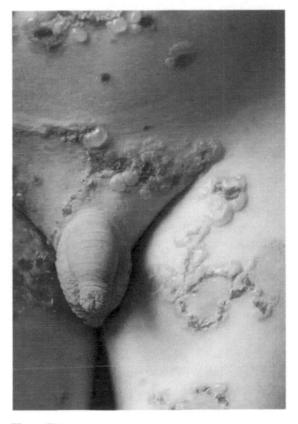

Figure 78.3

Linear immunoglobulin A dermatosis of childhood. Numerous tense vesicles are present, some in clusters, others in annular array. Residual hyperpigmentation is evident in the center of some of the rings. Note the hemorrhagic and yellowish crusts.

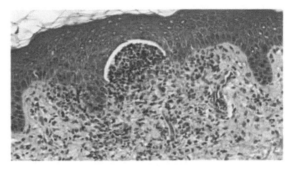

Figure 78.4

Linear immunoglobulin A dermatosis of childhood. The changes consist of a superficial perivascular and intersti-tial mixed cell infiltrate of neutrophils and eosinophils in focal collections at the tips of dermal papillae and in the subepidermal spaces.

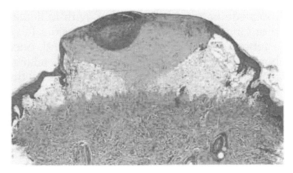

Figure 78.5

Linear immunoglobulin A dermatosis of childhood. The subepi-dermal blister has a necrotic epidermis as its roof and intact dermal papillae as its base. Within the blister itself and in the dermal papillae are collections of neutrophils.

Lupus erythematosus (LE) is a heterogeneous autoimmune disorder that includes a broad spectrum of clinical and laboratory findings. LE can be classified into four main forms: chronic LE with two varieties (discoid LE and lupus panniculitis), subacute cutaneous LE, systemic LE and neonatal LE.

DISCOID LUPUS ERYTHEMATOSUS

EPIDEMIOLOGY

Discoid LE is unusual in childhood. Its incidence in children ranges from 1 to 3%.

CLINICAL FINDINGS

The lesions may be located only on the face and external ear (localized discoid LE) or they may be diffuse (generalized discoid LE). They are characterized by well-defined erythematous, edematous, scaly patches with follicular plugging (Figs 79.1 and 79.2). The lesions have a tendency toward central clearing and, once healed, they usually leave atrophic, telangiectatic and pigmented scars. Lesions of the mucous membranes and scarring alopecia are extremely rare. The course is chronic, with remissions and relapses.

LABORATORY FINDINGS

The deposition of immunoglobulins and complement as a band or granular line along the dermoepidermal junction (lupus band

test) can be seen by direct immunofluorescence in more than 90% of specimens taken from affected areas, but not in clinically uninvolved skin.

HISTOPATHOLOGICAL FINDINGS

Discoid LE is characterized by typically thinned epidermis, vacuolar alteration of dermoepidermal junction, perivascular and periadnexal lymphocytic infiltrate and, often, deposits of mucin in the reticular dermis (Fig. 79.3).

MANAGEMENT

The treatment is similar to that for adults. Photoprotection by sunscreens together with topical or intralesional corticosteroids are recommended. Patients who do not respond to these measures may benefit from low doses of oral prednisolone (0.1–0.4 mg/day in the morning). Hydroxychloroquine has been used safely in pediatric patients at a dose of 7 mg/kg/day. An accurate ophthalmological examination is mandatory.

LUPUS ERYTHEMATOSUS PANNICULITIS (LUPUS PROFUNDUS)

EPIDEMIOLOGY

This form of discoid LE is typically a disease of middle age. No more than 20 cases have been reported in patients younger than 18 years.

CLINICAL FINDINGS

Lesions in the early stage of the disease consist of recurrent, deep, subcutaneous, small, non-tender nodules that arise primarily on the proximal portion of the limbs, the buttocks and the lower part of the back. The scalp, the face, and, more rarely, the legs may also be involved. Usually, the overlying skin is normal or slightly erythematous. Once healed, the lesions may leave cup-like depressions, attributable to subcutaneous atrophy, and considerable disfigurement (Fig. 79.4).

LABORATORY FINDINGS

Anti-nuclear antibodies can be detected in about 66% of pediatric cases and anti-nDNA antibodies in about 72%. Anti-cytoplasmic antibodies to Ro and La antigens are usually negative. The lupus band test of affected areas is positive in 70% of cases.

HISTOPATHOLOGICAL FINDINGS

LE panniculitis consists of patchy infiltrate of lymphocytes and plasma cells with lymphocytic nuclear 'dust' in concert with necrosis of adipocytes in fat lobules (Fig. 79.5).

MANAGEMENT

The treatment for patients with isolated LE panniculitis or with LE panniculitis associated with discoid lesions is similar to that for patients with chronic discoid DLE. Treatment with thalidomide was successful in a child in whom standard treatment failed.

SUBACUTE CUTANEOUS LUPUS ERYTHEMATOSUS

EPIDEMIOLOGY

Subacute cutaneous LE represents about 10% of all cases of LE with females affected more often than males.

CLINICAL FINDINGS

This LE subset may appear as erythematous, papular, scaly lesions (psoriasiform subacute cutaneous LE) or as annular erythematous, slightly scaling, polycyclic lesions. Atrophic scarring and follicular plugging are never observed; telangiectasia is often present. The disease is widespread, affecting the face, the shoulders, the upper trunk, the extensor part of the arm and the dorsum of the hand. Usually, photosensitivity is prominent. More than 50% of patients develop mild extracutaneous manifestations, such as fever, malaise and arthralgia. The systemic involvement is usually mild, so for the majority of patients the cutaneous manifestations represent the most important problem.

LABORATORY FINDINGS

Anti-dsDNA antibodies are present in low concentrations in the serum of about 30% of patients. Anti-Ro/SSA antibodies, a marker of neonatal LE, have been found in more than 65% of cases. Hypocomplementemia is rare. Lupus band test results are positive in only 50% of lesions and in 30% of uninvolved skin.

HISTOPATHOLOGICAL FINDINGS

The histological changes in subacute cutaneous LE are indistinguishable from those of early lesions of discoid LE, namely superficial, perivascular, lymphocytic infiltrates that partially obscure the dermoepidermal junction at the site of vacuolar alteration (Fig. 79.6). The epidermis is thinned, sometimes focally, but the cornified layer may be unaffected.

MANAGEMENT

Systemic therapy is required for most patients. The choice between antimalarial agents or moderate doses of oral prednisone in more severe cases, alone or in association, depends on the extent of the skin lesions, the severity of visceral involvement and the tolerance and responsiveness of the patient. Photoprotection and sun avoidance are also important to prevent worsening of skin lesions.

SYSTEMIC LUPUS ERYTHEMATOSUS

EPIDEMIOLOGY

The mean age of onset of systemic LE in children is 10 years. The disease is noted in people of all races and it is eight times more common in females than males.

CLINICAL FINDINGS

Cutaneous lesions of systemic LE can be classified as specific or non-specific. Specific lesions are characterized by an erythematous malar rash, commonly known as facial butterfly erythema, or by a scattered maculopapular edematous eruption (or both) (Figs 79.7 and 79.8). These lesions frequently arise after exposure to the sun and do not leave any skin atrophy. Telangiectasia of the palms, the fingers and mucous membranes may develop. Non-specific skin lesions are also important because they may be related to the degree of systemic LE activity. They consist of vasculitis, Raynaud's phenomenon (which affects about 33% of systemic LE patients), livedo reticularis, rheumatoid nodules, thrombophlebitis, diffuse non-scarring alopecia and calcinosis cutis. Vesicobullous eruptions are rare cutaneous manifestations of systemic LE (Fig. 79.9), but they may be the presenting and predominant skin lesions. Vesicles and bullae appear mostly on sites of sun exposure and the V portion of the chest, the upper part of the back, the hairline and the face. When skin lesions are present, evidence of multisystem involvement is prominent (arthritis, polyserositis, neurologic disorders and psychosis). Hematological and renal involvement are common. Fever,

malaise and weakness are frequent findings. The course of the disease is more aggressive in children than in adults.

LABORATORY FINDINGS

The erythrocyte sedimentation rate is consistently elevated. Polyclonal gammopathy, elevation of gammaglobulins and hypocomplementemia are frequent findings. Hemolytic anemia and leukopenia with lymphocytopenia or pancytopenia are common. Proteinuria, erythrocyturia and several types of urinary cellular casts may be present, their severity depending on the extent of renal disease. A high-titre anti-nuclear antibody test may be the most sensitive laboratory test for systemic LE, the nuclear fluorescence creating a homogeneous or peripheral pattern. Anti-dsDNA antibodies, often in high concentrations, are found in 60–80% of patients, whereas anti-Ro/SSA antibodies are found in only 25%. False-positive tests for syphilis and anti-cardiolipin antibodies also are noted. The lupus band test is positive in 95% of cases when using involved skin and in 75% of cases when using normal skin.

HISTOPATHOLOGICAL FINDINGS

The histological changes of systemic LE are indistinguishable from those of early lesions of subacute LE. In bullous systemic LE the blister is subepidermal and associated with neutrophils, neutrophilic nuclear dust and deposits of mucin in the reticular dermis (Fig. 79.10).

MANAGEMENT

The therapeutic schedule should be tailored to the severity of systemic involvement. For patients with less severe disease, anti-malarial and non-steroidal anti-inflammatory agents represent the first step in treatment. Prednisone (0.2–0.5 mg/day) given in a single morning dose or every other day to reduce toxicity, may be the second step. In the most severe cases, high doses of prednisone or oral immunosuppressive agents (or both) are used. Intravenous methylprednisolone pulses (15–30 mg/kg), intravenous cyclophosphamide, cyclosporine and plasmapheresis have been suggested as alternative therapeutic approaches in severe forms of systemic LE.

NEONATAL LUPUS ERYTHEMATOSUS

Neonatal lupus erythematosus is characterized by transient lupoid skin lesions or congenital heart block in an infant whose mother is affected by an autoimmune disorder or who bears anti-cytoplasmic antibodies and anti-Ro/SSA antibodies.

CLINICAL FINDINGS

Cutaneous lesions are present in approximately 85% of patients. They occur on exposed sites, such as the face (mainly the circumocular and temporal areas) and the scalp, often in response to ultraviolet light. Several kinds of lupoid lesions have been reported. The lesions are large, annular or circinate, sharply demarcated, erythematous macules, with no scaling or only light scaling (Figs 79.11 and 79.12). Healing leaves telangiectatic or dyschromic areas. Cardiac conduction defects (mainly congenital heart block) are present in about 54% of patients and begin *in utero*. Twenty-five per cent of patients with cardiac involvement have associated transposition of the great vessels and structural congenital heart defects. Other extracutaneous manifestations are autoimmune hemolytic anemia, thrombocytopenia, and hepatosplenomegaly. The eruption is self-limited, usually resolving within the first 6 months of life.

LABORATORY FINDINGS

Infants often fail to demonstrate serological abnormalities that are classically associated with systemic LE (including anti-nuclear antibodies and the LE cell test), despite the fact that they have anti-Ro/SSA antibodies and anti-La/SSB antibodies in their serum. These antibodies are also present in the mother. In affected infants, these antibodies disappear after about 12 months. The detection of these antibodies in the sera of newborns with lupoid cutaneous lesions or isolated congenital heart block is considered diagnostic of neonatal LE. The lupus band test is positive in only 50% of cases.

HISTOPATHOLOGICAL FINDINGS

The histopathological changes in neonatal LE are those of early discoid LE.

MANAGEMENT

No treatment is necessary in the absence of cardiac involvement. It is not known whether treatment of mothers during gestation is useful or harmful to fetuses with severe cardiac disease.

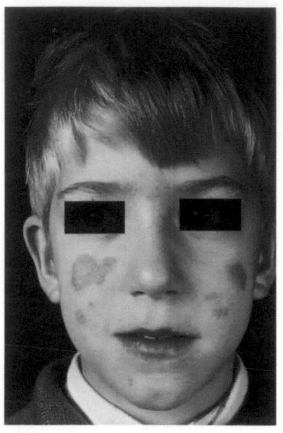

Figure 79.1
Discoid lupus erythematosus. Erythematous scaling plaques on the face of a 10-year-old boy.

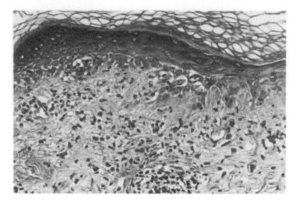

Figure 79.3
Discoid lupus erythematosus. This lesion can be inferred to be in its early stage because the infiltrate is superficial only, the cornified layers maintain its basket-woven configuration and the dermoepidermal junction is only slightly smudged by vacuolar alterations.

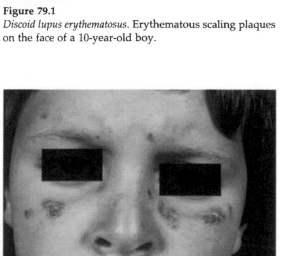

Figure 79.2
Discoid lupus erythematosus. Reddish papules covered by scaly crusts are present on the malar eminence and the forehead. Some of the crusts are hemorrhagic.

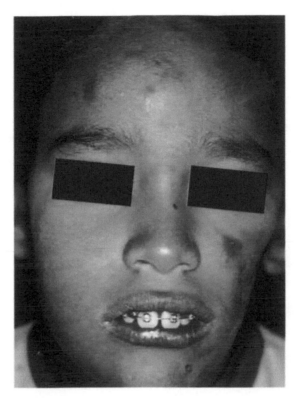

Figure 79.4
Lupus erythematosus panniculitis. Indurated plaques with central deeper atrophy are present on the left part of the face. The depression induced by the lesion is disfiguring. The erythematous scaling plaques on the forehead are characteristic of discoid LE.

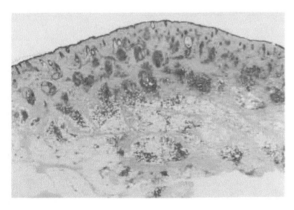

Figure 79.5
Lupus erythematosus panniculitis. The lesion involves both the dermis and the subcutaneous fat. In the latter location, patchy infiltrates of lymphocytes and plasma cells are associated with necrosis of adipocytes.

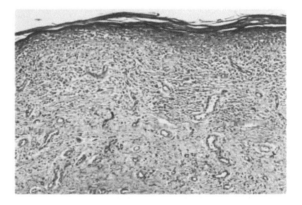

Figure 79.6
Subacute lupus erythematosus. Superficial and perivascular lymphocytic infiltrate partially obscure the dermoepidermal junction at the site of vascular alteration.

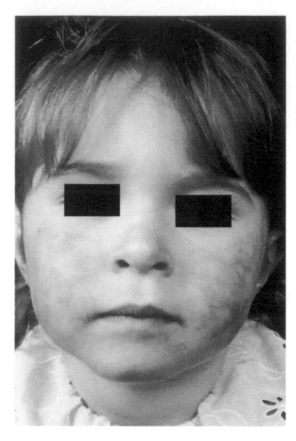

Figure 79.7
Systemic lupus erythematosus. The lesions consist of erythematous, slightly edematous, poorly demarcated patches. Scaling and atrophy are absent.

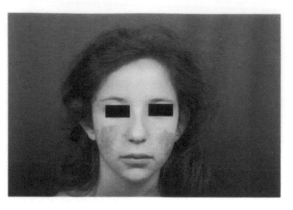

Figure 79.8
Systemic lupus erythematosus. Typical malar rash.

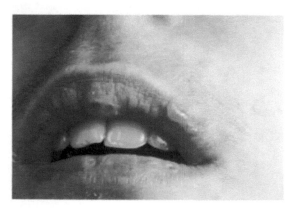

Figure 79.9
Systemic lupus erythematosus. Vesicles and small blisters appeared on the lips of this patient after sun exposure.

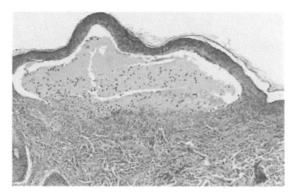

Figure 79.10
Bullous systemic lupus erythematosus. The subepidermal blister houses abundant plasma cells and many neutrophils. Neutrophils and neutrophilic nuclear 'dust' are also present in dermal papillae and at the base of the blister.

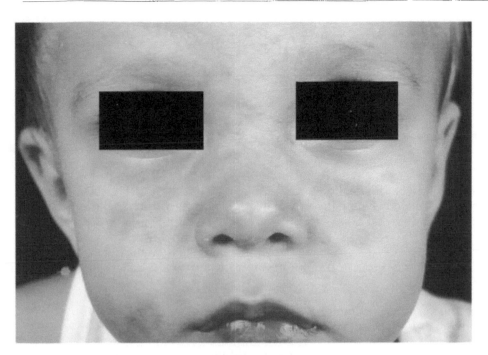

Figure 79.11
*Neonatal lupus erythe-
matosus.* Irregular
erythematous telang-
iectatic patches are
evident on the nose,
periorbital tissue and
cheeks.

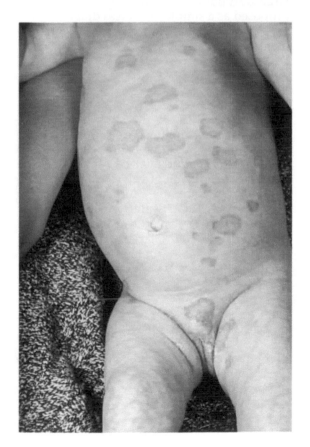

Numerous, somewhat
e trunk and are charac-
periphery and clearing

80

LYMPHANGIOMA

Lymphangiomas are hamartomatous malformations that consist of dilated lymphatic channels lined by normal endothelial cells.

EPIDEMIOLOGY

Lymphangiomas are much more uncommon than capillary hemangiomas but are not rare.

CLINICAL FINDINGS

Lymphangioma circumscriptum is the commonest type. It consists of numerous, grouped or scattered clear papules that range in size from minute to 5 mm in diameter. These papules have traditionally been compared morphologically to frog spawn (Fig. 80.1). The translucent papules contain clear fluid that is occasionally tinged with blood. The fluid color then changes from pink to dark red. A warty hyperkeratosis may cap the papules, some of which coalesce to form plaques. Lesions occur on almost any part of the body, but sites of predilection are the proximal parts of the limbs and the adjacent parts of the limb girdles, such as the buttocks, the upper part of the thighs and the shoulder region. The area of affected skin ranges from less than 10 mm^2 (localized lymphangioma circumscriptum) to several square centimeters. The tongue and oral mucosa can also be involved (Fig. 80.2). The condition is usually asymptomatic.

Lymphangioma cavernosum appears as an ill-defined, painless, soft swelling of the skin and subcutaneous tissue (Fig. 80.3). It may involve large areas of the face, the neck, the trunk, and the extremities. The surface of the skin is usually normal.

Lymphangiomas may be visible at birth or appear afterwards.

LABORATORY FINDINGS

High-resolution ultrasonogaphy has been proposed as a simple, harmless diagnostic aid to the clinical examination of lymphangiomas.

HISTOPATHOLOGICAL FINDINGS

Lymphangioma circumscriptum consists of a proliferation of numerous, thin-walled vessels lined by thin endothelial cells and, in some instances, protrusion of valves from the lining endothelium into the lumen. The entire dermis may be affected (Fig. 80.4). Lymphangioma cavernosum usually is characterized by large, muscle-coated lymphatic vessels situated in the subcutaneous fat.

ETIOLOGY AND PATHOGENESIS

Lymphangiomatous lesions are considered to be circumscribed developmental defects of lymphatic tissue of unknown origin.

MANAGEMENT

If treatment is necessary for cosmetic reasons, weeping and crusting, or recurrent infections, it is advisable to attempt complete surgical excision. The excision must encompass all affected tissue, including the caverns in the underlying subcutaneous structures in some cases. Recurrence or persistence is common and manifests itself most often within 3 months of the attempted excision.

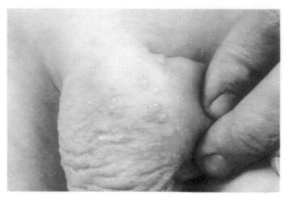

Figure 80.1
Lymphangioma circumscriptum. Clear papules, some of which tend to coalesce, resemble vesicles but are not vesicles. Each papule represents a widely dilated, lymph-containing vessel in the uppermost part of the dermis. These clear papules that tend to merge have been compared to frog spawn.

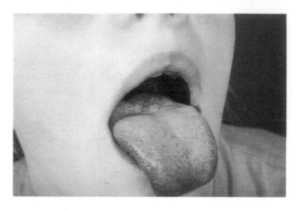

Figure 80.2
Lymphangioma circumscriptum. Papules are densely packed in the posterior part of the tongue.

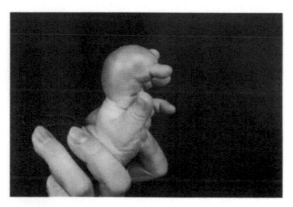

Figure 80.3
Lymphangioma cavernosum. This pink–gray swelling of a finger is a congenital form of this malformation.

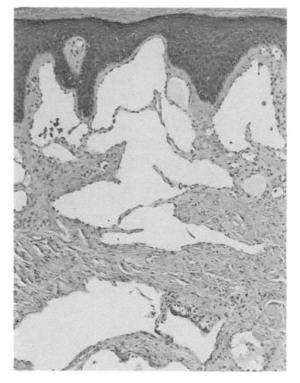

Figure 80.4
Lymphangioma cavernosum. The numerous vacuolar structures in the upper half of the dermis are lymphatics, the most superficial of which are situated just beneath the epidermis.

81

LYMPHOMA

Primary cutaneous non-Hodgkin's lymphoma is characterized by isolated or multiple skin lesions or by a diffuse erythroderma in the absence of any clinical or laboratory sign of systemic involvement.

EPIDEMIOLOGY

Primary cutaneous non-Hodgkin's lymphomas are rare in children, accounting for about 1% of all non-Hodgkin's lymphomas.

CLINICAL FINDINGS

The most common skin manifestations in children affected by low-grade cutaneous T-cell lymphomas are erythematous, scaling, roundish patches and plaques ('parapsoriasis *en plaque*) (Fig. 81.1) or erythroderma. These lesions are usually asymptomatic or mildly pruritic. Tumors may subsequently develop, as in classic mycosis fungoides of adults. Cutaneous lesions of high-grade lymphoblastic lymphomas and CD30+ lymphomas are fast growing, painful, red–violaceous nodules and ulcerated tumors, which sometimes show simultaneous satellite lymphadenopathy. The skin of the head and the neck (Fig. 81.2) is the commonest site of involvement. Generalized systemic involvement occurs rapidly. The course of low-grade cutaneous T-cell lymphomas is usually prolonged, with partial or complete remission, whereas lymphoblastic or large T-cell lymphomas run an aggressive course.

LABORATORY FINDINGS

Skin biopsy, physical examination, blood investigations (red blood cells, leukocytes, platelet count, lactate dehydrogenase, alkaline phosphatase and evaluations for calcemia), chest radiographs, abdominal computed tomography scans, bone marrow biopsy and aspirate, and biopsy of enlarged lymph nodes are essential staging investigations for cutaneous lymphomas. In the early stage of mycosis fungoides, however, bone marrow biopsy and aspiration are not necessary Lymphangiography, scintigraphy, and spleen and liver biopsy are performed only in cases of high-grade lymphoma.

Immunohistochemical studies are important means by which to confirm the diagnosis of cutaneous lymphomas. In mycosis fungoides, the most frequent phenotype of infiltrating proliferating cells is characterized by the expression of the helper T-cell markers CD3, CD4 and CD45RO. Lymphoblastic lymphomas, pre-pre-B-cell or pre-B-cell phenotypes (TDT+, CALLA+, Ig+/-) or T-cell phenotypes (CD3+) have been demonstrated. Large infiltrating cells in primary cutaneous CD30+ lymphomas show T-cell markers similar to those of lymphomatoid papulosis cells (CD2+, CD3+ and CD4+). Genotypic analysis may also be used to demonstrate the presence of a clonal infiltrate into the skin lesions or in the blood and bone marrow of patients affected by cutaneous lymphomas.

HISTOPATHOLOGICAL FINDINGS

Patch and plaque lesions (Figs 81.3 and 81.4) are characterized by a band-like, patchy lymphocytic infiltrate in the upper dermis extending to skin appendages and by the presence of lymphocytes in the context of spongiotic epidermis (Pautrier's microabscesses). Many lymphocytes have cerebriform outlines. Nodular lesions show dense infiltrates of atypical lymphocytes, many of which are in mitosis, throughout the dermis and often in the subcutaneous fat. CD30+ lymphomas mostly consist of large mononuclear cells with oval or reniform nuclei and abundant amphophilic cytoplasm accompanied by a variable number of multinucleated cells and Reed–Sternberg-like cells. The nuclei are often eccentrically placed in the cytoplasm and many of them are in mitosis. Cells of lymphoblastic lymphoma have large, convoluted or round–oval nuclei. The chromatin pattern is fine and dust-like and nucleoli are rarely seen. The cytoplasm is scant and the cell outlines are ill-defined. In hematoxylin and eosin sections, the diagnosis of lymphoblastic lymphoma may be difficult. Therefore, the diagnosis and classification of primary cutaneous lymphomas other than mycosis fungoides must be confirmed by immunohistochemical studies.

ETIOLOGY AND PATHOGENESIS

Primary cutaneous lymphoproliferative disorders are caused by the neoplastic infiltration of lymphoid cells, with a particular pattern of homing receptors causing their preferential migration into the skin compartment.

MANAGEMENT

Sun exposure, ultraviolet-B therapy, psoralen and ultraviolet-A therapy and local radiotherapy can be used to control the evolution of mycosis fungoides in children. For high-grade malignant lymphoblastic or large cell lymphomas, extensive polychemotherapy and local radiotherapy are required. Photopheresis, retinoids and interferon-alpha-2 can also be considered.

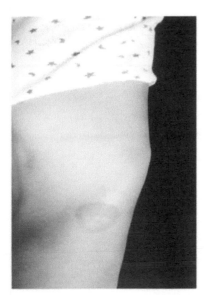

Figure 81.1

Cutaneous T-cell lymphomas. An oval, sharply demarcated erythematous to scaly patch (parapsoriasis *en plaque*) on the trunk can be seen.

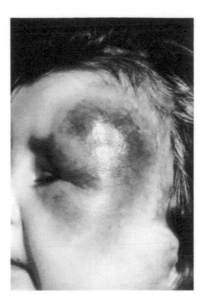

Figure 81.2

High-grade lymphoblastic lymphoma. This large tumor has shades of pink, orange and brown and is covered by telangiectases.

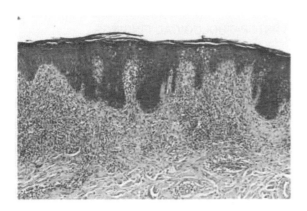

Figure 81.3

Figures 81.3 and 81.4

Mycosis fungoides. The psoriasiform lichenoid pattern is that of mycosis fungoides because the papillary dermis is thickened by a patchy lichenoid infiltrate of lymphocytes together with wiry bundles of collagen in haphazard array. Lymphocytes arranged as solitary units and in collections can be seen within the hypoplastic epidermis.

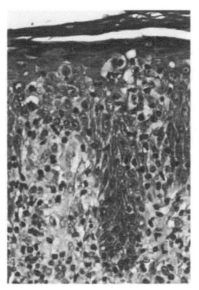

Figure 81.4

82

LYMPHOMATOID PAPULOSIS

Lymphomatoid papulosis is a continuing, self-healing, cutaneous eruption. Clinically it is a benign pathological process. Histopathologically, strikingly atypical lymphocytes are seen.

EPIDEMIOLOGY

Lymphomatoid papulosis is extremely rare in children and exceptional in infants.

CLINICAL FINDINGS

The clinical features of the condition in children are similar to those in adults. The predominant lesions of lymphomatoid papulosis consist of a few to more than 100 pink to reddish-brown papules that range in size from 2 to 12 mm. The papules are situated mainly on the trunk (Fig. 82.1) and the limbs, and they often form typical groups (Fig. 82.2). Lesions arise less often on the face, the scalp, the palms, the soles and the genitalia. In time, central hemorrhage, necrosis and ulceration or central hyperkeratosis and scaling may develop. Lesions regress in 3–4 weeks, leaving hyperpigmented or hypopigmented macules and atrophic scars, but the lesions may continue to come and go for months to many years. The general health remains good.

LABORATORY FINDINGS

No abnormalities are detected in the blood. Staging of the disease reveals no tendency for extracutaneous involvement.

HISTOPATHOLOGICAL FINDINGS

Fully developed lesions are characterized by dome-shaped surfaces and dome-shaped, superficial and deep, perivascular and interstitial mixed-cell infiltrates of atypical lymphocytes, neutrophils and eosinophils. Some atypical lymphocytes are in mitosis, and some of these mitoses are atypical (Figs 82.3 and 82.4). The infiltrate may involve the edematous papillary dermis, as well as the slightly hyperplastic epidermis, which may be focally ulcerated and covered by scaly crusts. A variable number of extravasated erythrocytes may be found in the upper part of the dermis.

Cytologically, the atypical lymphocytes of lymphomatoid papulosis are of two types. Large cells with abundant, amphophilic cytoplasm, bi- or multi-nucleation and prominent nucleoli are called histiocytoid cells or large atypical cells; these cells may closely resemble Reed–Sternberg cells of Hodgkin's disease. By contrast, smaller atypical lymphocytes with scant cytoplasm and cerebriform, hyperchromatic nuclei are called convoluted mononuclear cells, and they may be indistinguishable from the Lutzner cells of mycosis fungoides. Immunopathologically, a majority of both large atypical cells and convoluted mononuclear cells react with pan-T-cell monoclonal antibodies CD3 and CD2, specifically the CD4 T-helper subset, and rarely with the CD8 suppressor–cytotoxic subtype. Large atypical cells are also positive for Hodgkin's disease-associated antigen, CD30, in 50–80% of cases.

ETIOLOGY AND PATHOGENESIS

The etiopathogenesis of lymphomatoid papulosis is unknown.

MANAGEMENT

Because the disease is self-healing, systemic treatments are inadequate. Ultraviolet-B irradiation and psoralen and ultraviolet-A therapy are the methods of choice for exacerbations.

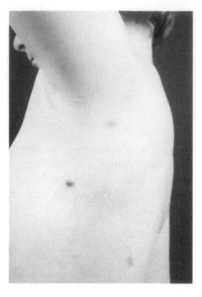

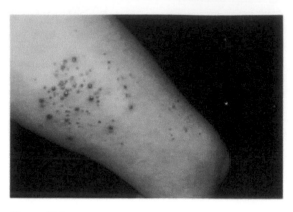

Figure 82.2
Lymphomatoid papulosis. A cluster of reddish, smooth and shiny papules of different sizes on a thigh of a 12-year-old boy.

Figure 82.1
Lymphomatoid papulosis. A few reddish-brown papules are present on the trunk of this 8-year-old boy.

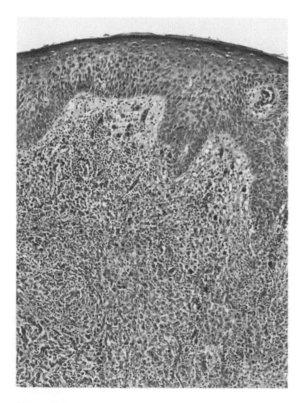

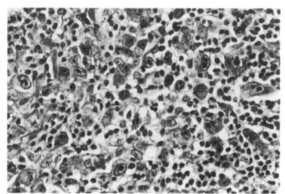

Figure 82.4

Figures 82.3 and 82.4
Lymphomatoid papulosis. This wedge-shaped, superficial and deep, perivascular and interstitial mixed-cell infiltrate is characterized by atypical lymphocytes. The lymphocytes have large nuclei dotted by prominent nucleoli and are associated with abundant amphophilic cytoplasm. In addition to atypical lymphocytes, note also numerous small lymphocytes and, in some fields, plasma cells, eosinophils and neutrophils. The architectural pattern of the lesion and the assembly and distribution of cells is diagnostic of this condition.

Figure 82.3

83

MALIGNANT MELANOMA

Malignant melanoma is a malignant neoplasm that originates from melanocytes. Malignant melanoma usually begins as a proliferation of atypical melanocytes in the epidermis that extends into the dermis and subcutaneous tissue, sites from which it may metastasize.

EPIDEMIOLOGY

About 0.4% of malignant melanomas occur in prepubertal children. They may appear at any age and may be present at birth.

CLINICAL FINDINGS

Malignant melanomas in infants and children arise mainly in association with pre-existing congenital types of melanocytic nevi, especially the large, hairy kind (Fig. 83.1). Only rarely do these lesions arise *de novo* (i.e. in the absence of a melanocytic nevus). Malignant melanoma may evolve from macules to patches (Fig. 83.2) or from macules to papules to nodules and tumors. Whatever the anatomical site, melanomas tend to be asymmetrical, scalloped or notched at the periphery, and variegate in color, especially in nuances of brown, ranging from tan to black. When this neoplasm undergoes regression, zones of white or off-white appear, followed by a patch or plaque. It is exceedingly difficult to recognize the development of malignant melanoma within a large, hairy congenital nevus because such lesions usually do not have the features of malignant melanomas that arise *de novo*. By the time it is detected, the lesion is usually an indistinct nodule or tumor in the substance of the nevus.

The course of malignant melanoma is as unpredictable in children as it is in adults. Some malignant melanomas grow rapidly and metastasize quickly, whereas others are more indolent and do not metastasize for many years. Thick malignant melanomas with large volumes of neoplastic cells tend to metastasize more readily.

HISTOPATHOLOGICAL FINDINGS

The diagnostic findings of malignant melanoma, whatever the anatomical site, are asymmetry, poor circumscription, failure of maturation of melanocytes with progressive descent into the dermis, nests of melanocytes within the epidermis that vary in size and shape, and nests in the epidermis that have become confluent at least in some foci (Figs 83.3 and 83.4). Cytologically, features of importance are nuclear atypia, an increased number of mitotic figures (especially near the base of the neoplasm) and the presence of necrotic neoplastic cells. Another diagnostic clue is the presence of atypical pagetoid melanocytes arranged in a pagetoid pattern within the epidermis (i.e. neoplastic cells with large atypical nuclei and abundant pale-staining cytoplasm that contain dusty melanin). Pagetoid melanocytes in a pagetoid pattern are virtually diagnostic of malignant melanoma.

ETIOLOGY AND PATHOGENESIS

Racial traits such as fair skin and a tendency to sunburn rather than to tan, together with intense sunlight exposure have been advocated as risk factors for malignant melanomas in adults. The importance of these factors on the development of malignant melanoma in children has not been determined. Many malignant melanomas in children arise in large congenital melanocytic nevi, and according to various studies, the lifetime expected frequency of development of malignant melanoma in such nevi ranges from 4.6 to 14%. The mechanism whereby malignant melanomas develop in pre-existing melanocytic nevi has yet to be delineated. The familial occurrence of melanoma is well established. Children in these melanoma-prone families typically develop more acquired melanocytic nevi (Clark's nevi) than is common in children their age.

MANAGEMENT

Therapy for primary cutaneous melanoma is complete excision of the neoplasm. If excision occurs before the melanoma has metastasized, no matter how narrow the margin, the patient is cured. If, however, metastasis occurs before the definitive surgical procedure, the patient is likely to die of metastatic melanoma, no matter how wide and how deep the blade of the surgeon is carried. No evidence supports the contention that wider excisions for thicker lesions has merit. The usefulness of studying a regional lymph node (sentinel lymph node) is controversial.

Chemotherapy and various forms of immunotherapy have proven as ineffective in children as they are in adults. The inadequacy of available treatment for metastatic melanoma underlines the importance of early diagnosis and prompt surgical treatment of malignant melanomas in children.

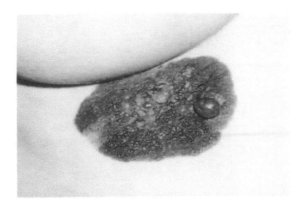

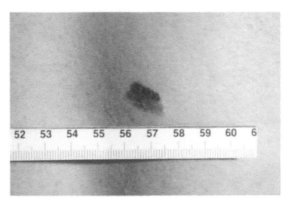

Figure 83.1

Malignant melanoma arising in a congenital nevus. The malignant melanoma is visible on the right of this lesion as an irregularly surfaced, rust-brown nodule. It is on a brownish plaque of a congenital nevus. Note the papillated surface of the congenital nevus.

Figure 83.2

Malignant melanoma. This lesion on the back of a 13-year-old girl appears as an asymmetrical, broad, pigmented plaque with notched borders and variegations of color.

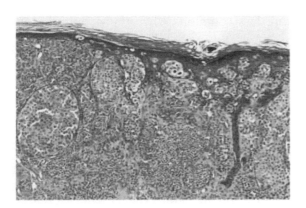

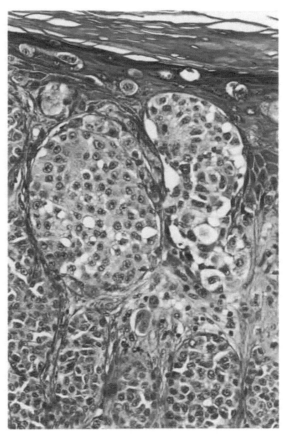

Figure 83.3

Figures 83.3 and 83.4

Malignant melanoma. This neoplasm of melanocytes fulfils all the criteria for melanoma – asymmetry and poor circumscription; failure of maturation of melanocytes with progressive descent into the dermis; nests of melanocytes within the epidermis that are not equidistant from one another, vary in size and shape, and have become confluent; atypical pagetoid melanocytes in a pagetoid pattern within the epidermis and epithelial structures of adnexa; and nests of melanocytes within the dermis that have become confluent to form sheets.

Figure 83.4

Mastocytosis is the collective name for a spectrum of clinical disorders that are characterized by an abnormal proliferation of mast cells in the skin or other organs. Mastocytosis is, in most cases, a pediatric, benign and self-healing condition.

EPIDEMIOLOGY

Mastocytosis occurs in between 1 in 1000 and 1 in 8000 patients. It usually begins in the first years of life. In 50% of patients, lesions are visible at birth or in the first 3 months of life.

CLINICAL FINDINGS

Although the cutaneous manifestations of mastocytosis are polymorphous, they are all marked by whealing of the lesions after rubbing (Darier's sign). Mastocyosis occurs in cutaneous and systemic forms; the latter is almost exclusively confined to adults. The clinical expressions of cutaneous mastocytosis are solitary mastocytoma, urticaria pigmentosa and diffuse mastocytosis.

Solitary mastocytoma, which is usually present at birth, represents about 10% of all forms of mastocytosis. It consists of a round or oval plaque or nodule of a few centimeters in diameter. The color varies from that of the surrounding skin to yellowish or brownish, and its surface usually resembles the pitted skin of an orange. Solitary mastocytomas may occur on the trunk, the neck or the wrist, where they are rubbed easily, producing a serous or hemorrhagic bulla (Fig. 84.1). The

lesions tend to regress spontaneously within a few years.

Urticaria pigmentosa is the most common form of cutaneous mastocytosis. The eruption consists of monomorphic, pigmented, maculopapular or plaque-like lesions distributed symmetrically on the trunk (Fig. 84.2). Papules are the most frequent type of lesion. They vary in color, have a smooth or shagreen-like surface, and are firm. Macules are less common. When the papular lesions have a yellowish hue, the disease is called mastocytosis xanthelasmoidea. Vesicles and bullae are less common in urticaria pigmentosa than in solitary mastocytoma.

The urticaria-like aspect of the lesions is characteristic of mastocytosis. A brownish lesion becomes red and swollen, losing its chromatic characteristics and becoming an urticarial lesion. This change can be spontaneous or it can occur after confrication of dressing objects, trauma to the lesion, or heating of the skin. Lesions tend to fade in thickness with time, and Darier's sign becomes more difficult to evoke. Residual hyperpigmentation may be long-lasting.

Diffuse cutaneous mastocytosis can be observed early in life. The two forms of the disease are urticarial and pachyerythrodermic, the difference being attributed to a quantitative degree of infiltration of the skin by mast cells. In the urticarial form (Fig 84.3), the skin appears normal but wheals easily, either spontaneously or after minor trauma. In the pachyerythrodermic form (Fig. 84.4), the skin is thickened, marked by deep furrows, and red–brown in color. Discrete or grouped urticarial plaques and serous bullae (Fig. 84.3) are common and are associated with severe and generalized itching. Diffuse mastocytosis seems to run a slower course with mild improvement.

Cutaneous mastocytosis is usually asymptomatic except when lesions are rubbed. In this situation, localized pruritus is the major symptom and is related to the extent or number of lesions involved.

Blushing crises are another characteristic sign of mastocytosis. They begin suddenly, most often involving the face and the upper trunk.They last for 10–30 minutes and resolve naturally. These crises seem spontaneous, but they sometimes correlate with an exogenous or endogenous stimulus that causes the degranulation of mastocytes. In diffuse forms of the disease, general symptoms can be severe and identical to those seen in anaphylaxis.

HISTOPATHOLOGICAL FINDINGS

In nodular lesions, there is a monomorphous dense diffuse infiltrate of mast cells involving the whole dermis (Fig. 84.5). In macular lesions, mast cell infiltration is sparse and located around blood vessels and between collagen bundles (Fig 84.6).

ETIOLOGY AND PATHOGENESIS

The cause of mastocytosis is unknown. The various clinical forms of mastocytosis are considered benign proliferative disorders of the reticuloendothelial system. The degranulation of mast cells is responsible for the disturbances caused by the disease.

MANAGEMENT

Before deciding on a form of treatment in children with cutaneous mastocytosis, the length of the disease and its tendency to spontaneous regression must be considered.

Although H_1 and H_2 antihistamines, in combination or alone, are the drugs of choice, symptomatic therapy is not necessary in most cases. The continuous use of antihistamines can be dangerous because of a rebound effect, with great release of histamine, when the treatment is stopped. Antihistamines must be given only for short periods in patients with diffuse bullous mastocytosis. Gradual sun exposure in summer is useful, especially after the 2nd year of life. Photochemotherapy, on the contrary, can be dangerous in children.

Some experts have used disodium cromoglycate, cimetidine and nifedipine, but the results are contradictory. The efficacy of ketotifen seems good. Especially in the forms of mastocytosis that cause massive concentration of mast cells, counselling must be given to avoid exposure to histamine-releasing substances (e.g. aspirin, morphine, codeine, polymyxin B, adenosine triphosphate). For the same reason, hot baths must also be avoided.

Adrenaline (epinephrine) remains the drug of choice in severe crises characterized by diffuse red flushing and shock.

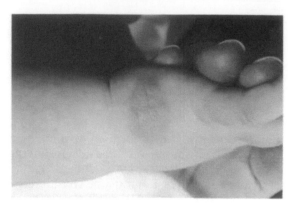

Figure 84.1
Solitary mastocytoma. This solitary plaque is tan, relatively well circumscribed and devoid of scales. Its surface resembles the pitted skin of an orange.

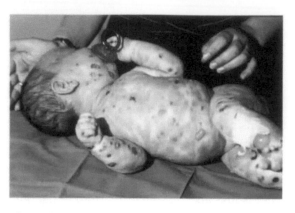

Figure 84.3
Diffuse cutaneous mastocytosis. Reddish papules and plaques accompany vesicles and bullae. Some of the blisters have ruptured and are covered by yellow and deep-red crusts.

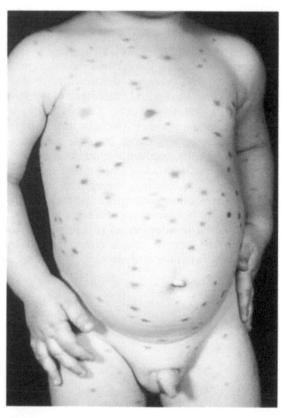

Figure 84.2
Urticaria pigmentosa. These widespread copper-colored and brownish papules become urticarial when rubbed.

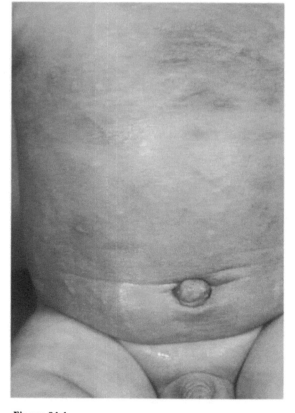

Figure 84.4
Diffuse cutaneous mastocytosis (pachyerythrodermic form). In addition to diffuse redness, note the urticarial lesions at sites that have been scratched and the thickening where the skin has been rubbed.

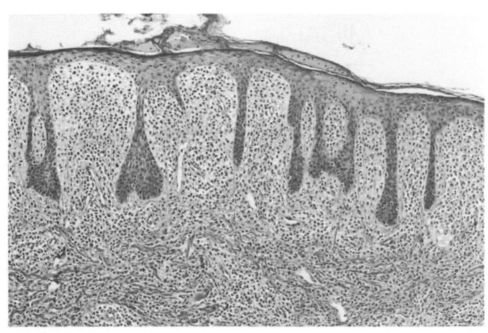

Figure 84.5
Mastocytosis (nodular lesion). There is a monomorphous infiltrate of mononuclear cells throughout the dermis. Mast cells are identified in sections stained by hematoxylin and eosin by their dark-staining nuclei, oblong and round contours and delicate granules within abundant amphophilic cytoplasm.

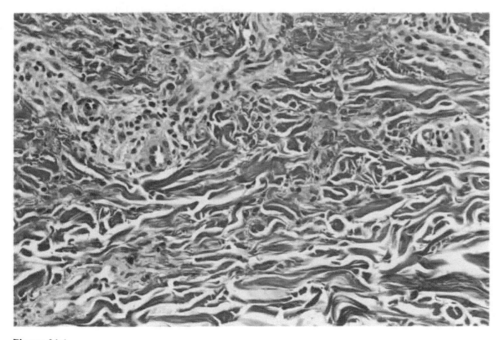

Figure 84.6
Mastocytosis (macular lesion). There is a subtle monomorphous infiltrate around widely dilated venules of the superficial plexus and between collagen bundles in the upper part of the dermis.

85

MILIARIA

Miliaria is a common dermatosis caused by the obstruction of the eccrine sweat glands.

EPIDEMIOLOGY

Miliaria is a common dermatosis in the first few years of life, especially in hot and humid climates

CLINICAL FINDINGS

Two main clinical forms of miliaria are observed – miliaria crystallina (sudamina) and miliaria rubra (prickly heat). In miliaria crystallina, the lesions are represented by small, clear vesicles that spread on the head, the neck and the trunk without symptoms (Fig. 85.1).

In miliaria rubra, small papules or vesicles appear in the same locations, but they are surrounded by an erythematous halo (Fig. 85.2). Itching is always present and is sometimes disturbing. In both forms, the palms and the soles are spared.

HISTOPATHOLOGICAL FINDINGS

Miliaria rubra is a subtle spongiotic dermatitis that is differentiated from other types of spongiotic dermatitis by the presence of spongiosis centered around one or more acrosyringia (Fig. 85.3).

Miliaria crystallina, by contrast is a subcorneal vesicular dermatitis. The tense epidermal vesicle is situated immediately beneath the cornified layer and contains few inflammatory cells; similarly, the dermis contains few inflammatory cells.

ETIOLOGY AND PATHOGENESIS

Miliaria is the result of an inability to eliminate sweat through the duct after thermal stimulus or placement of an occlusive dressing. The augmented sweat production first infiltrates the horny layer or the area just below the horny layer, and then enhances the bacterial resident flora. Finally, obstruction occurs. When the obstruction is superficial (intracorneal), the clinical appearance is that of miliaria crystallina. In miliaria rubra, sweat invades the epidermis and induces an inflammatory reaction. The immaturity of eccrine ducts in children is another factor that favors sweat retention.

MANAGEMENT

The focus of treatment is on the avoidance of excessive sweating. It is therefore important to avoid wool, silk or synthetic clothes in favor of those made of cotton or linen, probably because cotton and linen act as a sponge. It is also useful to increase evaporation from the skin and, if it is possible, to diminish the temperature and humidity. If not, wet compresses applied three to four times a day or cool baths may be useful. Systemic antihistamines may be used when itching is disturbing.

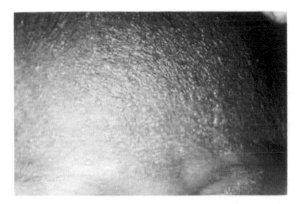

Figure 85.1
Miliaria crystallina. A few drop-like lesions cover the forehead of this infant. Unlike other forms of miliaria, the blisters form directly beneath the cornified layer.

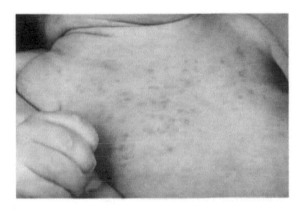

Figure 85.2
Miliaria rubra. Papules and vesicles are surrounded by an erythematous halo.

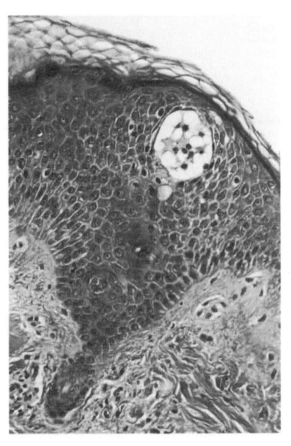

Figure 85.3
Miliaria rubra. The crucial finding for diagnosis of miliaria is spongiosis around acrosyringium.

86 MOLLUSCUM CONTAGIOSUM

Molluscum contagiosum is a common and benign infectious disease of the skin and mucous membranes caused by a DNA poxvirus.

EPIDEMIOLOGY

The condition is common and worldwide in distribution. It can occur at any age but is more common in childhood.

CLINICAL FINDINGS

The incubation period ranges from 2 to 7 weeks. Typical lesions of molluscum contagiosum are smooth, pearly or flesh-colored, hemispheric, firm papules 3–6 mm in diameter with umbilicated centers (Fig. 86.1). Giant lesions may reach a diameter of 20–30 mm. A milk-like material can be expressed from the umbilications. These benign lesions are usually numerous and have a tendency to group (Fig. 86.2). Extensive eruptions have been observed in immunodepressed and atopic patients. Lesions are asymptomatic and may be situated on any area of the skin and, occasionally, on the mucous membranes. In children, lesions occur mainly on the face, the trunk and the limbs, whereas in adults, the genital area is more frequently affected. In 10% of patients, and especially atopic patients, an inflammatory reaction develops around the lesions. This molluscum dermatitis represents a delayed hypersensitivity reaction to the molluscum contagiosum virus. Lesions may persist for months to a few years. Spontaneous resolution occurs after inflammation.

HISTOPATHOLOGICAL FINDINGS

The lesion is characterized by its exoendophytic character and its domed shape. At the center of the papule is a crater formed by widely dilated, contiguous infundibula that house orthokeratotic cells (Fig. 86.3). Within the cytoplasm of these cells are large ovoid bodies (molluscum bodies), which are amphophilic in the spinous and granular zones, and basophilic in keratinocytes of the cornified layer.

ETIOLOGY AND PATHOGENESIS

The causative agent is a large DNA virus (200–300 μm) in the poxvirus group.

MANAGEMENT

Removal of the lesions by gentle curettage after medication with EMLA® or application of liquid nitrogen is simple and effective.

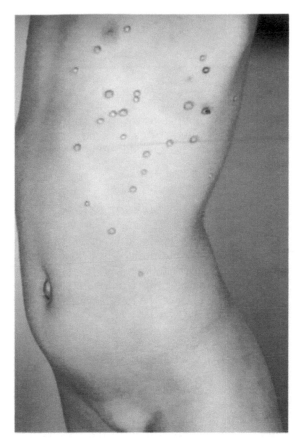

Figure 86.1
Molluscum contagiosum. These reddish-brown, discrete papules have a central dell that contains cornified cells.

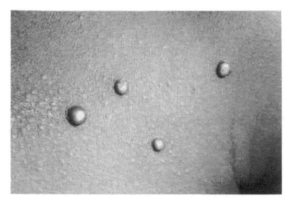

Figure 86.2
Molluscum contagiosum. These hemispheric brownish papules have a distinct central umbilication.

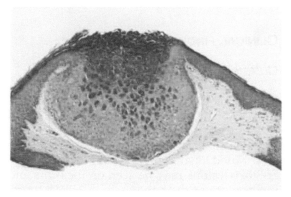

Figure 86.3
Molluscum contagiosum. This dome-shaped lesion consists of a hyperplastic infundibulum, the ostium of which is plugged by corneocytes. Within the majority of epithelial cells in this bulbous epithelium are molluscum bodies. These structures, which are confined to the cytoplasm, are ovoid and consist of amphophilic granular material. Note that molluscum bodies in the cornified layer stain more darkly than those in the viable epithelium.

87

MUCINOSIS

The cutaneous mucinoses consist of a hetero-geneous group of diseases characterized by accumulation of mucin in the dermis, either focally or diffusely.

EPIDEMIOLOGY

Primary cutaneous mucinoses are extremely rare in the pediatric population.

CLINICAL FINDINGS

Cutaneous mucinosis of infancy

Cutaneous mucinosis of infancy is character-ized by the eruption of multiple, small (1–2 mm), pale, opalescent, firm papules. These lesions, which are densely grouped, are distributed symmetrically on the elbows. Solitary lesions may be seen on the arms and the dorsum of the hands.

Self-healing juvenile cutaneous mucinosis

Self-healing juvenile cutaneous mucinosis (Fig. 87.1) consists of the rapid onset on the face, the trunk and the limbs of asymptomatic papules that merge into infiltrated, non-tender plaques. Deep nodules may be observed on the face and periarticular regions. Signs of arthritis are present in the knees, the elbows and the fingers. Regression occurs in a few months.

Follicular mucinosis

Follicular mucinosis appears as follicular papules mimicking chronic folliculitis. Frequently, papules merge into erythematous plaques (Fig. 87.2) that may or may not be alopecic, and their surface may show empty follicular openings. Sites of predilection are the face and the neck. The lesions may persist for years.

Acral persistent papular mucinosis

Acral persistent papular mucinosis is identi-fied by the asymptomatic eruption of multi-ple, white, translucent persistent papules of 2–5 mm in diameter that are located symmet-rically on the back of the hands (Fig. 87.3), the forearms and the wrists.

HISTOPATHOLOGICAL FINDINGS

Cutaneous mucinosis of infancy, self-healing juvenile cutaneous mucinosis and acral persistent papular mucinosis are character-ized by deposits of mucin in the papillary or upper reticular dermis, which leads to separa-tion and fragmentation of collagen bundles.

The main histological changes in follicular mucinosis are deposits of mucin that are located mainly in the outer root sheet together with a mixed inflammatory cell infiltrate around and within the follicular epithelium (Fig. 87.4).

ETIOLOGY AND PATHOGENESIS

The initial stimulus that induces an increase and accumulation of acid glycosaminoglycans (mucin) and fibroblast proliferation remains unknown in primary cutaneous mucinoses. In these diseases, mucin appears to consist of hyaluronic acid and dermatan sulfate.

MANAGEMENT

No treatment is effective.

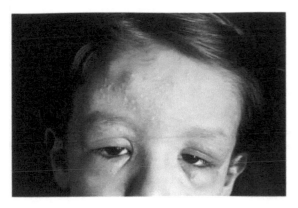

Figure 87.1
Cutaneous self-healing mucinosis. The upper part of the face is covered by tiny, skin-colored papules, some in linear array. Two deep nodules are evident on the forehead, and the eyelids are swollen.

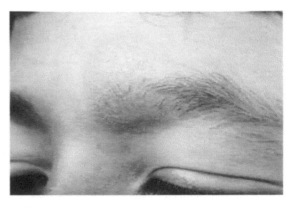

Figure 87.2
Follicular mucinosis. A nummular erythematous plaque involves the forehead and the eyebrows, inducing partial alopecia.

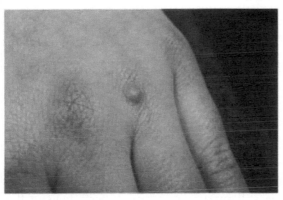

Figure 87.3
Acral persistent papular mucinosis. A white, translucent, persistent papule on the back of the hand of a 13-year-old girl.

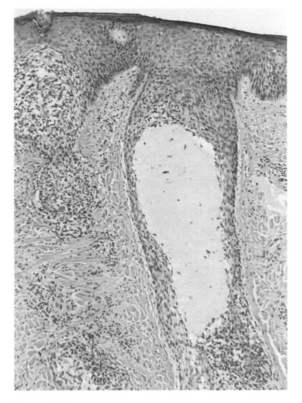

Figure 87.4
Follicular mucinosis. Abundant deposits of mucin are observed in the outer root sheet of most of the follicles in this section. A moderately dense, mixed inflammatory cell infiltrate composed mostly of lymphocytes and histiocytes is present around and within the follicular epithelium.

88

NECROBIOSIS LIPOIDICA

Necrobiosis lipoidica is a degenerative disease of the connective tissue characterized by asymptomatic, slightly depressed, atrophic plaques that are usually located over the anterior surface of the legs.

EPIDEMIOLOGY

Necrobiosis lipoidica is uncommon in the pediatric age group and is closely associated with diabetes mellitus. The disease is three times commoner in women than men.

CLINICAL FINDINGS

Skin lesions of necrobiosis lipoidica demonstrate a distinctive evolution. The process begins with 1–3 mm, red–brown, firm papules that coalesce and expand slowly to form large, oval or irregular plaques. The border of the plaques is often violaceous, slightly elevated and sharply demarcated; the center is depressed or atrophic with a waxy, yellow, translucent surface (Figs 88.1 and 88.2). Multiple telangiectases are easily seen through the atrophic epidermis. Variable amounts of scaling may be present. These plaques are alopecic, hypohidrotic and sometimes partially or completely anesthetic. In 85–90% of patients, lesions arise on the pretibial area and are often bilateral. In the remaining patients, necrobiosis lipoidica may occur on the scalp, the face, the arms or the trunk. The commonest complication is recurrence of ulceration after trauma. The disease has a chronic course with periods of waxing and waning of the lesions. Spontaneous resolution has been reported in about 15% of cases.

HISTOPATHOLOGICAL FINDINGS

Fully developed lesions are characterized by the involvement of the entire reticular dermis with a lymphoplasmocytic perivascular infiltrate, histiocytes arrayed in palisades and extensive degeneration of collagen in the center of the granuloma (Figs 88.3 and 88.4). In advanced lesions, sclerosis replaces the collagen degeneration and the number of inflammatory cells decreases.

ETIOLOGY AND PATHOGENESIS

The etiopathogenesis of necrobiosis lipoidica is still unknown. Many experts believe that the primary event is diabetic microangiopathy, resulting in collagen degeneration attributable to vascular occlusion. The demonstration of immunoglobulin M, immunoglobulin A and complement (C3) deposition in vessel walls raises the possibility that the primary event is an antibody-mediated vasculitis. Trauma is considered a triggering factor rather than a causative factor.

MANAGEMENT

Treatment of necrobiosis lipoidica is usually not satisfactory. It is useful to protect the legs with occlusive bandaging to avoid trauma. Corticosteroid injections into active areas may clear some lesions, but atrophy may occur.

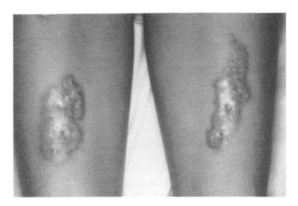

Figure 88.1
Necrobiosis lipoidica. Bilateral, irregular, yellow–red atrophic plaques with a waxy translucent surface, coursed by telangiectatic vessels and with violaceous borders are present on the anterior surface of the legs.

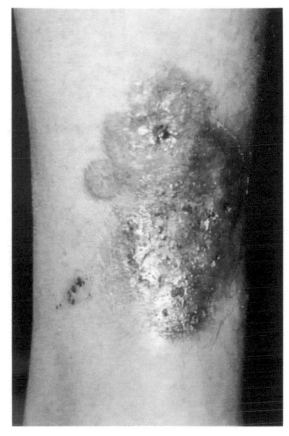

Figure 88.2
Necrobiosis lipoidica. These plaques have different sizes and shapes and tend to confluence. Some borders are scalloped and sharply circumscribed. The plaques situated superiorly have a yellowish cast as well as zones that are pink and purple. The plaque found inferiorly is dark purple and ulcerated.

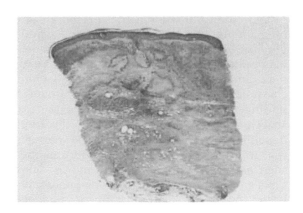

Figure 88.3

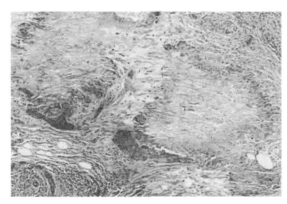

Figure 88.4

Figures 88.3 and 88.4
Necrobiosis lipoidica. At scanning magnification the patchy pink zones represent degeneration of collagen. At the periphery of these zones, histiocytes are arrayed in a palisade (Fig. 88.4). A lymphoplasmocytic infiltrate is present around blood vessels in the dermis and the subcutaneous fat.

Neurofibromatosis is an autosomal-dominant disease. It is characterized by changes in the skin, the nervous system, the bones and the endocrine glands. Four forms are now recognized: peripheral neurofibromatosis (von Recklinghausen's disease or NF1), acoustic neurofibromatosis (NF2), segmentary neurofibromatosis, and multiple café-au-lait spots without associated findings.

EPIDEMIOLOGY

Neurofibromatosis is one of the commonest genodermatoses, with an estimated incidence of 1 in 3000 live births. Males are slightly more often affected than females.

CLINICAL FINDINGS

Von Recklinghausen's disease is characterized by three hallmark features – multiple café-au-lait spots, multiple neurofibromas, and Lisch nodules. Café-au-lait macules are present in 99% of patients. They are usually present at birth or become apparent during the first months of life and frequently represent the first sign of the disease. The spots are regularly circumscribed, light or dark brown patches. They vary in diameter from 2 mm to more than 150 mm, and are randomly distributed over the body surface. The presence of at least six café-au-lait macules that exceed 5 mm before puberty or 15 mm after puberty in broadest diameter are considered pathognomonic for neurofibromatosis. Freckling, with clusters of hyperpigmented macules about 2 mm in diameter in intertrigi-nous areas such as the axillary vault (Crowe's sign), is an important sign (Fig. 89.1).

Neurofibromas occur in childhood independent of café-au-lait spots; they are usually widespread except for the palmoplantar surfaces. They may be superficial or subcutaneous. The superficial tumors are soft, pink, sessile or pedunculated lesions that vary in size and number. The subcutaneous tumors may occur as violaceous nodules along a peripheral nerve or as deeper, large plexiform masses (Fig. 89.2).

Pigmented hamartomas of the iris (Lisch nodules) are present in 90% of patients over 12 years of age and in more than 30% of patients of 6 years of age or older. They are asymptomatic but increase in number with age and are important for diagnosis, especially when other clinical manifestations are not prominent. Additional cutaneous signs include hypopigmented lesions and xanthogranulomas.

Neurological involvement is present in 40% of patients. Neural crest tumors include gliomas, meningiomas, astrocytomas, neuromas, pheochromocytomas, neurofibrosarcomas and malignant schwannomas. Optic chiasmatic glioma is a particularly frequent finding in children. Intellectual handicaps, speech impediments and seizure disorders depend on the degree of central nervous system involvement. Skeletal abnormalities such as macrocephaly, kyphoscoliosis, bone cysts and pseudoarthroses of long bones have been found in almost 50% of patients. Endocrinological dysfunctions of various types and vascular deformities may complete the clinical picture. The course is variable, but usually it is slowly progressive.

Acoustic neurofibromatosis is characterized by bilateral acoustic neuromas, the frequent presence of other central nervous system tumors such as astrocytomas, the paucity of café-au-lait spots (which are seen in less than 50% of cases) and peripheral neurofibromas (which are seen in less than 20% of cases), and the absence of Lisch nodules and skeletal abnormalities.

Segmental neurofibromatosis is characterized by café-au-lait spots or cutaneous neurofibromas localized to a segment of the body with a unilateral dermatomal distribution.

Multiple café-au-lait spots is a subtype of neurofibromatosis. Affected patients have only multiple café-au-lait spots, which are more than 15 mm in broadest diameter, inherited as an autosomal-dominant trait. There are no associated Lisch nodules, neurofibromas, skeletal problems or any of the other characteristic features described above.

HISTOPATHOLOGICAL FINDINGS

Neurofibromas are sharply circumscribed, benign neoplasms that consist of delicate fibrillary bundles of collagen accompanied by cells with wavy nuclei (Figs 89.3 and 89.4). Café-au-lait spots consist of typical melanocytes in normal numbers situated at the dermoepidermal junction.

ETIOLOGY AND PATHOGENESIS

Von Recklinghausen's disease is an autosomal-dominant disease with no race predilection, a penetrance that approaches 100%, and extremely variable expression. About 50% of cases represent spontaneous mutations. The von Recklinghausen's disease gene has been localized to the proximal long arm of chromosome 17 (NF1 gene) and the gene of acoustic neurofibromatosis has been localized to the long arm of chromosome 22. Segmental neurofibromatosis probably results from a postzygotic somatic mutation, with minimal risk of familial transmission of the disease. The pathogenesis of lesions in all forms of neurofibromatosis is still unknown.

MANAGEMENT

The two most important aspects of treatment are genetic counselling and surgical excision of neurofibromas when necessary (because of rapid growth, pain or functional or esthetic problems) and possible.

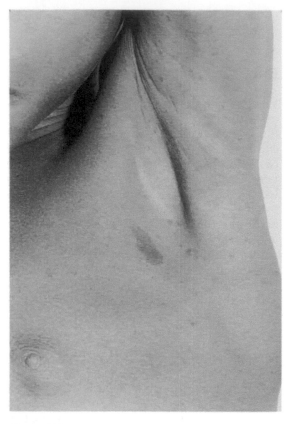

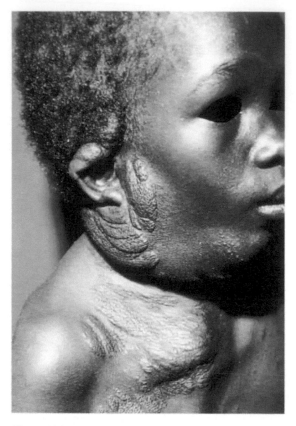

Figure 89.1
Neurofibromatosis. Crowe's sign: hyperpigmented macules and a café-au-lait spot in the axilla. These lesions are sometimes referred incorrectly as axillary freckles.

Figure 89.2
Neurofibromatosis. The cerebriform lesions around the ear are characterized histologically by the changes of a plexiform neurofibroma.

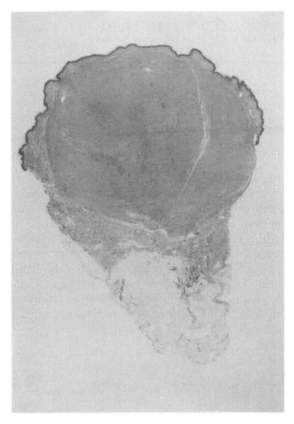

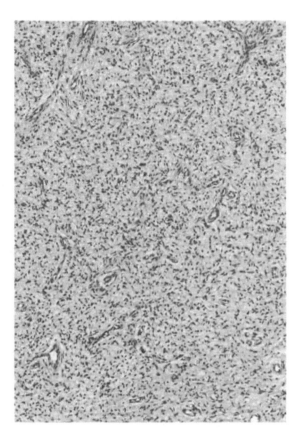

Figure 89.3

Figure 89.4

Figures 89.3 and 89.4

Neurofibroma. This neoplasm is benign; it is symmetrical and well circumscribed, and it has smooth borders. It is a neurofibroma because its numerous cells have oval and wavy nuclei, the collagen associated with it is fibrillary, and numerous venules course throughout it. Abundant mucin, seen as granular basophilic material, is present within the stroma (Fig. 89.4).

90   NEVUS ACHROMICUS

Nevus achromicus (also called nevus depigmentosus) is a rare, congenital, non-familial, stationary, hypomelanotic macular lesion. The lesion is often located on the trunk.

EPIDEMIOLOGY

The incidence of nevus achromicus is difficult to estimate because the clinical problems are often not sufficient to induce patients to contact a dermatologist. In the authors' opinion it is common.

CLINICAL FINDINGS

Nevus achromicus consists of hypopigmented areas that are irregular in shape and size, have geographical margins, and change from pale to white (Fig. 90.1). Lesions usually involve the trunk and the proximal extremities, but the face and the neck may also be affected. The nevus is often unilateral or circumscribed, or has a dermatomal pattern, but it may be systematized. Theoretically present at birth, it may become evident only after several months or even years of life.

The systematized variant of nevus achromicus corresponds to incontinentia pigmenti achromians or hypomelanosis of Ito. This disorder may be subdivided into a cutaneous form, in which the disease is limited to pigmentary changes and sweating abnormalities, and a neurocutaneous form, with severe nervous system defects and bony abnormalities in addition to hypopigmentation. In the systematized variant, lesions manifest themselves as a hypopigmented band and whorl on the trunk and extremities, with a bizarre pattern similar to that of incontinentia pigmenti (i.e. following Blaschko's lines). These lesions tend to progress initially and then remain stable.

HISTOPATHOLOGICAL FINDINGS

Normal melanocytes are present in the epidermis, which is normal except for decreased amounts of melanin within keratinocytes (Fig 90.2).

ETIOLOGY AND PATHOGENESIS

Nevus achromicus seems to be the consequence of decreased synthesis and abnormal transfer of melanosomes.

MANAGEMENT

No effective treatment is available.

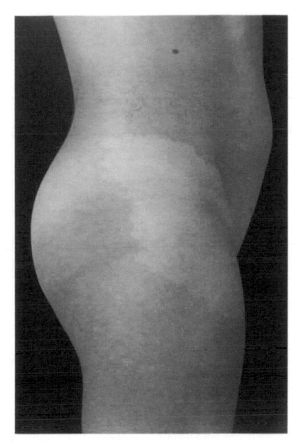

Figure 90.1
Nevus achromicus. This broad, irregularly shaped, hypopigmented patch is congenital and unilateral and has not enlarged.

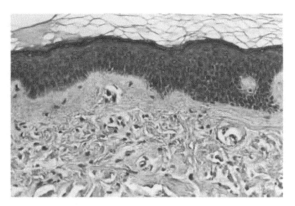

Figure 90.2
Nevus achromicus. This patch is clinically dramatic but histopathologically unremarkable. In fact, no abnormalities are detectable.

91

NEVUS LIPOMATOSUS CUTANEOUS SUPERFICIALIS

Nevus lipomatosus cutaneous superficialis is an idiopathic hamartoma characterized by mature ectopic adipose tissue in the dermis.

EPIDEMIOLOGY

Nevus lipomatosus cutaneous superficialis is very rare.

CLINICAL FINDINGS

Two clinical variants have been described, a solitary form and a multiple form. The multiple form (the classic form originally described by Hoffman and Zurhelle) consists of aggregates of soft, asymptomatic, skin-colored or yellow, elevated papules or nodules that sometimes coalesce into plaques with cerebriform surfaces (Fig. 91.1). Such plaques vary in size up to 80 mm by 150 mm. The predominant sites for lesions is the pelvic girdle, particularly the gluteal, sacral, and coccygeal regions, and the upper part of the posterior aspects of the thighs. In a few cases, lesions are confined to the abdominal, thoracic, and lumbar regions, the extremities and the scalp. Only rarely do the nodules extend across the midline. Solitary lesions may be dome-shaped, sessile or pedunculated, and solitary lesion have been reported at sites other than those of the classic form, including the knee, the axilla, the arm and the scalp. Onset is at birth, during childhood or in adolescence. Once formed, the lesions remain unchanged or enlarge for many years.

HISTOPATHOLOGICAL FINDINGS

Nevus lipomatosus cutaneous superficialis is characterized by sheets of adipocytes through the dermis and caricatures of them in the subcutaneous fat, which is intersected by thickened, haphazardly arranged septa. These septa consist of thickened bundles of collagen, which are sometimes associated with deposit of mucin (Fig. 91.2)

ETIOLOGY AND PATHOGENESIS

The cause of nevus lipomatosus cutaneous superficialis is unknown.

MANAGEMENT

Treatment, if required, is by surgical excision.

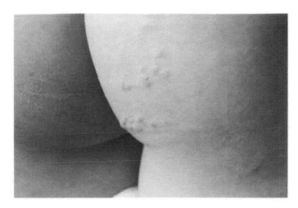

Figure 91.1
Nevus lipomatosus cutaneous superficialis. Some of the numerous skin-colored papules are arranged in clusters. The buttocks is a site of predilection.

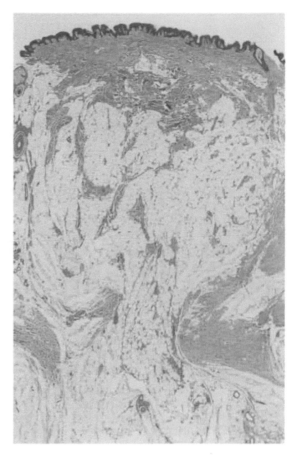

Figure 91.2
Nevus lipomatosus cutaneous superficialis. Much of the lower half of the dermis has been replaced by collections of adipocytes that vary in size and shape. The subcutaneous fat is also altered by an increased number of haphazardly arranged septa. Lobules of adipocytes are not intersected by thin fibrous septa in the manner of normal subcutaneous fat; instead, the connective tissue elements, both fibrous and adipose, are organized in a way that has completely changed the architecture of the subcutaneous fat. The collagen bundles that form aberrant septa are thicker than those within normal fibrous septa, and many of the lobules of adipocytes are accompanied by abundant mucin, seen as granular, probably basophilic material.

92

NEVUS SEBACEUS

Nevus sebaceus is a localized hamartoma of the epidermis and the pilosebaceous units and, occasionally, of the ectopic apocrine glands.

EPIDEMIOLOGY

The lesion is present in 0.3% of all neonates, with an equal incidence in males and females. In most cases nevus sebaceus is seen at birth but it may be apparent later in life.

CLINICAL FINDINGS

Nevus sebaceus is a unilateral, circumscribed, raised, usually solitary, yellow or yellow–brown, hairless plaque with a smooth, velvety surface (Fig. 92.1). The lesion may be rounded, linear or irregular, and it varies in size from small papules to large areas of involvement. In rare instances, the lesions are extensive and multiple. The most common sites are the scalp, the face, the forehead and the cheeks, but lesions may be located elsewhere. Nevus sebaceus may enlarge gradually.

Associations

The association of extensive sebaceus nevi with other conditions such as epilepsy, mental retardation, neurological defects, and skeletal deformities is known as 'nevus sebaceus syndrome' (Fig. 92.2).

Complications

After puberty, various secondary neoplasms develop secondarily within nevus sebaceus in about 10% of patients. Most of these lesions are trichoblastomas (Fig. 92.3) (which in the past were considered basal cell epitheliomas) or syringocystadenoma papilliferum. Less common are nodular hidradenomas, syringomas, sebaceous epitheliomas, chondroid syringomas, trichilemmomas and proliferating trichilemmal cysts.

HISTOPATHOLOGICAL FINDINGS

Prepubescent lesions appear as clusters of tiny, pyriform, sebaceous lobules associated with vellus follicles, often together with follicular germ cells and papillae, usually on the scalp (Fig. 92.4).

Post-pubescent lesions appear as papillated or digitated epidermis in association with numerous large, pyriform, sebaceous lobules, follicular germ cells and papillae. These lesions are characterized by the absence, or near absence, of terminal follicles within the lesion. Again the lesions are usually on the scalp.

ETIOLOGY AND PATHOGENESIS

The cause of nevus sebaceus is not known.

MANAGEMENT

Because of the risks of malignant change, surgical excision during childhood is recommended.

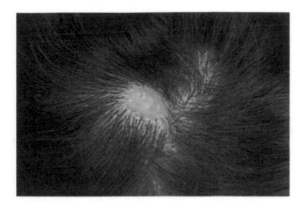

Figure 92.1
Nevus sebaceus. A well-circumscribed, raised, smooth, yellowish, alopecic plaque on the vertex of the scalp.

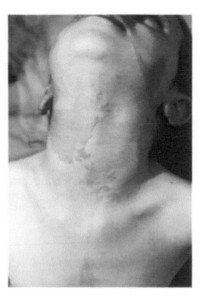

Figure 92.2
Nevus sebaceus syndrome. These large lesions are characterized by yellowish plaques composed of discrete and confluent papules. The surface of the lesion in some foci is cobblestone-like. The extensive nature of these lesions suggests they are cutaneous manifestations of other congenital vascular, skeletal or neural abnormalities, which in fact proved to be the case.

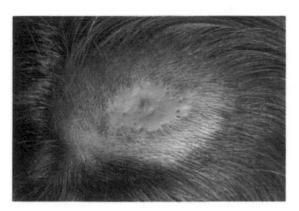

Figure 92.3
Nevus sebaceus. The blue–gray nodule that appeared at puberty within this hairless yellow plaque is a trichoblastoma. This neoplasm is frequent complication of a sebaceous nevus.

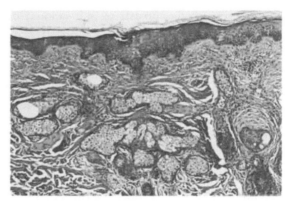

Figure 92.4
Nevus sebaceus. The diagnostic features of nevus sebaceus in this child are the cluster of sebaceous lobules in association with vellus follicles, many of these lobules are pyriform, and several structures resemble follicular germs and papillae. This lesion has a relatively flat expanse rather than the prominently papillated surface that develops at puberty. Note also that the sebaceous lobules are smaller than those in postpubescent patients.

93

NEVUS VERRUCOSUS

Nevus verrucosus is a localized hamartoma that is made up almost exclusively of keratinocytes.

EPIDEMIOLOGY

The lesion has been estimated to be present in 1 per 1000 live births, with equal incidence in males and females. In most cases nevus verrucosus is seen at birth but it may not be apparent until later in life.

CLINICAL FINDINGS

Nevus verrucosus consists of skin-colored or yellow–brown, keratotic papules that tend to merge to form a well-demarcated papillomatous plaque (Fig. 93.1). Their configuration is protean. Among the different shapes they assume are linear (Fig. 93.2), zosteriform (Fig. 93.3), rectangular and whorled. Such lesions often follow the Blaschko's lines and rarely cross the midline. The linear form is the commonest, especially for lesions on the limbs. When the lesions are distributed on one-half of the body, the nevus is termed nevus unius lateris. The surface of most verrucous nevi is rough and tends to become velvety and macer-ated in the folds. Lesions may gradually extend during childhood. The term 'epidermal nevus syndrome' has been given to the concurrence of an epidermal nevus and another malformation in at least one extracutaneous body system.

HISTOPATHOLOGICAL FINDINGS

Verrucous nevi may present several different histopathological patterns, of which the commonest is sharply demarcated hyperkeratosis, acanthosis and papillomatosis (Fig 93.4). In about 20% of cases, lesions assume features of epidermolytic hyperkeratosis, focal acantholytic dyskeratosis, seborrheic dermatosis and cornoid lamellation.

ETIOLOGY AND PATHOGENESIS

The cause of nevus verrucosus is unknown.

MANAGEMENT

The definitive therapy is surgical excision. Laser vaporization and dermoabrasion are alternative treatments.

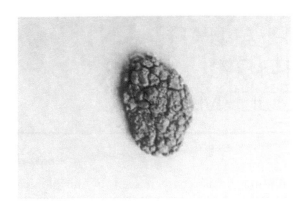

Figure 93.1
Nevus verrucosus. The lesions consist of closely set verrucous papules that coalesce to form a well-demarcated, papillomatous plaque.

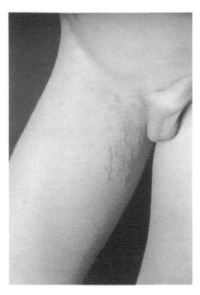

Figure 93.2
Nevus verrucosus. This unilateral lesion was present at birth and consists of pink keratotic papules, some in linear array.

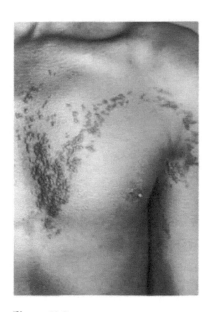

Figure 93.3
Nevus verrucosus. This unilateral nevus follows Blaschko's lines and stops sharply at the midline.

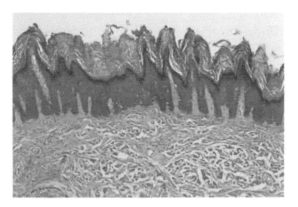

Figure 93.4
Nevus verrucosus. This epidermal nevus is characterized by a digitated thickened epidermis, hypergranulosis and a basket-woven appearance, and laminated and compact orthokeratosis.

94

PALMOPLANTAR HEREDITARY KERATODERMA

Palmoplantar hereditary keratodermas (PPHK) are a heterogeneous group of diseases characterized by erythema and hyperkeratosis of the palms and soles. They are distinguishable by other clinical features, associated abnormalities, and mode of inheritance. These conditions can be divided into two forms – diffuse and focal PPHK.

DIFFUSE PALMOPLANTAR HEREDITARY KERATODERMA

UNNA–THOST DISEASE

Unna–Thost disease is thought to be the most common type of PPHK. It usually manifests itself at 2–5 years of age with a diffuse erythema. Hyperkeratosis then commences at the margins of the soles and extends to the center. The disease is bilateral, symmetrical and has no tendency to spread to extensor surfaces (Figs 94.1 and 94.2). Initially, it has sharp borders surrounded by an erythematous halo. Marked hyperhidrosis is usual. Histologically, the disorder is characterized by compact hyperkeratosis, hypergranulosis and moderate acanthosis (Fig. 94.3). It is determined by an autosomal-dominant gene.

EPIDERMOLYTIC PALMOPLANTAR HEREDITARY KERATODERMA OF VORNER

Epidermolytic PPHK of Vorner may be present at birth or it may appear during the first months of life. It resembles Unna–Thost disease but hyperhidrosis is not a common finding. It is characterized by histological features of epidermolytic hyperkeratosis. The disease is inherited via an autosomal-dominant trait.

MAL DE MELEDA

Mal de Meleda is a very rare transgrediens disorder. It is a progressive form of PPHK comprising a glove and sock hyperkeratosis that does not usually have sharply defined margins. Hyperkeratotic plaques may occasionally appear, especially on the elbows and the knees. Hyperhidrosis with maceration and malodour is always present. This disease is very similar to progressive PPHK of Greither except that it is persistent and is inherited as a recessive trait. Histopathologically, mal de Meleda is characterized by epidermal hyperplasia, hyperkeratosis and inflammatory infiltrate around the dermal vessels.

PROGRESSIVE PALMOPLANTAR HEREDITARY KERATODERMA OF GREITHER

Progressive PPHK of Greither is an autosomal-dominant disorder that is characterized by diffuse keratoderma with hyperhidrosis extending to the dorsal aspect of the feet (transgrediens pattern). In addition, keratotic patches may develop on the limbs (progrediens pattern). The disease tends to improve spontaneously in middle age. It is essentially different from mal de Meleda in that it has a dominant mode of inheritance.

DIFFUSE PALMOPLANTAR HEREDITARY KERATODERMA WITH ASSOCIATED FEATURES

PAPILLON–LEFEVRE SYNDROME

Papillon–Lefèvre syndrome (or PPHK with periodontosis) is a recessively inherited disease characterized by a diffuse transgrediens palmoplantar keratosis, psoriasiform lesions on the knees and the dorsal aspect of the feet, and hyperhidrosis that causes an unpleasant odour (Fig. 94.4). These cutaneous lesions appear between 1 and 5 years of age. Severe gingivostomatitis and periodontitis occur later, with loss of teeth (Fig. 94.5). Patients suffering from the disorder frequently develop pyogenic skin infections. The histological features of the disease are similar to those of mal de Meleda (Fig. 94.6).

PALMOPLANTAR HEREDITARY KERATODERMA MUTILANS VOHWINKEL

Determined by an autosomal-dominant gene, PPHK mutilans Vohwinkel usually begins in infancy as a diffuse palmoplantar hyperkeratosis that has a honeycomb pattern and a violaceous border (Fig. 94.7). In addition, patients may develop distinctive starfish-shaped keratoses on the dorsal aspect of the lower limbs. The second main clinical feature is constricting fibrous bands, which commence in the second decade (Fig. 94.8). These bands lead progressively to mutilations of the digits. Mutilation of the digits may also occasionally occur in mal de Meleda, Olmsted syndrome and congenital pachyonychia. Histopathological findings are a hammock-shaped outline produced by the surface of viable keratinocytes, hypergranulosis, and tiny remnants of nuclei in the corneocytes of the stratum corneum (Fig. 94.9).

OLMSTED SYNDROME

Olmsted syndrome is an extremely rare disease that is probably transmitted in an autosomal-recessive manner. It is characterized by the unusual association of a well-defined, progressive, transgrediens palmoplantar keratoderma (Fig. 94.10) and perioreficial hyperkeratosis (Fig. 94.11). During childhood, flexion deformities of the digits may lead to constriction phenomena and, progressively, to the need for amputation. The disease is highly disabling because of the severe itching and the painful nature of the keratoderma.

HYDROTIC ECTODERMAL DYSPLASIA

Hydrotic ectodermal dysplasia (Clouston syndrome) consists of dystrophy of the nails, sparsity and defects of the hair, and palmoplantar keratoderma. Hyperkeratosis of the soles has a papillomatous appearance, which increases in severity with age. The disease has an autosomal-dominant pattern of inheritance.

FOCAL PALMOPLANTAR HEREDITARY KERATODERMA

PUNCTATE KERATODERMA

Punctate keratoderma is inherited via a regular dominant trait. It develops at puberty and is characterized by numerous yellow to dark brown, round, isolated keratotic papules with a central keratotic plug (Fig. 94.12). Hyperhidrosis does not occur.

TYROSINAEMIA TYPE II

Tyrosinaemia type II (Richner–Hanhart disease, oculocutaneous tyrosinosis) is a rare disease determined by an autosomal-dominant gene. It causes deficiencies in tyrosine aminotransferase, which leads to increased levels of serum tyrosine. The disorder is characterized by the triad of palmoplantar keratoderma, corneal dystrophies (bilateral ulcerative keratitis) and mental retardation. The cutaneous lesions typically consist of painful, discrete, hyperkeratotic plaques on the soles and the palms (Figs 94.13 and 94.14). Bullous lesions and hyperhidrosis may be observed. The discomfort is often proportional to the levels of serum tyrosine. The histopathological findings are characterized by compact hyperkeratosis, hypergranulosis and slight psoriasiform hyperplasia (Fig. 94.15).

CONGENITAL PACHYONYCHIA

Congenital pachyonychia is a rare genodermatosis that is transmitted via an autosomal-dominant trait. It is characterized by a combination of ectodermal defects. The main clinical features are hypertrophy and distortion of the nails (seen in all patients) (Figs 94.16 and 94.17), palmoplantar hyperkeratosis (seen in 60%) (Fig. 94.18), leukokeratosis (seen in 60%) (see Fig. 94.16) and follicular keratosis (seen in 37%). The palmoplantar keratoderma is symmetrical, non-progressive and non-transgrediens. It is mainly located at points of pressure. Hyperhidrosis is common.

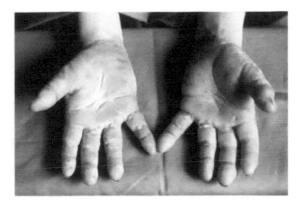

Figure 94.1

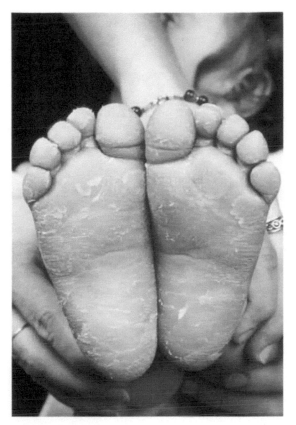

Figures 94.1 and 94.2
Unna–Thost disease. Diffuse involvement of palms and soles is manifest by yellowish hyperkeratosis. The lesions are most prominent at sites of trauma. Fissures are also seen on the palms. Note that lesions are also sharply marginated at the wrists.

Figure 94.2

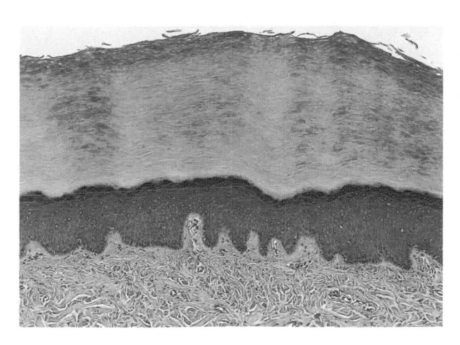

Figure 94.3
Unna–Thost disease. Lesions on the palms and the soles are remarkably hyperkeratotic, which is reflected in a cornified layer that is thicker than normal for volar skin. The remainder of the epidermis is not strikingly abnormal.

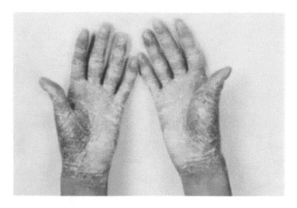

Figure 94.4
Papillon–Lefèvre syndrome. The palms and wrists have diffuse erythema and prominent scaling.

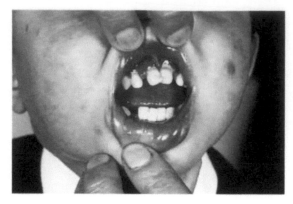

Figure 94.5
Papillon–Lefèvre syndrome. This condition is associated with gingival stomatitis. Teeth are lost as a consequence of periodontal disease.

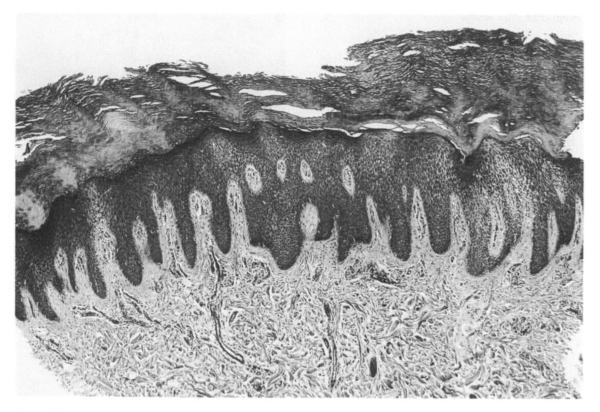

Figure 94.6
Papillon–Lefèvre syndrome. The cornified layer is almost ten times as thick as the cornified layer on the normal skin of the wrist. Note also striking psoriasiform hyperplasia, the foci of spongiosis and the sparse, superficial, perivascular lymphocytic infiltrate. This example of Papillon–Lefèvre syndrome is a spongiotic psoriasiform dermatitis with hypergranulosis and hyperkeratosis, and is similar to the findings observed in mal de Meleda.

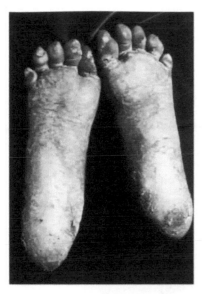

Figure 94.7
Mutilating keratoderma. The soles are covered by diffuse hyperkeratosis. Similar changes are present on the balls of the toes. Fissures have formed in hyperkeratotic zones. The process is associated with loss of digits.

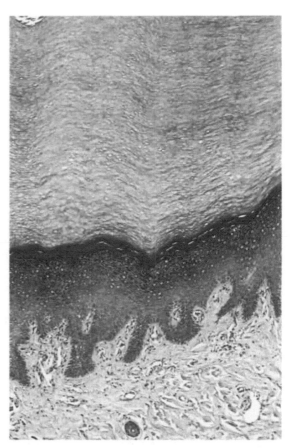

Figure 94.9
Mutilating keratoderma (Vohwinkel's disease). The granular zone is strikingly thickened and makes up almost one-half of the thickness of the viable epidermis. The configuration of the epidermis is psoriasiform. Diagnostic features of Vohwinkel's disease are that each corneocyte is punctuated by a small, round nucleus and that the parakeratotic cornified layer is associated with hypergranulosis. No other keratoderma of the palms and soles has such an affiliation.

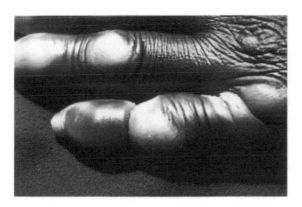

Figure 94.8
Mutilating keratoderma. Hyperkeratosis involves the dorsum of the fingers. Note also changes of pseudoainhum (i.e. focal constrictions of the digits).

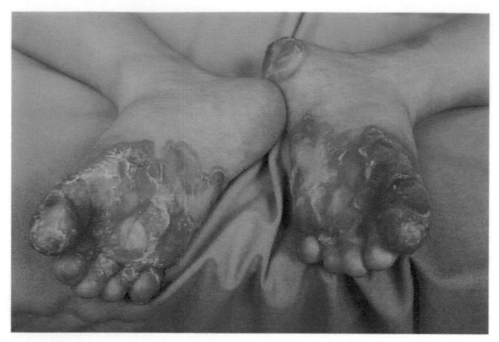

Figure 94.10
Olmsted syndrome. Progressive, well-defined painful plantar lesions can be seen.

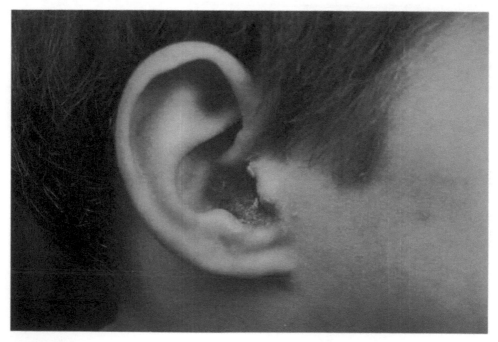

Figure 94.11
Olmsted syndrome. The perioreficial hyperkeratosis is a characteristic sign of the disease.

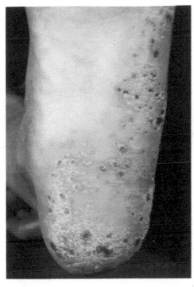

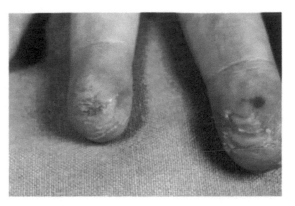

Figure 94.14
Tyrosinemia type II. Hyperkeratotic lesions tend to follow the dermatoglyphic lines and are whitish, yellowish or blackish.

Figure 94.12
Punctate keratoderma. More than one-half of the sole is involved by punctate keratotic lesions. Many of these areas are discrete and others tend to confluence. The lesions are not confined to the major skin creases, but are scattered diffusely.

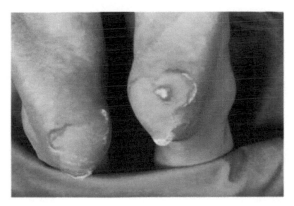

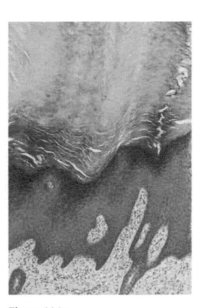

Figure 94.13
Tyrosinemia type II. Arcuate and nummular lesions are characterized by whitish and yellowish hyperkeratosis.

Figure 94.15
Palmoplantar keratoderma in tyrosinemia type II. This specimen was taken from a patient with clinically prominent hyperkeratosis. That change is reflected histopathologically in a cornified layer, thick even by standards of volar skin, slight papillation of the viable epidermis, hypergranulosis and epidermal hyperplasia.

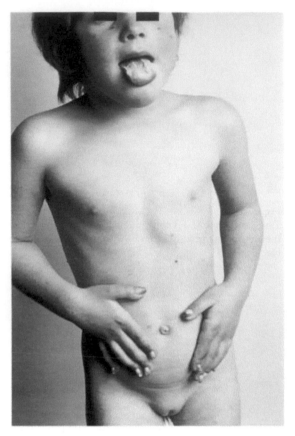

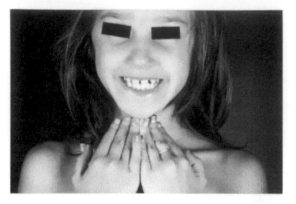

Figure 94.17
Congenital pachyonychia. Hypertrophy and distortion of nails are accompanied by hyperkeratotic changes on the lips and by dental abnormalities.

Figure 94.16
Congenital pachyonychia. The tongue is hyperkeratotic and all the nails are dystrophic.

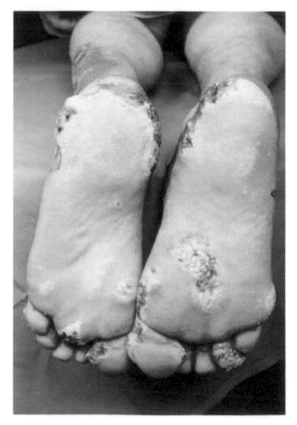

Figure 94.18
Congenital pachyonychia. Plantar keratoderma is symmetrical, non-transgrediens and mainly localized over pressure points.

95

PELLAGRA

Pellagra is a systemic disease caused by an inadequate dietary supply of nicotinic acid (niacin) and nicotinamide. These two substances are called pellagra-preventing factors, from which the term 'vitamin PP' is derived. The disease is characterized by the classic triad of dermatitis, diarrhea and dementia – the three Ds. Pellagra still exists in developing countries, affecting children and adults, whereas in the Western world the disease is rare and is observed almost exclusively in patients affected by chronic alcohol abuse, gastrointestinal diseases or severe psychiatric disturbances.

CLINICAL FINDINGS

Pellagra begins on sun-exposed areas, such as the face and the dorsum of the hands. It consists of erythema and scaling, sometimes accompanied by pruritus. The skin is smooth and edematous; vesicles and blisters may appear, with fissures and scales (Fig. 95.1). Scaly desquamation can be followed by wizened and glazed skin (Fig. 95.2). On the face, erythema predominates on the nose and cheeks, giving a symmetric 'butterfly' eruption (see Fig. 95.2). A well-marginated eruption, Casal's necklace, can be seen on the neck, closing in the back and going down to the sternal area. The erythema fades in winter and recurs in spring. With time, the skin becomes rougher, drier, and pigmented with a darker margin. The lips are dry and fissured (see Fig. 95.2). The oral mucosa is red, dry and smooth, with numerous aphthous lesions, which may be large. The tongue is usually swollen and magenta in color, but it can also be atrophic and black. Vulvar involvement is less common. The diaper area is particularly affected in infants.

Diarrhea is one of the symptoms that marks the severity of the disease. Feces are frequent, water-like at the beginning and then with a bloody aspect. Neurological signs consist of weakness, insomnia, and mental depression. Without significant improvement in the diet, the course is chronic.

LABORATORY FINDINGS

The mean serum values for serotonin and its metabolite 5-hydroxyindoleacetic acid (5–HIAA) are significantly higher in pellagra patients than in the general population.

HISTOPATHOLOGICAL FINDINGS

Evolving lesions are characterized by pallid, ballooned keratinocytes in the spinous and granular layers (Fig. 95.3) and foci of parakeratosis that contain neutrophils.

MANAGEMENT

The administration of oral nicotinamide at a dose of 100–500 mg/day is rapidly effective. Severe cases necessitate intravenous treatment. A protein-rich diet is highly recommended for all patients.

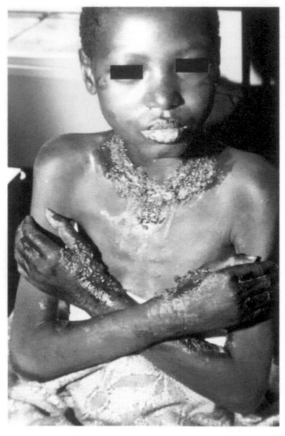

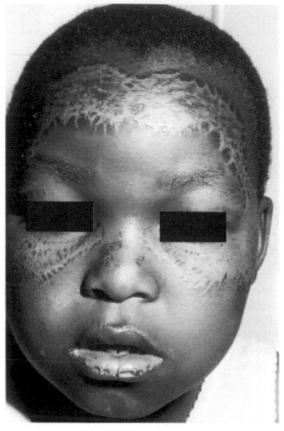

Figure 95.1
Pellagra. Acute changes (ulcerations and vegetations) involve the lips, the upper part of the chest and the hands. Post-inflammatory hyperpigmentation is also evident in these areas.

Figure 95.2
Pellagra. Ichthyosiform hyperpigmented plaques are present on the forehead, the nose and the intraorbital regions, giving a mask-like appearance. The lips are also affected by the process.

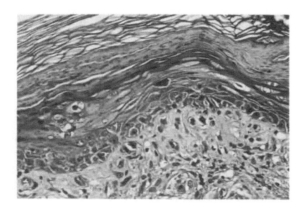

Figure 95.3
Pellagra. Note the confluent necrosis of the epidermis beneath a normal basket-woven cornified layer; the pallor of the granular and spinous zones; the focal thinning of the epidermis; and the sparse, perivascular lymphocytic infiltrate. These features are also manifestations of acrodermatitis enteropathica and necrolytic migratory erythema.

96

PEMPHIGUS

Pemphigus is a severe autoimmune disease characterized by intraepidermal blister formation on the skin and mucous membranes.

EPIDEMIOLOGY

Pemphigus is rare in children. The age of onset is between 1 and 15 years, except in neonatal pemphigus, which is present at birth or appears in the first hours of life.

CLINICAL FINDINGS

The most frequent form of pemphigus in children is pemphigus vulgaris. In pemphigus vulgaris, the primary lesion is a flaccid bulla, arising spontaneously on normal or erythematous skin, that breaks rapidly, leaving erosions with the tendency to enlarge peripherally and to become crusted (Fig. 96.1). Sites of predilection are the scalp, the face, the axillae and the oral mucosa, but the disease may be diffuse from the beginning. Nikolsky's sign is present. Itching is variable; burning pain is a common complaint. Each lesion heals spontaneously, leaving transient hyperpigmentation. In most childhood cases of pemphigus vulgaris, the lesions on the oral mucosa may precede the development of cutaneous lesions.

The sporadic form of pemphigus foliaceus in children may start as pemphigus erythematosus, which involves the sebaceous regions of the body, or it may start with a herpetiform appearance. The bullae are superficial, break easily and are continuously covered with scales and crusts (Fig. 96.2). An erythrodermic state may develop quickly. The oral mucous membranes are not involved.

The sporadic and endemic forms of pemphigus foliaceus in children are clinically identical; they are distinguished only by their epidemiology.

Neonatal pemphigus vulgaris has been described in children born of mothers with pemphigus vulgaris. The disease lasts for 4–6 weeks and resolves spontaneously. It usually involves the skin only, sparing mucous membranes. Typical bullous lesions are seen.

Immunoglobulin A pemphigus is characterized by a vesiculobullous eruption that simulates subcorneal pustular dermatoses or impetigo. The course of pemphigus in children is unpredictable. It is usually severe, and the severity depends not only on the disease itself, but also on the side effects of the drugs used for treatment.

LABORATORY FINDINGS

Direct immunofluorescence reveals immunoglobulin G and complement (C3) in the intercellular spaces of the epidermis. Indirect immunofluorescence shows immunoglobulin G autoantibodies. These autoantibodies are directed against a 130 kDa glycoprotein (desmoglein III) in pemphigus vulgaris and against a 160 kDa glycoprotein (desmoglein II) in pemphigus foliaceus. The titre of immunoglobulin G antibodies seems to be related to the severity of the disease.

HISTOPATHOLOGICAL FINDINGS

Common findings in pemphigus vulgaris and pemphigus foliaceus are acantholytic cells in the epidermis (keratinocytes that have lost their moorings, separated from adjacent keratinocytes and rounded up). This acantholytic process leeds to the formation of an intraepidermal blister, which is suprabasal in pemphigus vulgaris (Fig. 96.3) and subcorneal in pemphigus foliaceus (Fig. 96.4).

ETIOLOGY AND PATHOGENESIS

The etiology is unknown. Acantholysis occurs as a result of circulating autoantibodies of the immunoglobulin G class binding to the cell surface glycoproteins (pemphigus antigen).

MANAGEMENT

As a rule, the childhood forms of pemphigus are severe and require high doses of corticosteroids, sometimes in association with immunosuppressive drugs (e.g., cyclophosphamide, azathioprine) to decrease immunoglobulin G levels. Cyclosporin is variably useful. Alternative treatments include plasmapheresis to deplete immune complexes from the blood; this seems to be especially useful in association with corticosteroids. Dapsone, too, has been used with good results. Neonatal pemphigus usually is treated only topically.

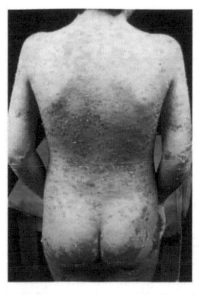

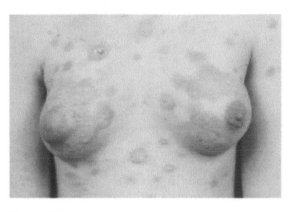

Figure 96.2
Pemphigus foliaceus. This 12-year-old girl has erythematous scaling patches and erosions on the trunk.

Figure 96.1
Pemphigus vulgaris. This severe case, which rapidly progressed to generalization with mucosal involvement, was particularly resistant to therapy. The back is completely covered with flaccid blisters, scales and crusts. Nikolsky's sign was easily induced.

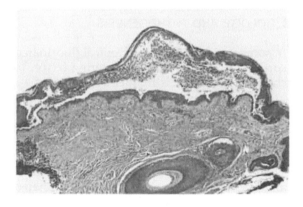

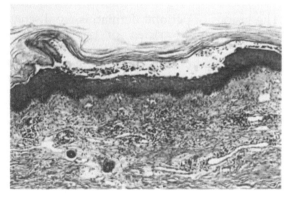

Figure 96.3
Pemphigus vulgaris. The blister within the epidermis is situated mostly above the basal layer; in foci, it is present in the mid-spinous zone. Within the blister itself are numerous acantholytic cells. This constellation of findings is diagnostic of this disorder. The mixed inflammatory cell infiltrate is a common finding.

Figure 96.4
Pemphigus foliaceus. The Intraepidermal separation occurs between the granular and the horny layers, and acantholytic cells and neutrophils are seen in the lumina of the blisters.

97

PERIORAL DERMATITIS

Perioral dermatitis is an uncommon, distinctive papular eruption that occurs on the face with a prominent distribution around the mouth.

EPIDEMIOLOGY

The condition is predominantly observed in young women. In 10% of patients, the onset is between 2 and 12 years of age.

CLINICAL FINDINGS

The lesions of perioral dermatitis are discrete papules, papulovesicles, or papulopustules (Fig. 97.1). A lupoid (granulomatous) aspect may be apparent on diascopy, especially in children. Some papules are arranged in clusters. The condition is symmetrical on the chin and in the nasolabial folds and characteristically spares a narrow area around the vermilion border of the lips. In about 20% of patients, a few papules may be situated on the glabella and eyelids. The course is chronic.

HISTOPATHOLOGICAL FINDINGS

Early papules of perioral dermatitis consist of lymphoplasmocytic infiltrates around dilated blood vessels in the upper half of the dermis and around vessels that surround vellus follicles. In time, the lymphoplasmocytic infilrate is joined by epithelioid histiocytes, some of which are multinucleate, to form collections, especially in the vicinity of follicles. As these collections of epithelioid histiocytes enlarge, they act as a core of granuloma enveloped by a mantle of lymphocytes and plasma cells (Fig. 97.2). Pustules of perioral dermatitis may develop independently of papules. When they do, they consist of suppurative folliculitis together with perivascular and perifollicular lymphoplasmocytic infiltrates.

ETIOLOGY AND PATHOGENESIS

In some patients, the use of topical fluorinated corticosteroids is surely a triggering factor. In children, the cause is frequently unknown.

MANAGEMENT

The first step in treatment is the avoidance of all topical preparations, especially fluorinated corticosteroids. In children erythromycin (250 mg twice a day for 4 weeks) is the drug of choice. In adolescents, tetracycline (250 mg twice a day for 4 weeks) is the drug of choice. Topical erythromycin or clindamycin solutions may be helpful.

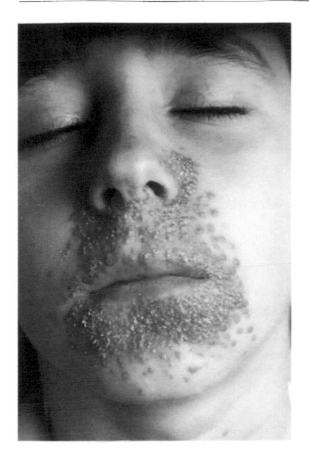

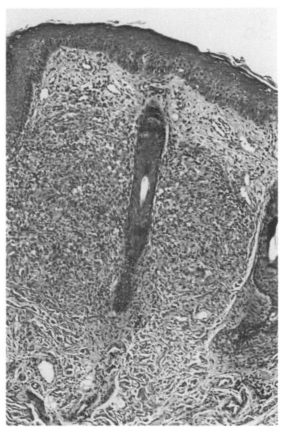

Figure 97.1
Perioral dermatitis. Scaly and crusted, reddish papules are present around the mouth and the lower portion of the nose.

Figure 97.2
Perioral dermatitis. This papular lesion is characterized by granulomatous perifollicutis together with lymphoplasmacytic infiltrates.

98

PILOMATRICOMA

Pilomatricoma is a benign adnexal tumor composed of cells resembling those of the hair matrix.

EPIDEMIOLOGY

Forty per cent of pilomatricomas begin before the age of 10 years, and more than 60% manifest themselves before the age of 20 years with a peak between 8 and 13 years of age.

Pilomatricomas represent 10% of nodules and tumors in children 16 years of age and younger. The neoplasm is more common in females than in males.

CLINICAL FINDINGS

Pilomatricomas typically manifest as solitary, irregularly shaped papules, nodules or tumors. Early lesions are cystic (Fig. 98.1), whereas more advanced lesions may develop flattened, polygonal outlines (the so-called 'tent sign') and are rock hard. In most instances, the epidermis is unaffected. Pilomatricomas often assume a blue or grayish hue, although shades of red and yellow, as well as normal skin tone, are also seen. In some certain fully developed lesions, chalk-white concretions (calcified or ossified foci) may be discerned within the nodule (Fig. 98.2). Affected people are often asymptomatic, although about 50% of patients report some tenderness when the lesion is palpated. Most pilomatricomas enlarge slowly over several months. Once the lesion has calcified, there is no tendency for regression. In about 70% of patients, lesions arise on the head (see Figs 98.1 and 98.2) (particularly the face) and the neck; other lesions are situated, in decreasing frequency, on the arms, the thighs and the trunk. The palms, the soles and the mucous membranes have not been reported to be involved to date.

Carcinomatous transformation, although rare, has been reported in pediatric patients.

Associations

Patients with myotonic dystrophy have a higher incidence of pilomatricoma than the general population.

LABORATORY FINDINGS

Radiographic examination demonstrates the presence of calcium salts. Calcification is common in pilomatricoma, occurring in about 80% of all cases.

HISTOPATHOLOGICAL FINDINGS

In the early stage pilomatricoma is characterized by a cystic structure that is lined by infundibular and matrical epithelium and that contains cornified cells, which may be 'shadow cells'. The shadow cells exhibit pale, eosinophilic ghosts of nuclei (Figs 98.3 and 98.4). These cells undergo progressive calcification. Subsequent ossification of shadow cells occurs as a consequence of metaplasia of fibrocytes and osteoblasts.

ETIOLOGY AND PATHOGENESIS

It is not known whether this tumor is derived directly from the hair matrix cells or from pluripotential cutaneous epithelial stem cells.

MANAGEMENT

Complete but conservative excision is curative.

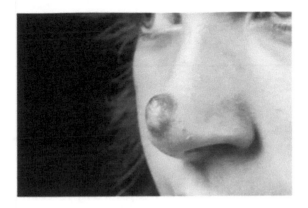

Figure 98.1
Pilomatricoma. The tumor is firm and yellow–brown, with whitish areas where the calcification is more superficial.

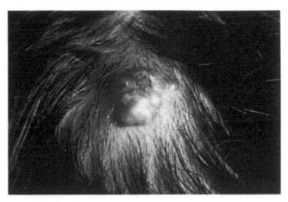

Figure 98.2
Giant pilomatricoma. This multilobulated nodule is ulcerated and crusted. Whitish zones at the periphery represent areas of calcification.

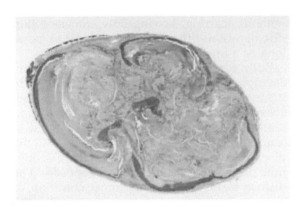

Figure 98.3

Figures 98.3 and 98.4
Pilomatricoma. Cystic stage (Fig. 98.3) – even a large lesion may be mostly cystic. The lining of the cyst consists entirely of matrical cells. As these cells mature, they become cornified in a faulty attempt to form hair shafts. Those cells demonstrate karyolysis; ghosts of nuclei have prompted the designation shadow cell (Fig. 98.4).

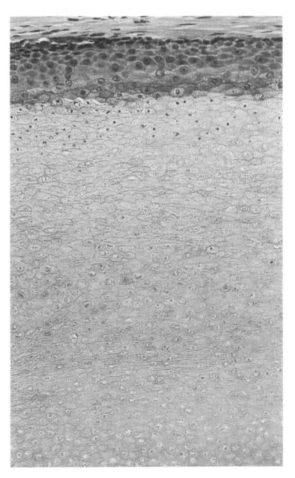

Figure 98.4

99

PITYRIASIS LICHENOIDES

Pityriasis lichenoides, also known as guttate parapsoriasis, is a self-limited, polymorphous skin disorder of unknown origin. It is characterized by erythematous papules that tend to evolve into scales, vesicles, pustules and crusts, sometimes with central necrosis. The disease is usually divided into an acute form (acute guttate parapsoriasis, parapsoriasis varioliformis, Mucha–Habermann disease, pityriasis lichenoides et varioliformis acuta) and a chronic form (pityriasis lichenoides chronica, guttate parapsoriasis of Juliusberg). A new classification based on the distribution of the lesions subdivides the disease into three forms – diffuse, central and peripheral.

EPIDEMIOLOGY

Pytiriasis lichenoides is an uncommon disorder that affects males and females with equal frequency. In about 20% of patients, it begins in childhood. The age distribution curve show two peaks, one at 5 years and one at 10 years.

CLINICAL FINDINGS

The acute form of pityriasis lichenoides is characterized by pink, orange or purpuric papules that may evolve into vesicles that resolve with hemorrhagic crusts (Figs 99.1 and 99.2). Some papules and vesicles ulcerate and heal to leave varioliform scars. The lesions tend to be numerous and to erupt in crops, and they are accompanied by fever and malaise in some patients. The course of the disease runs from a few weeks to several months.

In the chronic form (Figs 99.3 and 99.4) the lesions consist of reddish-brown papules with an adherent central scale that tends to separate spontaneously. The lesions clear without scarring, leaving only transient skin discolorations. The disease course may be as long as a few years.

Both forms of pityriasis lichenoides are asymptomatic or accompanied by slight itching. Because both types of lesions often coexist in the same patient and no correlation seems to exist between the severity of the skin lesions and the overall duration of the disease, a classification based on the distribution of the lesions has been proposed. The diffuse form, which is the most common, is characterized by acute and chronic lesions scattered over the entire body surface, except the palms, the soles, and the mucosae. The central form usually involves the trunk, whereas the less common peripheral form is limited to the limbs and buttocks and tends to last longer.

HISTOPATHOLOGICAL FINDINGS

Stereotypical changes of the lesions of pityriasis lichenoides are a wedge-shaped, superficial and deep, perivascular lymphocytic infiltrate; edema of the papillary dermis; extravasated erythrocytes in the papillary dermis and sometimes in the epidermis; lymphocytes aligned along the dermoepidermal junction together with vacuolar alteration; and necrotic keratinocytes disposed as solitary units in the lower half of the epidermis (Figs 99.5 and 99.6).

ETIOLOGY AND PATHOGENESIS

The etiopathogenesis of pityriasis lichenoides remains obscure.

MANAGEMENT

Topical treatment with cortisone, tars, salicylate creams and various vitamin ointments have been used as symptomatic therapy with modest improvement. Long-term treatment with oral erythromycin has been proposed, but further confirmation is needed. Ultraviolet-B irradiation seems to be effective in alleviating symptoms without major side effects.

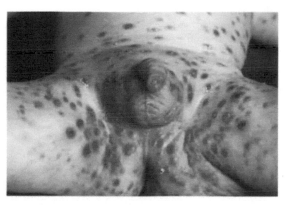

Figure 99.2
Acute pityriasis lichenoides (diffuse form). Pink macules, reddish papules and ulcerated papules covered by scaly crust are widespread. Note also the confluence of some papules to form plaques.

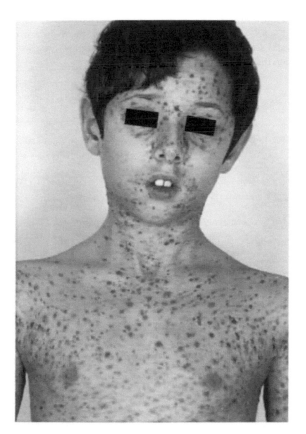

Figure 99.1
Acute pityriasis lichenoides (diffuse form). Purpuric macules, papules, and hemorrhagic, crusted papules involve the face, the neck, the trunk and the extremities.

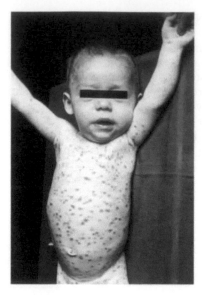

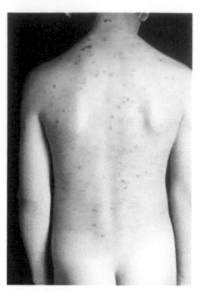

Figure 99.3
Chronic pityriasis lichenoides (diffuse form). Rust-brown macules and papules cover the trunk and extremities.

Figure 99.4
Chronic pityriasis lichenoides (central form). Reddish-brown and scaly papules are seen on the trunk, but few are seen on the extremities.

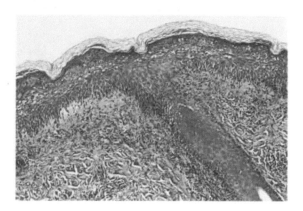

Figure 99.3

Figure 99.5 and 99.6
Acute pityriasis lichenoides. This lesion of Mucha–Habermann disease is of recent onset because the cornified layer is almost entirely of basket-weave design and parakeratotic cells have not yet emerged. The process is that of Mucha–Habermann disease because the infiltrate of lymphocytes is wedge-shaped, perivascular and interstitial, and because the infiltrate obscures the dermoepidermal junction focally. Within the epidermis are signs of spongiosis and ballooning as well as hints of scaly crusts.

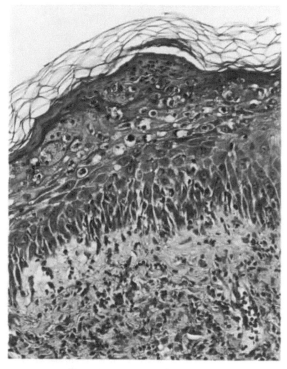

Figure 99.4

Pityriasis rosea is an acute, common, self-limited inflammatory disease of unknown cause characterized by a distinctive eruption.

EPIDEMIOLOGY

Pityriasis rosea is common during adolescence. Only 5% of patients are less than 5 years of age. It affects males and females equally. Seasonal incidence appears to vary according to geographical location. In temperate climates, it is more frequent in the spring.

CLINICAL FINDINGS

In about 80% of cases, the disease starts with a single isolated lesion, called the herald patch, which may appear anywhere on the body. This initial lesion is a round or oval, sharply defined plaque with a pink center and a slightly elevated and finely scaled border. It is 20–60 mm in diameter. After a few days or weeks, secondary lesions (Fig. 100.1) appear, usually on the trunk, the neck and the proximal parts of the extremities. These lesions are smaller, pink or light brown, with a center that has an appearance of cigarette paper, surrounded by a typical collar of scales.

Particularly in children, pityriasis rosea may be atypical in its morphology and distribution. Various types of lesions have been described in atypical variants, especially during the early stages of the eruption, as vesicular, urticarial, papular purpuric, and erythema multiforme-like. Pityriasis rosea may be unilateral and may occur on the face, the extremities and the oral mucous membranes. Subjective symptoms are usually absent or consist of slight pruritus. One-fifth of patients have had acute infections before the appearance of the disease. Spontaneous resolution generally occurs within 4–12 weeks.

HISTOPATHOLOGICAL FINDINGS

A superficial perivascular, predominantly lymphocytic infiltrate is associated with slight edema of the papillary dermis and extravasated erythrocytes, both in the papillary dermis and within the epidermis. Focal spongiosis, slight epidermal hyperplasia and mounds of parakeratosis are also seen (Fig. 100.2).

ETIOLOGY AND PATHOGENESIS

The etiology of pityriasis rosea is unknown. Many conditions have been suggested as possible causes or precipitating factors – viral or bacterial infections, the atopic state and seborrheic dermatitis.

MANAGEMENT

No treatment is required. If itching is present, a mild corticosteroid cream may be useful.

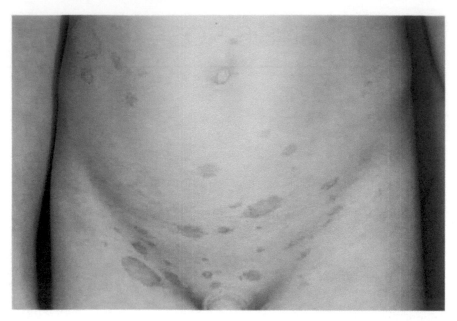

Figure 100.1
Pityriasis rosea. Oval papules and plaques have reddish-brown scales, mostly at their periphery.

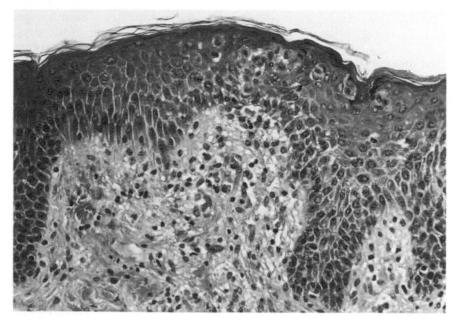

Figure 100.2
Pityriasis rosea. This lesion is in its early stages because of the absence of mounds of parakeratosis. The superficial perivascular lymphocytic infiltrate, the slight epidermal hyperplasia, the slight edema of the papillary dermis with extravasated erythrocytesm and the slight focal spongiosis are characteristic of this condition.

PITYRIASIS ROTUNDA

Pityriasis rotunda is an unusual disorder of keratinization characterized by persistent, round or oval, sharply demarcated, scaling patches, which are either darker or lighter than the surrounding skin.

EPIDEMIOLOGY

Although pityriasis rotunda may begin in infancy or childhood, the majority of patients who have been reported on have been 20–45 years of age. The condition has been described most often in Japanese people and in South African and West Indian blacks. In Italy, pityriasis rotunda is common among Sardinian people.

CLINICAL FINDINGS

Pityriasis rotunda is characterized by strikingly circular or occasionally oval, hypopigmented or hyperpigmented patches (Fig. 101.1) covered with fine scales. The edges of the patches are sharply demarcated from normal skin, and there is no evidence of inflammation. Lesions vary in size from 5 to 280 mm in diameter, and they may be numerous (as many as 30) and become confluent. Sites of predilection are the trunk and the limbs. The lesions are asymptomatic. The condition tend to be chronic.

HISTOPATHOLGICAL FINDINGS

Histological sections of pityriasis rotunda show laminated orthokeratosis, thinning of the granular layer and hyperpigmentation of the basal keratinocytes (Fig. 101.2), accompanied by a sparse superficial lymphohistiocytic infiltrate.

ETIOLOGY AND PATHOGENESIS

The etiopathogenesis is unknown. The clinical and microscopic features suggest that pityriasis rotunda is a special localized variant of acquired ichthyosis.

MANAGEMENT

Treatment with topical 'keratolytic' agents may ameliorate the condition.

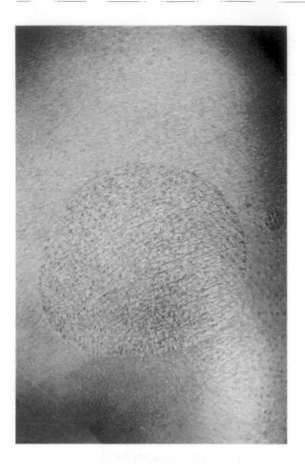

Figure 101.1
Pityriasis rotunda. This large nummular patch is markedly hyperpigmented and is covered by subtle scales.

Figure 101.2
Pityriasis rotunda. Histopathological features of pityriasis rotunda are basket-woven and laminar orthokeratosis together with a thin granular layer and hyperpigmentation of the basal keratinocytes.

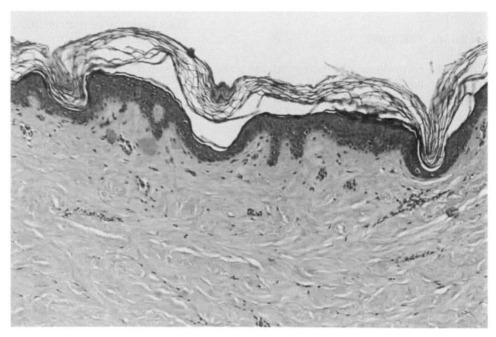

Pityriasis rubra pilaris is a benign, erythematous, squamous disorder. It is characterized by follicular plugging, perifollicular erythema, a cephalic rash and palmoplantar hyperkeratosis. It affects prepubertal children and young adults more commonly than others.

EPIDEMIOLOGY

Pityriasis rubra pilaris is a rare disorder. It occurs in one case in every 3500 new patients. Males and females are affected with equal frequency. In childhood there is a peak age of onset between 3 years and 6 years.

CLINICAL FINDINGS

The most characteristic clinical feature is a follicular verrucous papule, about 1 mm in diameter, with a central keratotic plug. This papule is surrounded by a classic yellow–orange ring. Initially these papules are discrete, but they soon coalesce to form hyperkeratotic plaques (Figs 102.1 and 102.2) that have a characteristic 'pachydermic' appearance with an exaggerated furrowing of the skin. In children, the elbows and the knees (see Fig. 102.2) are frequently affected, followed by, in decreasing order of frequency, the dorsal aspect of the feet and hands (Fig. 102.3) and the ankles; the involvement of the dorsal aspect of the proximal phalanges (see Fig. 102.3) is not as common as it is in adults.

The second important diagnostic element is a palmoplantar keratoderma, which is present in most cases. It can be distinguished from ichthyotic keratoderma by its salmon color and by the presence of edema that can sometimes be partially disabling. The dermatitis has a sharply demarcated border that is usually delimited by the dorsal aspect of the limbs. The Achilles tendon is frequently involved.

The third diagnostic element is a cephalic rash (see Fig. 102.1), which sometimes extends beyond the neck in a cape-like formation; again, this rash has sharp borders.

The unifying element of all lesions is their characteristic salmon color, which is therefore of particular diagnostic importance. Pruritus can occur but is usually mild. In a few cases there is a burning sensation. The disease usually resolves spontaneously after a variable period of time ranging from a few months to several years.

HISTOPATHOLOGICAL FINDINGS

The crucial findings are in the stratum corneum, where squares of orthokeratosis and parakeratosis alternate in chess board fashion (Fig. 102.4). Follicular plugging is not required to make the diagnosis of pityriasis rubra pilaris; in fact, in certain anatomic sites, such as the palms and the soles, the ostia of adnexal structures are not plugged.

ETIOLOGY AND PATHOGENESIS

Although a viral cause can be postulated by the fact that a febrile illness precedes the onset of pityriasis rubra pilaris in many cases, no specific etiology has been demonstrated.

Some papers claim a possible role for a serine protein, retinol binding protein, in the development of the disease.

MANAGEMENT

Topical treatment with cortisone, tars, salicylate creams and vitamin A have been used as symptomatic therapy with modest improvement. Synthetic retinoids such as isotretinoin and etretinate have also been used and seem to influence the course of pityriasis rubra pilaris positively even though the response to this treatment still remains unpredictable. Stanazolol has also been used, with inconstant results.

Phototherapy in its various forms is of little help in pityriasis rubra pilaris.

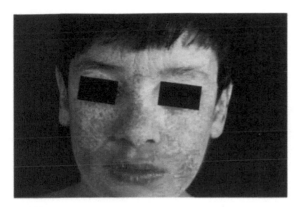

Figure 102.1
Pityriasis rubra pilaris. The face, including the lips and
eyelids of this young patient, is covered by whitish scales
situated on top of reddish bases.

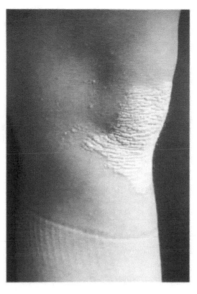

Figure 102.2
Pityriasis rubra pilaris. A plaque of pityriasis rubra pilaris
is sharply circumscribed and covered by chalky-white
scales. At the periphery of this plaque are satellite
keratotic papules.

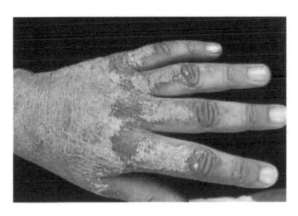

Figure 102.3
Pityriasis rubra pilaris. Hyperkeratotic plaque on the
dorsal aspect of a hand. Numerous keratotic papules are
present on the dorsal aspect of the proximal phalanges.

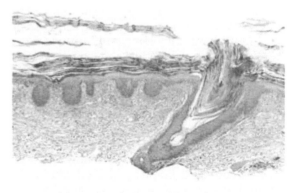

Figure 102.4
Pityriasis rubra pilaris. This fully developed lesion of pityriasis rubra pilaris is characterized by alternating orthokeratosis and parakeratosis, slight epidermal hyperplasia,
and a sparse lymphohistiocytic infiltrate around dilated
blood vessels of the superficial plexus. A follicular
infundibulum houses a large horny plug surrounded by
perifollicular parakeratosis.

Polyarteritis nodosa (PAN) is a nodular vasculitis of the medium and small muscular arteries. It involves the skin and several other organs. Two main forms have been described – benign cutaneous PAN and systemic PAN.

CLINICAL FINDINGS

Benign cutaneous polyarteritis nodosa

Benign cutaneous PAN may arise elsewhere, but the most frequent site is on the legs (Fig. 103.1). The arms (Fig. 103.2), the neck and the head may also be involved. Crops of a few or more than 100 painful red nodules, from 5 to 20 mm in diameter, are usually the first manifestation of benign cutaneous PAN. These nodules usually occur bilaterally. Deep nodules along the course of arteries have rarely been found. Often a starburst pattern (see Fig. 103.1) of persistent livedo reticularis follows the flare of nodules and prefers areas of pressure such as the feet, the legs, the buttocks and the scapulae. Punched-out ulcerations are frequently observed as a complication of ischemia, and extensive ulcerations are also seen. Arthralgia with swelling and stiffness is common. Edema and erythema of the overlying skin may be observed. Myalgia and painful neuritis with paresthesia of the involved extremities are common. Fever and malaise are usually accompanying signs of the cutaneous flares. In pediatric series, hypertension is described in about 50% of cases.

Benign cutaneous PAN has a chronic, relapsing, benign course.

Systemic polyarteritis nodosa

In infants and younger children the mode of presentation of systemic PAN and its course are very similar to Kawasaki's disease, so there is a high probability that they are in fact the same disease. Systemic PAN begins with high fever, malaise, conjunctivitis, skin eruptions of many types (a bright red rash confined to the diaper area, erythema multiforme-like eruptions or a scarlatiniform rash) and erythema and desquamation of the skin of the hands and the feet. The skin lesions are localized mainly in the legs. Purpura and bullae are the commonest types of lesions. Ulcers may develop as a consequence of acute infarction. Focal or extensive livedo reticularis with areas of acute hemorrhage and bright inflammation is also often observed. In younger children, there may also be lymphoadenomegaly, arthritis and involvement of the coronary arteries and sometimes the renal arteries. In older children, the systemic involvement is manifested mainly by weight loss, malaise, fever, arthralgia, myalgia and peripheral neuropathy. Hypertension is almost always seen in pediatric cases. Kidney involvement may be severe and may lead to irreversible renal failure. Nausea, vomiting and abdominal pain are frequent; bowel perforation may occur. The cardiac involvement may lead to congestive cardiac failure and pericarditis. Seizures and cerebral vascular accidents may occur. The prognosis for untreated patients is poor.

LABORATORY FINDINGS

Benign cutaneous polyarteritis nodosa

In benign cutaneous PAN, an elevated erythrocyte sedimentation rate is usually found in relation to acute flares of the skin lesions. Mild leukocytosis is often present. Thrombocytosis and elevated levels of immunoglobulin A and immunoglobulin M seem to be related to the severity of the disease. Direct immunofluorescence studies usually show deposition of immunoglobulin M and complement (C3) in vessel walls, sometimes only in small, uninvolved dermal vessels.

Systemic polyarteritis nodosa

In systemic PAN, anti-neutrophil cytoplasmic antibodies directed against myeloperoxidase can be found. This finding is typical of a systemic vasculitis and in the appropriate clinical setting it strongly suggests the presence of systemic PAN. Other non-specific laboratory findings include an elevated erythrocyte sedimentation rate, a significant leukocytosis with eosinophilia, and anemia with hypergammaglobulinemia. In pediatric series, elevated anti-streptococcal antibodies are common but the presence of circulating hepatitis B antigen is a rare occurrence, whereas it is positive in about 30% of adult cases. High blood urea nitrogen levels with hematuria and proteinuria reflect kidney involvement. Abdominal and cerebral arteriography often show aneurysms.

HISTOPATHOLOGICAL FINDINGS

The cutaneous lesions of PAN are characterized by a leukocytoclastic vasculitis that involves medium and small arteries (Figs 103.3 and 103.4). Within the wall of medium-sized arteries situated in the septa of the subcutaneous fat is abundant fibrin in a mixture of inflammatory cells (neutrophils, eosinophils, lymphocytes, plasma cells and histiocytes). This infiltrate is accompanied by variable amounts of nuclear 'dust' surrounding the fibrin-containing vessel and, eventually by fibroplasia.

ETIOLOGY AND PATHOGENESIS

The etiology of PAN is obscure. It has been hypothesized that the disease may be triggered by several infective agents (e.g. streptococcal, hepatitis B virus infection). It is considered an immune complex-mediated disease.

MANAGEMENT

In benign cutaneous PAN, treatment with non-steroidal anti-inflammatory drugs and moderate doses of prednisone is successful. In systemic PAN, combined therapy with prednisone and an immunosuppressive agent (e.g. cyclophosphamide, azathioprine) is indicated.

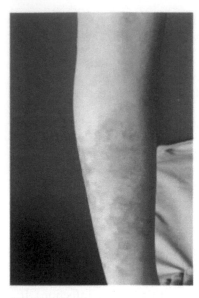

Figure 103.1
Benign cutaneous polyarteritis nodosa. Star-burst livedo reticularis and nodulation on a leg.

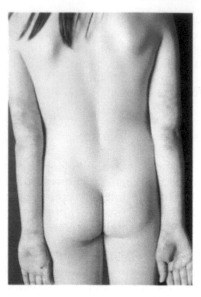

Figure 103.2
Benign cutaneous polyarteritis nodosa. Livedo reticularis with few nodules distributed bilaterally on the arms and the palms of an 11-year-old girl.

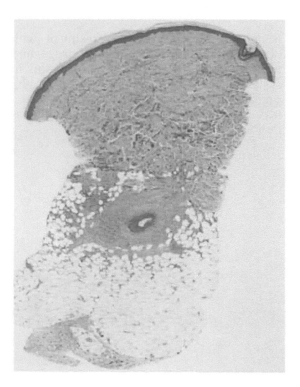

Figure 103.3

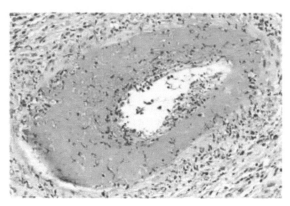

Figure 103.4

Figures 103.3 and 103.4
Polyarteritis nodosa. The histological findings of leuko-cytoclastic vasculitis (neutrophils, nuclear 'dust' and deposits of fibrin) are seen within and around a small artery situated in the subcutaneous fat. Secondary to the vascular changes there is a circumscribed lobular panni-culitis in the vicinity of the affected blood vessel.

104 POLYMORPHOUS LIGHT ERUPTION

The term polymorphous light eruption describes an acquired itching dermatosis of unknown origin. It is characterized by a delayed abnormal reaction to sunlight and it has heterogeneous morphological features.

EPIDEMIOLOGY

Polymorphic light eruption is the commonest photodermatosis – for example, it affects 10–20% of the population in the USA. All races may be affected, and females are more prone to develop the disease than males. Onset in early childhood or infancy is not infrequent in temperate areas.

CLINICAL FINDINGS

The disease typically starts in spring or early summer. The time of exposure necessary to induce the rash varies from a few minutes to some hours. In most cases the onset is acute. The distribution of the lesions is usually symmetrical on sun-exposed areas. The most frequent site is the face (Fig. 104.1), followed by the breast area, the dorsum of the hands, the arms and the limbs.

The morphological features of the eruption are very variable, and many different types of primary lesions have been described (vesicles, papules, erythema, edema, nodules, plaques and blisters) (Fig. 104.2). Moreover, several clinical patterns have been described. The commonest of these are a vesicopapular pattern (seen in 77% of patients), a prurigo-like pattern (seen in 24%), an eczematous pattern (seen in 13%) and a maculopapular pattern (seen in 11%). A combination of these lesions may be found, but usually one type predominates.

Itching is an important feature, being reported as present in percentages ranging from 51% to 100% of patients; a burning sensation has been reported in 66% of patients and tenderness to the touch in 34%. About 50% of patients have problems in the lips and the eyes, including light sensitivity of the eyes, redness of the conjunctiva, lacrimation, and drying and chapping of the lips. General malaise is present in about 69% of cases in relation to the skin outbreaks. However, general symptoms are usually mild; they include chills, fever, headache and nausea (the headache and nausea occurring some days after sun exposure). Lesions tend to involute spontaneously in 2–3 weeks if no further sun exposure occurs. The disease is chronic and tends to recur annually for many years.

LABORATORY FINDINGS

There is no laboratory parameter that is specific for polymorphous light eruption. Phototesting, using a broad spectrum of light in an area previously affected by early outbreaks of the disease may induce the lesions and may represent an important aid in establishing the diagnosis.

HISTOPATHOLOGICAL FINDINGS

Polymorphous light eruption is characterized by a superficial and deep, perivascular lymphocytic infiltrate together with edema of the papillary dermis (Fig. 104.3).

ETIOLOGY AND PATHOGENESIS

The etiopathogenesis of polymorphous light eruption is still unknown. However, a genetic predisposition undoubtedly has a role. A delayed hypersensitivity reaction to an antigen induced by ultraviolet light is a possible hypothesis.

MANAGEMENT

The therapy of polymorphous light eruption remains empirical. Avoidance of sunlight and broad-spectrum sunscreens are the prophylactic measures for milder forms of polymorphous light eruption. In children, beta-carotene (5–10 mg/kg per day) is the drug of choice because of its lack of side effects. Synthetic antimalarial agents are effective but must be used with caution and only in severe cases. In children it is better to avoid oral psoralen photochemotherapy, but ultraviolet-B therapy is safe and may be prophylactic, producing an increased resistance to sunlight ('hardening' phenomenon). Corticosteroid creams may help to shorten the duration of the cutaneous lesions and to relieve the itching.

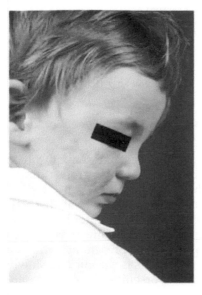

Figure 104.1
Polymorphous light eruption. Vesicopapular lesions with a tendency to confluence.

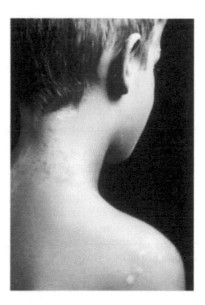

Figure 104.2
Polymorphous light eruption. The pink papules are both discrete and confluent on the neck.

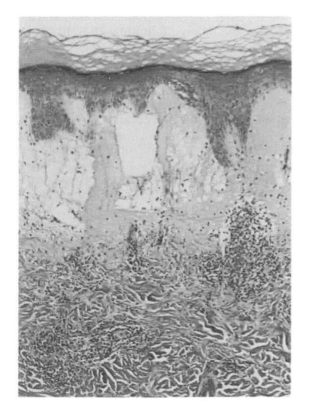

Figure 104.3
Polymorphous light eruption. The changes demonstrate a mostly lymphocytic infiltrate around the vessels of the superficial and deep plexus and marked edema of the papillary dermis that eventually form subepidermal vesiculation. These histological findings are seen in evolving lesions of polymorphous light eruption.

Porokeratosis is a chronic, progessive, asymptomatic keratoatrophoderma that takes various clinical forms. It is characterized histologically by columns of parakeratosis known as cornoid lamellae. Four clinical variants have been described in pediatric patients – the classical plaque porokeratosis of Mibelli, disseminated superficial porokeratosis (porokeratosis palmaris, plantaris et disseminata), porokeratosis punctata palmaris et plantaris, and linear porokeratosis.

EPIDEMIOLOGY

Porokeratosis is rare but not exceptional. In children the classical plaque type seems to be the commonest type. Porokeratosis usually occurs during childhood.

CLINICAL FINDINGS

In all forms of porokeratosis, the primary lesion is a small, hyperkeratotic papule that gradually enlarges to form a plaque with a raised, wall-like border that resembles a dike and an atrophic depressed center (Fig. 105.1). Classical porokeratosis of Mibelli (see Fig. 105.1) may have one or a few lesions of variable morphology located anywhere on the body, although the predilection is for the face and the extremities, including the palms and the soles. Mucous membrane may be involved. Rarely, lesions of 100–300 mm in diameter (giant porokeratosis) may be seen. In disseminated superficial porokeratosis, the lesions are uniform and widespread and do not exceed 10 mm in diameter. In porokeratosis punctata palmaris et plantaris, the lesions

present as numerous, seed-like keratotic plugs of 1–2 mm diameter that arise from rimmed crypts. In the linear variant, the lesions assume a zosteriform or unilateral distribution (Fig. 105.2), most commonly on the extremities, and resemble a linear verrucous nevus. This form may be present at birth. The course of all the variants is chronic and slowly progressive, with worsening after sun explosure.

HISTOPATHOLOGICAL FINDINGS

Although there are some differences among the types of porokeratosis, each is characterized by the following findings (Fig. 105.3):

- a cornoid lamella composed of a column of parakeratosis, beneath which the granular zone is thinned and the spinous zone contains vacuolated and dyskeratotic cells;
- a superficial perivascular infiltrate of lymphocytes;
- a lichenoid infiltrate of lymphocytes in evolving lesions;
- a thinned epidermis devoid of rete ridges together with muted dermal papillae in devolving lesions.

ETIOLOGY AND PATHOGENESIS

Porokeratoses are genodermatoses with an autosomal-dominant mode of inheritance. The linear form frequently occurs sporadically. The primary defect in porokeratosis seems to be the proliferation of abnormal clones of epidermal cells. A locus at chromosome 12q23.2-34 is responsible for disseminated superficial actinic porokeratosis only. Various triggering factors such as actinic radiation or immunosuppression may lead to the development of these dystrophic clones of epidermal cells.

MANAGEMENT

Treatment is generally unsatisfactory. Keratolytics and topical retinoids help to keep the lesions smooth and asymptomatic

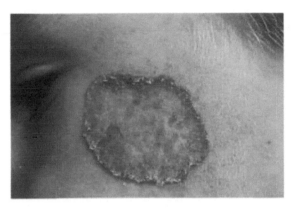

Figure 105.1
Porokeratosis of Mibelli. This somewhat annular, well-circumscribed lesion is characterized by a wall of hyperkeratosis and a central zone of post-inflammatory hyperpigmentation.

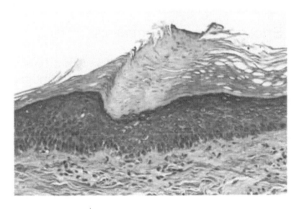

Figure 105.3
Porokeratosis of Mibelli. This lesion shows a cornoid lamella composed of a column of parakeratosis, underneath which the epidermis is devoid of the granular zone and the spinous layer contains vacuolated cells.

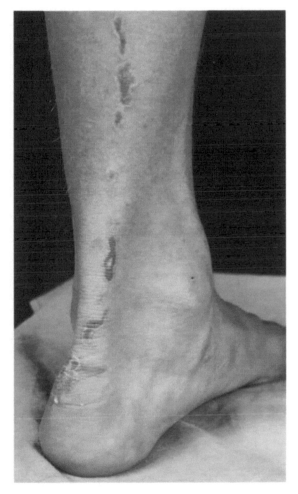

Figure 105.2
Linear porokeratosis. This linear streak is composed of numerous lesions of porokeratosis, which are characterized by a rim of hyperkeratosis and a center of hyperpigmentation.

The porphyrias are a heterogeneous group of disorders linked to enzymatic defects in the biosynthetic pathway of heme. They are characterized by excessive production of porphyrins or their precursors. Clinically, the porphyrias may be classified as:

- acute, when they cause acute visceral attacks without cutaneous manifestations;
- cutaneous, when only cutaneous manifestations are present;
- mixed, when acute attacks alternate with cutaneous manifestations.

All these variants are very rare. This chapter looks at the cutaneous porphyrias.

PORPHYRIA CUTANEA TARDA

CLINICAL FINDINGS

Porphyria cutanea tarda (PCT) is rare in children, in whom it is seen mainly in association with two conditions – familial PCT and PCT due to hexachlorobenzene.

PCT is characterized by moderate photosensitivity and fragility of the skin. Non-inflammatory serous or hemorrhagic vesicles and blisters develop on uncovered sites (mainly the dorsum of the hands and the face) (Fig. 106.1), after mechanical trauma (traumatic blisters), or after exposure to sunlight (actinic blisters). Sometimes itching may precede the onset of the lesions. Indolent erosions and serohematic crusts (see Fig. 106.1) rapidly follow and then heal to leave whitish scars, milia and areas of hyperpigmentation and hypopigmentation. Moreover, hypertrichosis, mainly of the malar areas, and hyperpigmen-

tation of sun-exposed areas are also common findings. Usually, all these lesions present are at the same time. Urine is brown in color. PCT is a chronic disease with seasonal worsening related to sunlight exposure.

LABORATORY FINDINGS

A high increase in plasma and urinary uroporphyrins, mainly isomer I, and 7-carboxylate porphyrin is typical of PCT. In most cases, the urine reveals coral-pink fluorescence when observed by Wood's lamp. High serum levels of transaminases and gamma-glutamyl transpeptidase are common and reflect hepatic involvement. Elevated amounts of serum iron and high levels of serum ferritin are found in one-third to one-half of patients.

ETIOLOGY AND PATHOGENESIS

PCT is due to a metabolic defect that halves the activity of hepatic uroporphyrinogen decarboxylase, the enzyme that catalyses decarboxylation of the four acetate groups to methyl. This reduction in enzyme activity may occur in familial PCT and non-familial PCT.

MANAGEMENT

Avoidance of exposure to sunlight and to exogenous triggers is mandatory. Applications of sunblock creams may be useful. Low doses of chloroquine given twice a week is the treatment of choice for the infantile form of PCT, whereas phlebotomy is contraindicated.

HEPATOERYTHROPOIETIC PORPHYRIA

CLINICAL FINDINGS

Hepatoerythropoietic porphyria is characterized by extreme photosensitivity with photophobia and fragility of the skin. Dark urine is an early and constant hallmark of the disease and is usually present from birth. Blistering with erosions and crusting usually occurs after exposure to the sun or mild trauma, during the 1st year of life (Fig. 106.2). Hyperpigmentation and pronounced hypertrichosis (see Fig. 106.2) are other features of the disease. Scarring may lead to severe sclerodermoid changes and, in extreme cases, to amputations of acral portions of the body and face. Erythrodontia has been reported only rarely. A general physical examination usually does not reveal pathological findings. However, hepatosplenomegaly is rarely found. The disease has a chronic course.

LABORATORY FINDINGS

The urinary porphyrins pattern is very similar to that observed in PCT. However, there are elevated levels of zinc-chelated protoporphyrin in red blood cells, and there are high levels of isocoproporphyrin and of coproporphyrin in the feces.

ETIOLOGY AND PATHOGENESIS

The disease is caused by a severe defect in the activity of uroporphyrinogen decarboxylase, which has 8–10% residual activity, in erythrocytes and hepatocytes.

MANAGEMENT

There is no specific treatment. Beta-carotene is not very effective, and hydroxychloroquine has been tried without any improvement of the clinical conditions. Strict avoidance of sunlight is advisable.

ERYTHROPOIETIC PROTOPORPHYRIA

CLINICAL FINDINGS

Erythropoietic protoporphyria usually begins early in childhood. Severe photosensivity is the clinical hallmark of the disease. Burning sensations develop after a few minutes of sun exposure in 91% of cases, and pruritus is present in 88% of cases and pain in 67%. Sometimes these sensations are not followed by any objective sign on the skin, so a correct diagnosis may be missed. Visible skin changes consist mainly of edematous urticaria-like plaques (seen in 94% of patients with skin manifestations) and erythema (seen in 69%). Papulovesicles and petechial lesions are found only in about 3% of cases. In 20% of patients, small varioliform scars may develop on the cheeks, the nose (Fig. 106.3) and the dorsum of the hands. Perioral pseudoragades and a typical thickening and furrowing of the skin over the knuckles and dorsum of the hands are other markers of the disease. Severe acute abdominal pain and jaundice accompanying hepatic damage have been reported in some cases. The course is chronic.

LABORATORY FINDINGS

High levels of free protoporphyrin are usually found in plasma, red blood cells and feces, but not in urine, owing to the insolubility of this porphyrin in water. Red blood cells show a characteristic transient coral-red fluorescence when examined by a fluorescence microscope under a lamp emitting a 400 nm wavelength. This test is so highly specific and sensitive that it is considered the screening test of choice.

ETIOLOGY AND PATHOGENESIS

The disease is caused by a biochemical defect in the activity of ferrochelatase (heme synthetase) in red blood cells, liver, and fibroblasts. This abnormality appears to be inherited in an autosomal dominant mode with variable penetrance.

MANAGEMENT

Applications of sunblock creams and avoidance of sun exposure must be recommended. Oral beta-carotene and canthaxanthine have been used but their effectiveness is controversial.

CONGENITAL ERYTHROPOIETIC PORPHYRIA

CLINICAL FINDINGS

Congenital erythropoietic porphyria (Gunther's disease) starts at birth or early in infancy. A typical discoloration of diapers, ranging from pink to brown, and extreme photosensivity are the first signs of disease. Recurring episodes of blistering appear on the face and the hands a few hours after sunlight exposure. Erosions and crusting follow and leave mottled hypopigmentation and hyperpigmentation (Fig. 106.4). Ulcerations cause severe scarring with loss of subcutaneous tissue and progressive sclerodermatous and mutilating changes (see Fig. 106.4). Scarring alopecia of the scalp is common, but hypertrichosis is seen in mildly involved areas, mainly on the face and the extremities. Photophobia is severe, and keratoconjunctivitis leads to scarring with ectropion, symblepharon and ultimately scleromalacia perforans. Teeth are brown–yellow and show a red fluorescence (erythrodontia) when observed with Wood's lamp. In addition, there is often hemolytic anemia and splenomegaly. The urine is pink. The course is chronic and progressive.

LABORATORY FINDINGS

The urine contains markedly increased levels of uroporphyrin I and mildly raised amounts of coproporphyrin I. In the faeces, coproporphyrin I is more prevalent than uroporphyrin I. Erythrocytes and erythroblasts contain high amounts of uroporphyrin I and have stable red fluorescence under Wood's lamp. Hemolytic anemia is characterized by normochromic anemia, shortened red blood cell survival time, and increased excretion of fecal urobilinogen.

ETIOLOGY AND PATHOGENESIS

Congenital erythropoietic porphyria is caused by an autosomal-recessively inherited deficiency of uroporphyrinogen synthetase.

MANAGEMENT

Treatment is inevitably anecdotal because of the rarity of the disease, and no controlled trial has been obtained. Chloroquine, beta-carotene, hematin and cyclophosphamide seem to be useful.

HISTOPATHOLOGICAL FINDINGS

All variants of cutaneous porphyria present similar findings and, of these, the most common are subepidermal blisters. These blisters are characterized by preservation of the dermal papillae and a dermis that is either entirely devoid of inflammatory cells or that contains a rather sparse infiltrate (Fig. 106.5 and 106.6). Venules and capillaries of the superficial plexus may be rimmed by homogeneous eosinophilic material that is periodic acid–Schiff-positive and diastase-resistant. These rims are most prominent in erythropoietic protoporphyria and least prominent in PCT.

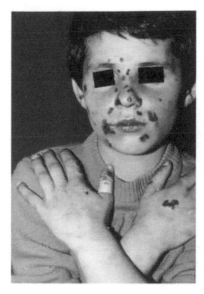

Figure 106.1
Porphyria cutanea tarda. Hemorrhagic crusts are present at sites of previous subepidermal blisters. Hemorrhagic crusts can be seen to heal with hypopigmented and hyperpigmented scars. All the lesions occur on sun-exposed sites.

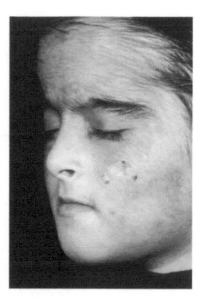

Figure 106.2
Hepatic erythropoietic porphyria. This varant of porphyria cutanea is characterized by subepidermal blisters, crusts and hypopigmented scars. Extensive hypertrichosis is often present on the face, as is commonly the case in PCT.

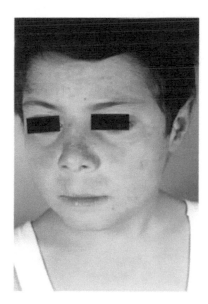

Figure 106.3
Erythropoietic protoporphyria. There are depressed, hyper-pigmented scars on the forehead, the nose, the cheeks and the upper lip.

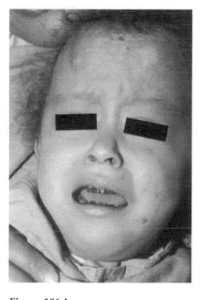

Figure 106.4
Congenital erythropoietic porphyria. The teeth are yellow–brown and show a red fluorescence (erythrodontia) when examined with Wood's light. Atrophic scars and crusts are present on the face.

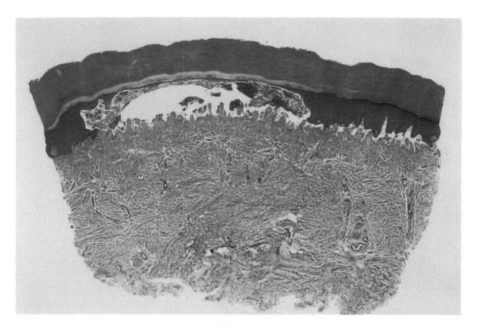

Figure 106.5

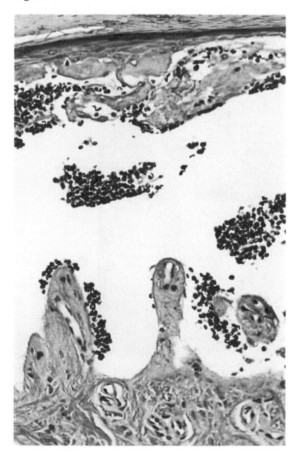

Figures 106.5 and 106.6

Porphyria cutanea tarda. At scanning magnification (Fig. 106.5), there is a subepidermal serohemorrhagic blister and a dermis that is nearly devoid of inflammatory cells. At high magnification (Fig. 106.6), the dermal papillae appear to be preserved, and thin rims of eosinophilic material are seen around the vessels of the papillary dermis.

Figure 106.6

PSEUDOLYMPHOMA

Cutaneous pseudolymphoma is a descriptive term for a heterogeneous group of benign inflammatory disorders characterized by reactive lymphoid infiltrates in the skin that simulate cutaneous lymphomas clinically or histologically. Numerous synonyms have been used for the designation of pseudolymphomas of the skin, including lymphocytoma cutis, lymphadenosis benigna cutis, Spiegler–Fendt sarcoid and cutaneous lymphoid hyperplasia.

EPIDEMIOLOGY

Pseudolymphomas are frequently seen in children and adolescents.

CLINICAL FINDINGS

Cutaneous pseudolymphomas can reveal various features. The lesions may be papules, nodules (Fig. 107.1), or plaques (Fig. 107.2). These lesions are generally firm but not hard, their surface is smooth, and their color ranges from pink to reddish brown; the most common color of pseudolymphomas in Caucasian skin is plum or rose. Pseudolymphomas practically never ulcerate. They may present as solitary lesions, multiple lesions confined to a particular part or, rarely, as widespread lesions. The localized forms are commoner in infants and children. Single lesions may expand peripherally and show a circinate arrangement. The face is the area of predilection (in 70% of cases), but other parts of the body may be affected. The course is unpredictable. Lesions may persists for months or years, they may resolve spontaneously, and they may recur.

HISTOPATHOLOGICAL FINDINGS

The least common denominator for diagnosis of pseudolymphomas is a nodular or diffuse infiltrate that consists mostly of small lymphocytes (Figs 107.3 and 107.4). In a small percentage of pseudolymphomas, germinal centers form within the infiltrate and tingible bodies (lymphocytic nuclear debris within macrophages) are present within them. Since these pseudolymphomas can mimic cutaneous B-cell lymphomas or cutaneous T-cell lymphomas histologically, they are divided into pseudo-B-cell lymphomas and pseudo-T-cell lymphomas. The application of monoclonal antibodies provides the basis for a more precise classification of cutaneous pseudolymphomas. According to the distribution of different compartments, four immunohistological types can be recognized:

- band-like T-cell pseudolymphomas;
- nodular T-cell pseudolymphomas;
- follicular B-cell pseudolymphomas;
- non-follicular B-cell pseudolymphomas.

The presence of a follicular B-cell pattern with polyclonal light chains and the absence of aberrant patterns of antigen expression (e.g. loss of some T-cell antigens) are the most important immunohistochemical findings in favor of cutaneous pseudolymphomas.

Recently, molecular analysis for the study of clonal rearrangements of the immunoglobulins or T-cell receptor genes was used to distinguish pseudolymphomas from true malignant lymphomas. In fact, most primary cutaneous B-cell or T-cell lymphomas show rearrangements of the heavy and light immunoglobulin chains and of the beta chain of the T-cell receptor, whereas no rearranged bands are usually detected in cutaneous pseudolymphomas.

ETIOLOGY AND PATHOGENESIS

The causes of cutaneous pseudolymphomas are largely unknown, but in some cases a triggering stimulus may be identified. In children, pseudolymphomas may develop in untreated scabies (nodular scabies), after insect bites (in particular tick bites that transmit a *Borrelia* infection), after antigen injections, and during treatment with antiepileptic drugs (e.g. phenytoin).

MANAGEMENT

Cutaneous pseudolymphomas can be treated with surgical excision, topical and intralesional corticosteroids, and cryosurgery.

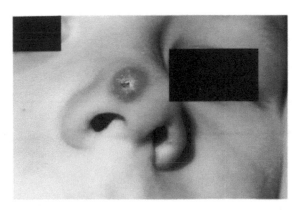

Figure 107.1
Pseudolymphoma. This dome-shaped, orange–pink nodule is covered by scales and crusts.

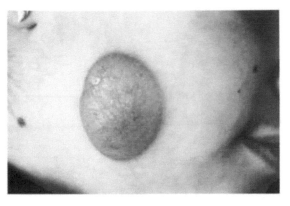

Figure 107.2
Pseudolymphoma. This slightly domed orange–brown plaque is well circumscribed.

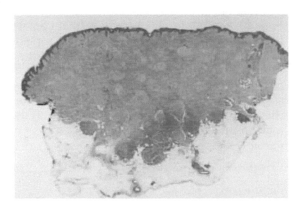

Figure 107.3

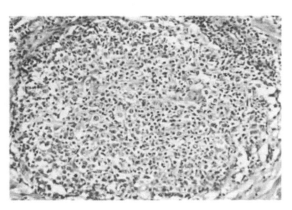

Figure 107.4

Figures 107.3 and 107.4
B-cell pseudolymphoma. This wedge-shaped lesion is made up of numerous well-defined lymphoid follicles that house germinal centers. At high magnification, tingible bodies are seen within macrophages sited in those centers. In short, these are the findings of follicular B-cell pseudolymphoma.

108 PSEUDOXANTHOMA ELASTICUM

Pseudoxanthoma elasticum is an hereditary connective tissue disorder that primarily affects the skin, the eyes and the cardiovascular system.

EPIDEMIOLOGY

The prevalence of the disease is considered to be about 1 in 100,000 persons. The disorder appears to be more common in women by a ratio of 2:1. The average age of onset of skin lesions is 13.5 years.

CLINICAL FINDINGS

Skin changes

The skin lesions are lemon yellow, xanthoma-like papules that join to form soft, lax plaques. These lesions give the affected area a 'pricked-chicken-skin' appearance (Fig. 108.1). The sites of predilection are the sides of the neck (see Fig. 108.1) and the flexural folds (the axillae and the antecubital, inguinal, abdominal and popliteal regions). Mucosal lesions may be present. Progression of the lesions from head to toe is the rule. Occasionally, and mainly in adults, spontaneous perforating lesions that present as well-demarcated, rough and hyperpigmented plaques with keratotic papules may be seen in the periumbilical and nuchal areas (perforating pseudoxanthoma elasticum). Pseudoxanthoma elasticum is a progressive disorder and the skin has a continuous cosmetic deterioration.

Ocular changes

The most characteristic ocular findings are angioid streaks, which first appear during adolescence in about 50–80% of patients but are not specific for the disorder. They consist of bilateral gray streaks radiating from the optic disk and lying behind the retinal vessels. Peculiar pigmentary retinal changes appearing as a speckled and yellowish mottled fundus may be an early finding. Eye abnormalities are slowly progressive, and may be associated with choroidal and retinal hemorrhages that lead to impairment of vision. If the macula is involved, central blindness of variable degree is the result.

Cardiovascular changes

Cardiovascular involvement is characterized by arterial calcification, which can lead to a systemic circulatory insufficiency. This process is evolved slowly, and it is very similar to atherosclerosis. The limbs are most commonly affected (30% of patients have intermittent claudication).

HISTOPATHOLOGICAL FINDINGS

The crucial histopathological changes in pseudoxanthoma elasticum reside in the reticular dermis and especially in the lower half. Tangles of decidedly abnormal elastic tissue can be discerned there (Fig. 108.2). In early lesions, no calcium is deposited on the abnormal elastic tissue, whereas in late lesions elastic fibers are completely obscured by abundant deposits of calcium. The appearance of the abnormal elastic tissue has been compared to steel wool and balls of yarn.

ETIOLOGY AND PATHOGENESIS

Pseudoxanthoma elasticum is a clinically and genetically heterogeneous disease. At least two autosomal-dominant and three autosomal-recessive subtypes have been recognized. These subtypes differ in the severity of the ophthalmological and vascular manifestations. The autosomal-recessive forms are the commoner types. The basic defect of pseudo-xanthoma elasticum remains unknown. It is unclear whether the deposition of calcium is a primary or a secondary event.

MANAGEMENT

The appearance of the skin of patients with pseudoxanthoma elasticum may be improved by plastic surgery. Periodic cardiovascular surveillance is absolutely necessary. Smoking should be discouraged. The usefulness of reducing calcium intake is debated, but it seems a reasonable measure. Ophthalmological examination should be undertaken annually. Laser photocoagulation is a procedure of great benefit in preventing retinal hemorrhage. Genetic counselling should be offered.

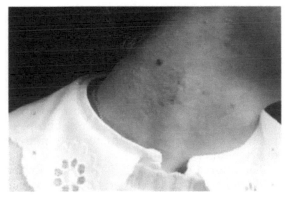

Figure 108.1
Pseudoxanthoma elasticum. Yellowish and xanthoma-like papules are confluent in plaques, giving the affected area a 'pricked-chicken-skin' appearance. The sides of the neck are a site of predilection.

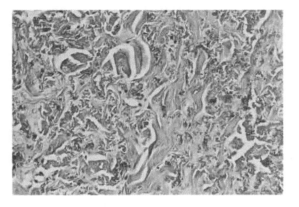

Figure 108.2
Pseudoxanthoma elasticum. In the reticular dermis, the distinctive finding is accumulation of irregularly clumped basophilic elastic fibers whose appearance resembles steel wool or balls of yarn. Abnormal elastic fibers are demonstrated vividly by orcein stain.

Psoriasis is a common chronic skin disease characterized by sharply demarcated erythematous scaling lesions that especially involve the scalp and the extensor surfaces in adolescents and adults, and the scalp and the skin folds in infants.

EPIDEMIOLOGY

The prevalence of psoriasis differs greatly from country to country. Available findings show a range between 0 and 5% in the general population. Psoriasis in childhood is not so common as in adults, but there are no definitive epidemiological studies. Psoriasis seems to have earlier onset in females than in males.

CLINICAL FINDINGS

Many clinical forms of psoriasis may occur in children. Guttate psoriasis is the commonest form of psoriasis in children. It is characterized by a sudden appearance, usually after an upper respiratory tract infection of streptococcal origin. Drop-like, round or oval lesions are scattered over the body, sparing the face (Fig. 109.1). The eruption is asymptomatic and lasts for several weeks, showing the tendency to heal spontaneously, at least in part.

Nummular psoriasis is less common in children than in adults but it presents the same clinical features. Sharply demarcated erythematous scaling lesions (Fig. 109.2) are usually located on the elbows, the knees, the scalp and the lumbosacral areas. The diaper area is involved in almost all infants. Not infrequently in children the disease involves the folds (inverse psoriasis), the genitalia, the eyelids and the palms and the soles. Large plaques may form by coalescence of several lesions. An isomorphic response (the Koebner phenomenon) may appear at sites of trauma.

Erythrodermic psoriasis arising *de novo* is occasionally observed in the neonatal period. Generalization of pre-existing cutaneous lesions (Fig. 109.3) may occur in association with drug allergy, atopic dermatitis, sunburn and leukemia.

Pustular psoriasis in children is rare and presents in three main clinical forms. The generalized form (von Zumbush variety) is characterized by an explosive, diffuse eruption of sterile, pinhead pustules associated with high fever, malaise, anorexia and pain (Fig. 109.4). This form is not usually preceded by psoriasis vulgaris. The annular form is commoner and less severe; it is characterized by erythema and pustules in circinate patterns.

The localized palmoplantar form (Barber variety) is characterized by recurrent crops of pustules of 2–4 mm in diameter within areas of erythema and scaling.

The course of psoriasis is usually chronic with remissions and exacerbations. Seasonal variations are common. Erythrodermic and pustular psoriasis appear to be less severe in children than in adults.

Associations

In all of the juvenile forms of psoriasis, the involvement of nails is rather common (seen in about 50% of patients). Involved nails display pitting, discoloration, onycholysis and subungueal hyperkeratosis. Whereas psoriatic arthritis was in the past believed to be extremely rare in children, recent literature reports several new cases quite regularly. Pustular psoriasis in children may be associated with geographic tongue, but this symptom is now considered to be a reactive phenomenon that can occur in many conditions.

LABORATORY FINDINGS

During the acute flare of pustular psoriasis there is leucocytosis, an elevated erythrocyte sedimentation rate, hypocalcemia and hypoalbuminemia. Elevated antistreptolysin-O titer may or may not accompany guttate psoriasis; thus, the presence of streptococci must be excluded with multiple swabs.

HISTOPATHOLOGICAL FINDINGS

The psoriatic lesion is characterized by mounds of parakeratosis adorned by neutrophils at their summits, a focal decrease in the thickness of the granular zone, small collections of neutrophils within the spinous and granular layer (spongiform pustules or microabscesses of Munro–Sabouraud), slight epidermal hyperplasia, dilated tortuous capillaries in dermal papillae, extravasated erythrocytes in the papillary dermis and in foci within the epidermis, and a sparse superficial perivascular infiltrate composed mostly of lymphocytes but with a sprinkling of neutrophils (Fig. 109.5). There are an increased number of mitotic figures above the basal layer.

Pustular psoriasis is merely an acceleration of the psoriasic process and, as consequence, spongiform, subcorneal and intracorneal pustules are present throughout the epidermis, which is only slightly hyperplastic (Fig. 109.6). Because the process is so rapid, the epidermis does not have time to become psoriasiform.

ETIOLOGY AND PATHOGENESIS

The cause of psoriasis is unknown. Genetic factors seems to play a crucial role in the etiology of the disease. To date, however, the inheritance pattern is unclear. Increased epidermal proliferation is the prime pathogenic fault. Hyperproliferation of epidermal cells may be influenced by many factors such as abnormal dermal-epidermal interactions, shortening of the reproductive cell cycle, defects in cyclic adenosine monophosphate, loss of the contact between keratinocytes, inhibition of growth, and lack of T-suppressor cells. Infections of the urinary tract and of the upper respiratory tract, stress and certain photosensitizing medications may precipitate psoriatic episodes.

MANAGEMENT

Treatment of psoriasis vulgaris in children must take into consideration the chronicity of the disease and should be as simple as possible. In the case of diaper-induced psoriasis, the treatment will be the same as for any uncomplicated diaper rash, so that the primary goal is to reduce local maceration and rubbing with frequent changing, superabsorbent diapers, and protective absorbent paste. A general course of a specific antibiotic is needed whenever an infective focus is discovered. The topical use of keratolytics and tar preparations, local calcipotriol, exposure to sunlight and the Goeckerman regimen are often sufficient to induce remission of the lesions and to keep patients in good cutaneous condition. Topical corticosteroids should be used only on limited areas and for short periods of time. Systemic corticosteroids and psoralen and ultraviolet-A therapy as well as antimetabolites are contraindicated in childhood psoriasis. In the pustular forms, one should start with mild local treatment. The use of oral retinoids should be preferred to methotrexate, except in cases of very severe manifestations.

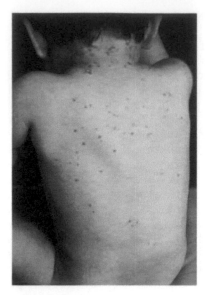

Figure 109.1
Guttate psoriasis. Drop-like, orange–brown papules covered by scales are scattered over the trunk.

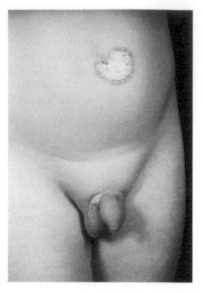

Figure 109.2
Nummular psoriasis. Psoriasis commonly involves the umbelicus and the genitalia, as seen here. The umbilical lesion is characterized by central whitish scales and an elevated orangish border.

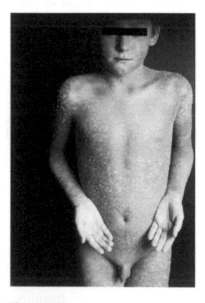

Figure 109.3
Erythrodermic psoriasis. The generalization of erythematous scaling lesions is the consequence of prolonged corticosteroid treatment. The palms and soles are spared.

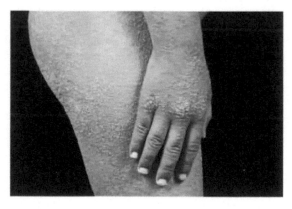

Figure 109.4
Pustular psoriasis (von Zumbush type). Myriad pustules are widespread and many have become confluent. In time, there will be 'lakes' of pus. These pustules are sterile.

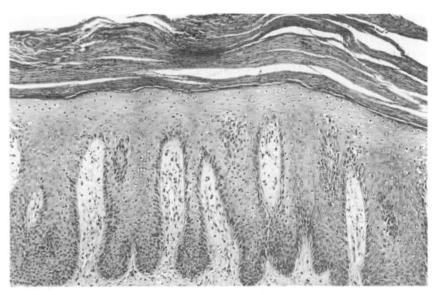

Figure 109.5
Psoriasis. This fully developed psoriatic lesion is characterized by marked psoriasiform epidermal hyperplasia with thin but club-shaped rete ridges of approximately equal length, confluent parakeratosis, absence of the granular layer, pallor of the upper part of the epidermis, thin edematous dermal papillae within which are dilated and tortuous capillaries, and a sparse inflammatory infiltrate composed of lymphocytes, histiocytes and neutrophils. Small collections of neutrophils appear to be staggered throughout a thickened parakeratotic horny layer.

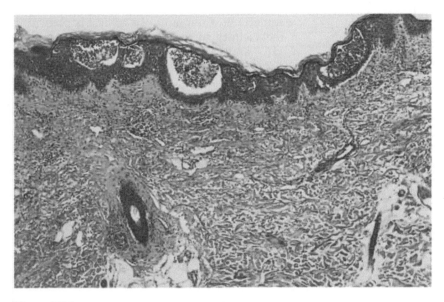

Figure 109.6
Pustular psoriasis. With low-power magnification a few spongiform pustules can be seen within the epidermis. Spongiform pustules form when neutrophils migrate from the capillary of the papillary dermis to the spinous and granular layers, where they group in small collections within the interstices of a sponge-like network caused by degeneration and thinning of epidermal cells. As the size of the pustule increases, a single large cavity develops in the centre of the pustule, whereas the spongiform network persists at the periphery. In pustular psoriasis, spongiform pustules form quickly and the epidermis has no time to become hyperplastic as in plaque lesions of psoriasis.

110

PYODERMA GANGRENOSUM

Pyoderma gangrenosum is an uncommon, inflammatory, ulcerative chronic skin disorder that frequently occurs in association with systemic diseases.

EPIDEMIOLOGY

The condition is extremely rare in the pediatric age range. The average age of onset is 40 years. The youngest reported patient was 7 months old.

CLINICAL FINDINGS

The lesions may start as vesicopustules or erythematous nodules, and subsequently evolve into distinctive, indolent, necrotizing ulcerations. The ulcers are round or polycyclic with bluish violet undermined borders surrounded by peripheral zones of erythema (Figs 110.1 and 110.2). When pressed, the borders issue purulent drops. Pyoderma gangrenosum occurs more frequently on the limbs, but any area of the body may be involved. Lesions may be single or multiple. Adjacent lesions may coalesce. The development of lesions at the sites of minor trauma (pathergy phenomenon) has been noted in many of the cases in children. The course is chronic and erratic. The average duration of cutaneous lesions is 20 years. Some lesions may enlarge rapidly and also regress rapidly; others may remain unchanged for months. When healing occurs, atrophic scars are left.

Associations

In children, pyoderma gangrenosum is nearly always associated with systemic abnormalities such as inflammatory bowel diseases (the most common association), arthritis, cardio-vascular diseases, Takayasu's arteritis, sarcoidosis, hypogammaglobulinemia and leukemia. The prognosis of the disease depends on these associated disorders.

LABORATORY FINDINGS

There are no specific laboratory findings for this disorder. Elevated erythrocyte sedimentation rate, leukocytosis and mild anemia are common findings.

HISTOPATHOLOGICAL FINDINGS

Histopathology is not diagnostic and consists of abscesses in the dermis or subcutaneous fat devoid of granulomatous inflammation; sometimes a remnant of a follicle is present in the vicinity of the zone of suppuration (Figs 110.3 and 110.4).

ETIOLOGY AND PATHOGENESIS

The cause and the precise pathogenic mechanism of this disorder remain unknown. A derangement in humoral or cell-mediated immunity or neutrophil functions is considered the most likely cause of pyoderma gangrenosum. Pyoderma gangrenosum may be caused by the same immunological disorder responsible for the development of an underlying disease, or it may represent a hypersensitivity reaction secondary to the underlying disease.

MANAGEMENT

The treatment of pyoderma gangrenosum in childhood is often difficult. Many drugs, such as corticosteroids, sulfapyridine or dapsone, thalidomide, cyclophosphamide, clofazimine and minocycline, may be tried.

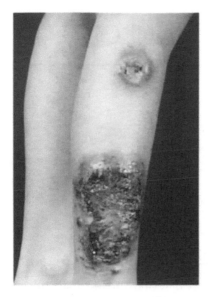

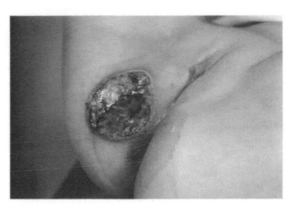

Figure 110.2
Pyoderma gangrenosum. A large, deep ulcer surrounded by an elevated border in the perineal area of a little girl.

Figure 110.1
Pyoderma gangrenosum. There are discrete pustules, boggy plaques on reddish bases, and a large, deep ulcer surrounded by a boggy border with evidence of hemorrhage and necrosis.

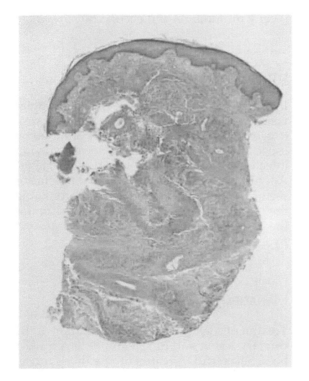

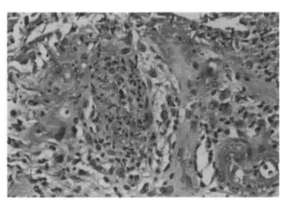

Figure 110.4

Figures 110.3 and 110.4
Pyoderma gangrenosum. The section that comes from the peripheral border of a lesion of pyoderma gangrenosum shows a neutrophilic abscess within the dermis and subcutaneous tissue accompanied by hemorrhagic areas. As a consequence of the acute inflammatory process a vasculitis in the form of fibrin and nuclear 'dust' in the wall of small vessels is evident at the periphery of the suppurative area.

Figure 110.3

111

PYOGENIC GRANULOMA

Pyogenic granuloma is a rapidly developing, sessile or polypoid, vascular nodule that tends towards ulceration and bleeding.

EPIDEMIOLOGY

Pyogenic granuloma is common and represents 0.5% of all skin nodules in children. The commonness of this lesion seems to decline almost linearly with age. The majority of pyogenic granulomas appear within the first 5 years of life.

CLINICAL FINDINGS

A pyogenic granuloma is a solitary, firm, bright red to reddish–brown, pedunculated or sessile vascular tumor of diameter 5–20 mm (Fig. 111.1). The lesion is usually painless and bleeds easily after trauma. It occurs most commonly on the hands and the face and in the mouth (Fig. 111.2). There is a type of pyogenic granuloma that recurs with several satellites. Satellite lesions erupt between 1 and 4 months after irritation or attempted destruction of the original lesion. In children they occur most frequently on the trunk, especially around the scapular regions. Such lesions are more abundant in the vicinity of the original lesions and appear as smooth, shiny, red, vascular tumors (Fig. 111.3). The initial growth of the lesions is rapid; this period of rapid growth is followed by a period of stability in which little change in size occurs. Epidermal breakdown, bleeding and crusting are reasonably common. The bleeding is often refractory to pressure and caustic solutions.

Spontaneous involution following infarction occurs rarely.

HISTOPATHOLOGICAL FINDINGS

The dome-shaped lesion, occasionally ulcerated, consists mostly of a proliferation of blood vessels of the caliber of venules, together with a highly edematous stroma replete with a mixture of inflammatory cells, especially neutrophils and lymphocytes (Fig. 111.4). Granulation tissue is embraced partially by collarettes of adnexal epithelium (i.e. by infundibula and eccrine ducts).

ETIOLOGY AND PATHOGENESIS

Pyogenic granuloma is a disorder of angiogenesis of unknown cause. Hypothetical triggering or predisposing factors are trauma, especially puncture wounds, localized viral infections and underlying port-wine stains. An unknown vascular stimulating factor seems to play an important role in promoting the rapid growth of the tumor. The reason for the development of 'satellite' lesions around pyogenic granuloma is obscure.

MANAGEMENT

Treatment consists of electrodesiccation of the primary lesion and of satellite lesions if need be. Successful treatment with surgical excision, cryotherapy and pulsed-dye laser has been reported.

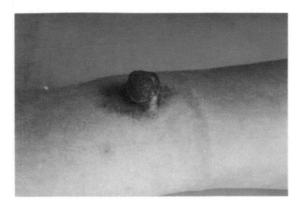

Figure 111.1
Pyogenic granuloma. This sessile lesion is sharply circumscribed and reddish, an indication that is vascular. The lesion is ulcerated and glistens because it is covered by plasma.

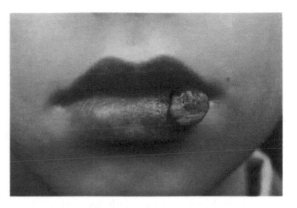

Figure 111.2
Pyogenic granuloma. This vascular tumor appeared on the lower lip of an 8-year-old child 1 week after a local trauma. The growth of the lesion was rapid (2 weeks).

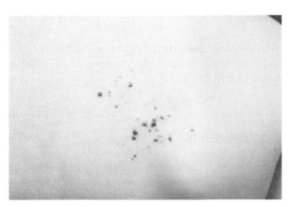

Figure 111.3
Pyogenic granuloma with sutellitosis. These asymptomatic, red, papulonodular lesions developed 2 months after the cauterization of a small vascular nodule. Such lesions occur most frequently on the trunk, especially around the scapular region.

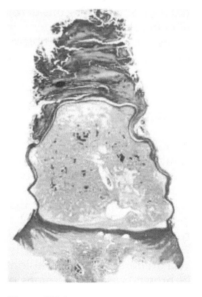

Figure 111.4
Pyogenic granuloma. The nodular exophytic lesion shown here is characterized by a proliferation of endothelial cells that form vessels of different sizes and shapes within an edematous stroma. Collarettes of adnexal epithelium completely embrace the lesion.

Pyogenic infections include a variety of conditions mainly caused by staphylococci or streptococci.

IMPETIGO CONTAGIOSA

Impetigo contagiosa is a highly contagious, superficial bacterial infection. It is considered to be the commonest skin infection in children, accounting for 10% of skin problems in dermatology clinics.

CLINICAL FINDINGS

Two clinical forms of impetigo may be observed, the bullous and the non-bullous forms, based on a different bacterial etiology. The bullous form of impetigo is a disease of infancy and begins as small vesicles that rapidly develop into large bullae (Fig. 112.1) that lack a surrounding erythematous zone. The thin roof of the bullae breaks easily, leaving a thin collarette scale. These lesions evolve into light brown crusts. The lesions of bullous impetigo may occur anywhere, with an irregular distribution.

The earliest sign of non-bullous impetigo is a circular erythematous macule, which soon develops into a small, superficial vesicle. Vesicles later become pustular and are replaced by soft crusts that are the color of honey (Fig. 112.2). Non-bullous impetigo is more likely to be seen on the face, especially around the nose and mouth, and on the limbs. It may develop at any time in childhood and adolescence.

The lesions of both forms of impetigo are usually asymptomatic. The natural course of untreated impetigo is extension locally and then spontaneous resolution in a few weeks, but lesions may be recurrent. Impetigo contagiosa usually heals without scars.

Association

Underlying inflammatory conditions of the skin, notably atopic dermatitis, may predispose to impetigo.

Complications

Bullous impetigo contagiosa may be diffuse all over the body and, in rare cases, it progresses into a scalded skin staphylococcal syndrome (see below). Furthermore, in newborns, the staphylococcal impetigo may be followed by serious secondary infections such as osteomyelitis, pneumonia or septic arthritis. Streptococcal impetigo may be complicated by urticaria and erythema nodosum. Certain strains of streptococci can induce acute glomerulonephritis, but this is rare.

LABORATORY FINDINGS

Examination by Gram stain of skin scrapings after removal of crusts or unroofing the bullae will reveal the presence of Gram-positive streptococci or clusters of *Staphylococcus aureus*. In resistant forms, culture is useful.

HISTOPATHOLOGICAL FINDINGS

Bullous impetigo

The dominant change in bullous impetigo is a blister situated in the uppermost part of the spinous zone, the granular zone, or the subcorneal zone. Within the blister, a few acantholytic cells and neutrophils are usually apparent (Fig. 112.7). Only a sparse infiltrate of lymphocytes and neutrophils is seen around the vessels of the superficial plexus.

Non-bullous impetigo

A discrete collection of neutrophils is housed beneath the stratum corneum in the upper part of the spinous zone and in the granular zone. There may be slight edema of the papillary dermis and a sparse superficial perivascular and interstitial infiltrate of lymphocytes and neutrophils (Fig. 112.8).

ETIOLOGY AND PATHOGENESIS

Impetigo contagiosa and the other skin diseases dealt with in this chapter are caused by bacteria. The commonest cause of non-bullous impetigo contagiosa is group A beta-hemolytic streptococci. *Staphylococcus aureus* is the major cause of bullous impetigo. In impetigo contagiosa caused by streptococci and staphylococci, the bacteria produce toxins, which are responsible for the clinical features of the disease, in that they function as exfoliatin, causing keratinocytes to separate from one another (acantholysis) at the level of the granular layer.

MANAGEMENT

Localized impetigo contagiosa may respond to topical antibiotics such as mupirocin (pseudomonic acid), bacitracin ointment or erythromycin. In addition to the topical treatment, it is always advisable to give a systemic antibiotic, although it is questionable whether this prevents the rare poststreptococcal glomerulonephritis. If streptococci are known to be the etiological agent, then oral penicillin or erythromycin is curative. When a specific bacterial cause is not known, or if lesions are bullous, then oral therapy with erythromycin, cephalosporins, dicloxacillin, or other antibiotics with effective antistaphylococcal activity should be given.

SCALDED SKIN STAPHYLOCOCCAL SYNDROME

Scalded skin staphylococcal syndrome is a rare, extensive, exfoliative form of pyogenic skin infection produced by *Staphylococcus aureus*. The onset is under 5 years of age; the median age at onset is 2 years.

CLINICAL FINDINGS

Clinically, the disease starts during or after a rhinitis, a conjunctivitis or a purulent otitis. It begins with a scarlatiniform erythema, accompanied by cutaneous tenderness (Fig. 112.3). It involves folds and periorificial regions. The toxic syndrome is characterized by high fever, malaise and vomiting. Within 24–48 hours the disease usually progresses from the scarlatiniform eruption to wrinkling with large, flaccid blisters. The Nicholsky sign is positive, even in apparently uninvolved skin. The rupture of the roofs of blisters causes large erosions that are red, wet and bordered by remnants of the roofs of blisters (see Fig. 112.3). The skin looks scalded. Severe mucosal involvement does not usually occur. If antibiotic therapy is given quickly, rapid post-inflammatory desquamation occurs, with complete restitution of epithelium. Recovery is the rule and occurs in 6–12 years.

Complications

Complications of scalded skin staphylococcal syndrome are the same as those of an extensive burn, as well as sepsis, pneumonia or other internal localizations.

LABORATORY FINDINGS

In scalded skin staphylococcal syndrome, the white blood cell count is augmented and the erythrocyte sedimentation rate is elevated. *Staphylococcus aureus* may be isolated from the exudate.

HISTOPATHOLOGICAL FINDINGS

There are sparse, superficial, perivascular mixed cell infiltrates of neutrophils and lymphocytes, subcorneal pustules that contain variable numbers of acantholytic cells, and epidermal necrosis in varying degree.

ETIOLOGY AND PATHOGENESIS

The syndrome is caused by an exotoxin produced by staphylococci of phage group 2. The exotoxin cleaves the epidermis beneath the stratum granulosum.

MANAGEMENT

Treatment consists of isolation of the patient, administration of penicillinase-resistant penicillin analogs, local disinfection with silver nitrate (1:1000 aqueous) or potassium permanganate solution, and restoration of the electrolyte balance.

FURUNCLES

Furuncles, also known as boils, are acute, deep-seated perifollicular abscesses caused by bacteria. They are not usually seen in infants and are commonest in the postpubertal period and in later childhood.

CLINICAL FINDINGS

Furuncles are tender and painful, red nodules, which may become fluctuant and enlarge to about 10 mm or more in diameter. From the nodules, purulent blood-tinged material may discharge (Fig. 112.4). The confluence of many furuncles is called a carbuncle. Furuncles typically heal with hyperpigmentation, and some of them may scar. They may be recurrent.

HISTOPATHOLOGICAL FINDINGS

Histopathologically, neutrophils not only clog widely dilated infundibula, they are present within walls of infundibula and in the periinfundibular dermis together with lymphocytes and a variable number of histiocytes. In furuncles, the suppuration always spreads along the lower segment of follicles as well as the upper segment. Gram staining may reveal bacteria within the cytoplasm of some neutrophils. A carbuncle develops when suppuration involves the infundibula of adjacent follicles and also extends far down along the inferior segments of a follicle to the level of the deep reticular dermis or the subcutaneous fat (Fig. 112.9).

ETIOLOGY AND PATHOGENESIS

The most important etiological agent is *Staphylococcus aureus*, but the strains differ from those of impetigo (e.g. a different range of groups, including phage type 80/81). The pathogenesis of furuncles is thought to be the production of factors that attract polymorphonuclear leukocytes and determine whether a particular strain of *Staphylococcus aureus* will elicit an inflammatory response on invasion of the hair follicle.

MANAGEMENT

Furuncles respond well to topical antibacterial treatment. Incision and drainage are indicated, too.

ECTHYMA

Ecthyma is a rare, deeper form of bacterial infection of the skin.

CLINICAL FINDINGS

Ecthyma is characterized by an initial vesicle or pustule on an erythematous base, most often located on the buttocks and lower extremities, which is followed by the development of induration and ulceration. The ulcers may be topped by a thick, circular, adherent crust (Fig. 112.5). The lesions of ecthyma may be painful, unlike those of impetigo contagiosa, and lymphadenopathy may be present. Pigmentary changes are common on healing of ecthyma, and scars may sometimes remain.

HISTOPATHOLOGICAL FINDINGS

Ecthyma is characterized by a superficial ulcer beneath which there is a dense infiltrate of neutrophils that may extend to the upper part of the reticular dermis.

ETIOLOGY AND PATHOGENESIS

Group A beta-hemolytic streptococci are the most frequent cause of ecthyma. Poor living conditions and poor hygiene are predisposing factors.

MANAGEMENT

The disease responds well to topical and systemic treatment with antibiotics with effective antistaphylococcal activity, such as erythromycin, dicloxacillin or benzathine penicillin.

ERYSIPELA

Erysipela (streptococcal cellulitis) is rarely seen in children. It is caused by group A beta-hemolytic streptococci.

CLINICAL FINDINGS

Erysipela is characterized by a superficial, acute, well-demarcated inflammation. In newborns, it lacks the typical border and the commonest localization is the periumbilical area, but the face may also be involved. In children, the lower extremities may be involved and may have superficial bullae. In a few cases, perianal and even genital streptococcal cellulitis (dermatitis) (Fig. 112.6) has been reported, which is accompanied by painful defecation and secondary constipation, rectal bleeding and brown mucoid discharge. Systemic signs and symptoms, such as fever, chills and prostration, may be present and variably severe. Recurrences are common.

HISTOPATHOLOGICAL FINDINGS

Erysipela is characterized by sparse perivascular and interstitial infiltrate composed mostly of neutrophils, extravasation of erythrocytes and edema of the papillary dermis.

MANAGEMENT

Treatment includes topical and oral antibacterial drugs, mainly penicillin, to be continued for at least 2 weeks.

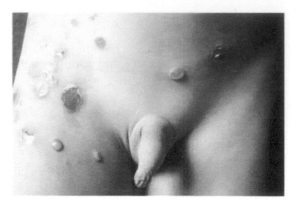

Figure 112.1
Bullous impetigo. The tense blisters rupture to leave erosions that soon are covered by scaly crusts.

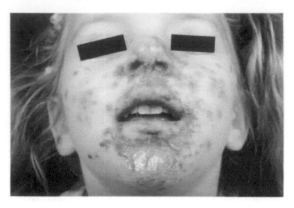

Figure 112.2
Non-bullous impetigo. The face is a site of predilection, especially around the mouth and nasal orifices. Lesions are characteristically covered by soft crusts that are the color of honey.

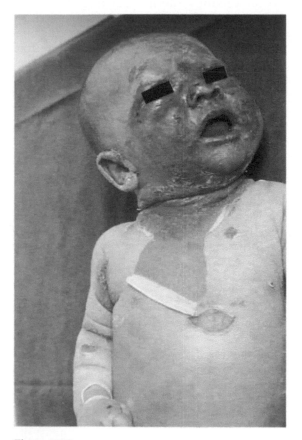

Figure 112.3
Staphylococcal scalded skin syndrome. This condition resembles scalded skin because the epidermis is gray as a consequence of necrosis and the skin is diffusely blistered.

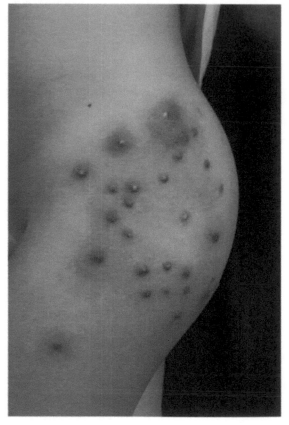

Figure 112.4
Furuncles. Typical nodulopustular lesions surrounded by an erythematous halo.

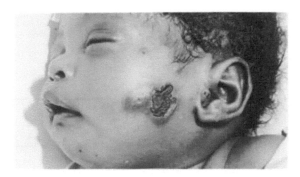

Figure 112.5
Ecthyma. Irregular, well-demarcated, adherent crust on an erythematous base.

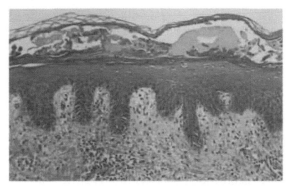

Figure 112.7
Bullous impetigo. In this section (stained by hematoxylin and eosin), there is an intracorneal blister containing several neutrophils. A sparse infiltrate of lymphocytes and neutrophils is present in the superficial dermis.

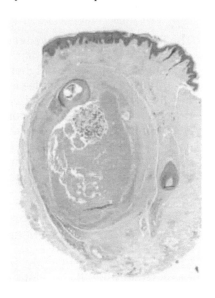

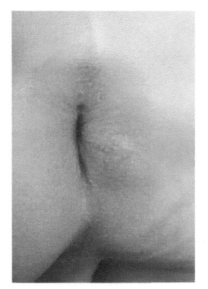

Figure 112.6
Perianal streptococcal cellulitis. Perianal erythema and edema cause painful defecation.

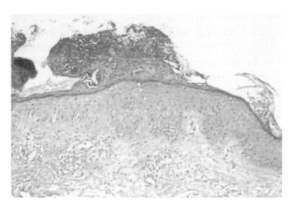

Figure 112.8
Impetigo. This lesion is characterized by slight epidermal spongiosis and collections of neutrophils within the horny layer. Note that numerous bacteria can be observed within the intracorneal pustule, where they appear as basophilic dots.

Figure 112.9
Furuncle. This section shows a nodular suppurative and granulomatous infiltrate that has led to the destruction of the lower part of adjacent hair follicle.

RESPONSE TO FLYING INSECT ASSAULTS

The term 'response to flying insect assaults' denotes the skin reactions that result from the bites of flying insects. Insect bites are most frequently seen in children who live in tropical climates or during the summer in temperate climates.

CLINICAL FINDINGS

The clinical features of flying insect bites are extremely variable, because of the great number of biting and stinging flying insects and their different feeding habits, the wide variation in patients' capacity to react to injected venom, and the nature of the venom. The skin reaction to bites may be immediate or delayed. The immediate reaction consists of erythema and wheal associated with pruritus or a burning sensation. The delayed reaction may occur several hours after the bite and consists of papules, papulovesicles and even bullae that persist for several days. Often either wheals and papules may show a central hemorrhagic punctum (Figs 113.1 and 113.2). Bullae are common on the lower legs, especially in children. They usually appear on wheals or papules. Because of the intense pruritus that often accompanies these lesions, there may be erosions, ulcerations and purulent hemorrhagic crusts (Fig. 113.3). An insect bite may be solitary, or there may be several bites or widespread bites. Lesions are often grouped in a linear fashion at irregular intervals (see Fig. 113.2). When the lesions are widespread, the feature of papular urticaria is realized. Papular urticaria (or strophulus) occurs mainly in children between the age of 2 and 7 years and is characterized by the eruption of numerous,

dome-shaped, red, pruritic papules that persist for weeks or months. This clinical entity is considered to be a hypersensitivity reaction to insect bites. Uncomplicated insect bites usually last a few days, but persistence of the lesions for months is possible, especially when a part of the sting apparatus is retained in the skin.

Complications

In highly sensitive people, fever and malaise may be present. Secondary infections, such as cellulitis or lymphangitis, and eczematization are common complications. In allergic subjects, anaphylactic shock may be induced, mainly by Hymenoptera stings.

HISTOPATHOLOGICAL FINDINGS

The lesion consists of a wedge-shaped, superficial and deep, perivascular and interstitial mixed cell infiltrate. At higher magnification, the infiltrate around venules is seen to consist mostly of lymphocytes and eosinophils, and the interstitial infiltrate to consist mostly of eosinophils. Early in the course of evolution of an insect bite, the papillary dermis may be edematous. In time, the edema may develop into subepidermal vesiculation (Fig. 113.4).

ETIOLOGY AND PATHOGENESIS

The flying insects that are most frequently responsible for bites in children and adolescents belong to the order of Diptera. Mosquitos, blackflies, horseflies, deerflies and soundflies are all bloodsuckers, which produce their effects on the skin by a variety of mechanisms. Skin reactions may be caused directly by the injection of irritant or by pharmacologically active substances contained in the delivery secretions that are necessary to dilute blood or to digest tissues. More frequently, skin manifestations depend on an immunological response to components of the salivary secretions by a previously sensitized host. Finally, some granulomatous reactions may be induced by retained mouth parts. Atopic dermatitis may represent a predisposing factor for long-lasting skin reactions.

MANAGEMENT

The treatment of Diptera bites requires cleansing with antiseptics, local application of combinations of steroid–antibiotic ointments and eventually oral antihistamines to relieve the itching. For severe reactions, such as those induced by Hymenoptera bites, subcutaneous adrenaline (epinephrine) and intravenous corticosteroids may be needed. Prevention with insect repellent creams may be useful.

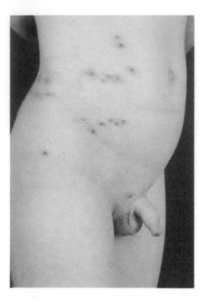

Figure 113.1
Insect bites. There are several papulovesicular lesions, which are grouped in a linear fashion. Few of these lesions show a central hemorrhagic crust.

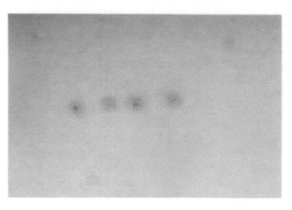

Figure 113.2
Insect bites. These papular lesions are typically distributed in a linear fashion, an indication that a single insect may have taken numerous bites in sequence. Their center is eroded or has a central hemorrhagic crust.

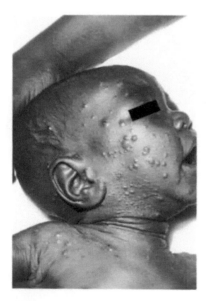

Figure 113.3
Insect bites. There are papules, papulovesicles, papulopustules, vesiculopustules and excoriated papules.

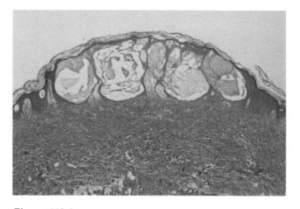

Figure 113.4
Insect bite. Characteristic findings are a superificial and deep perivascular and interstitial mixed cell dermatitis and marked edema of the papillary dermis that develops into subepidermal and intraepidermal vesiculation at the site of the bite. Note that the infiltrate is composed mostly of lymphocytes and eosinophils.

Reticulohistiocytosis of the skin covers a spectrum of rare clinical entities ranging from the solitary cutaneous form through the diffuse cutaneous form without systemic involvement to multicentric reticulohistiocytosis with systemic involvement. The skin lesions of all these conditions demonstrate an identical histological pattern that is characterized by the presence of numerous mononucleated or multinucleated histiocytes with abundant, eosinophilic, homogeneous to finely granular cytoplasm with a ground-glass appearance.

EPIDEMIOLOGY

All the variants of reticulohistiocytosis are extremely rare in children. Pediatric cases have been observed in patients aged from 6 to 13 years.

CLINICAL FINDINGS

Solitary cutaneous reticulohistiocytosis (reticulohistiocytoma cutis) is characterized by a single, firm, rapidly growing nodule that varies in color from yellow–brown to dark red (Fig. 114.1). This tumor most commonly involves the head and the neck, but it may be found on almost any cutaneous site. The lesion, which is often clinically misdiagnosed, occurs without evidence of systemic involvement. The onset may be preceded by a trauma and the lesion is usually self-healing in few years.

Diffuse cutaneous reticulohistiocytosis is a purely cutaneous form characterized by the eruption of firm, smooth, asymptomatic papules and nodules scattered diffusely on the skin. The color of new lesions is pink–yellow, while the older lesions show a red–brown color (Fig. 114.2). Joint or visceral lesions are absent. The lesions may involute spontaneously, but it is possible that they represent an early stage of multicentric reticulohistiocytosis before the appearance of joint and visceral manifestations.

Multicentric reticulohistiocytosis exclusively involves adults over 40 years of age and is always associated with a severe polyarthritis, which may precede the cutaneous eruption. The skin lesions are papulonodular, ranging in diameter from a few millimeters to 20 mm; they are round, translucent, and yellow–rose or yellow–brown in color. They do not tend to ulcerate and preferentially affect the fingers, the palms and the backs of the hands, the juxta-articular regions of the limbs and the face. Oral, nasal, and pharyngeal mucosa are involved in 50% of cases. Osteoarticular manifestations symmetrically involve the hands (in 80% of patients), knees (in 70%), and wrists (in 65%). There is no parallelism between the mucocutaneous and articular courses. The mucocutaneous lesions have a highly variable course and may remit spontaneously. The osteoarticular manifestations in half of the patients become stable; in the other half there is a progressive destructive course. Fever, weight loss and weakness may be present. The term 'lipoid dermatoarthritis' indicates a particular form of multicentric reticulohistiocytosis that is characterized by familial occurrence, ocular involvement (glaucoma, uveitis and cataract) and xanthomatous lesions.

Associations

In adults there is an association with an internal malignancy in 15–20% of cases. Solid tumors are the most common type of malignancy. Reticulohistiocytosis may occasionally occur in association with autoimmune diseases, systemic vasculitis and thyroid diseases.

HISTOPATHOLOGICAL FINDINGS

The histopathological findings in the three types of reticulohistiocytosis and in the various involved tissues are identical. The lesions of reticulohistiocytosis usually present as dome-shaped papules or nodules characterized by a dense diffuse infiltrate that is composed mostly of mononuclear, binucleate and multinucleate histiocytes (Figs 114.3 and 114.4). The histiocytes have a distinctive appearance, with roundish nuclei, abundant amphophilic cytoplasm, a finely granular, dark eosinophilic center and a light eosinophilic periphery ('ground-glass' cytoplasm). The number of giant cells may vary and the nuclei may be arranged haphazardly or they may align along the periphery or cluster in the center. In addition to the predominant infiltration of histiocytes, the lesions may be sprinkled with lymphocytes, eosinophils and, sometimes, neutrophils. A distinctive histochemical finding is the presence of a few fine granules that react with periodic acid–Schiff reagent after pre-treatment with diastase.

ETIOLOGY AND PATHOGENESIS

The etiopathogenesis is unknown. Reticulohistiocytoses may represent an abnormal histiocytic reaction to different stimuli. In solitary forms of reticulohistiocytosis, local trauma may play a role; in diffuse forms, the association with internal malignancies and autoimmune disease suggests an immunological basis for the initiation of the reaction.

MANAGEMENT

The solitary form is surgically excised. In multicentric reticulohistiocytosis, therapy is usually not helpful. Anti-inflammatory drugs are ineffective. Systemic corticosteroids have a short-lasting favorable effect on articular lesions only. Azathioprine has proved to be of no benefit. Antimitotic agents (mainly cyclophosphamide) have been reported to induce regression of mucocutaneous lesions in only a few cases.

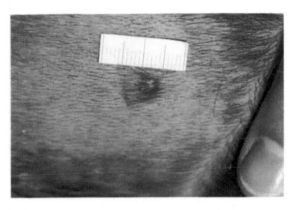

Figure 114.1

Solitary reticulohistiocytosis. An asymptomatic, dark, red, firm, dome-shaped nodule on the scalp. The patient was sent to a surgeon with the suspected diagnosis of a Spitz nevus.

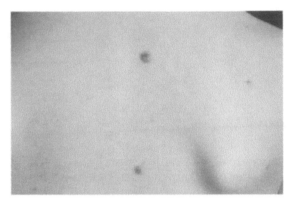

Figure 114.2

Diffuse cutaneous reticulohistiocytosis. There are many papules and nodules on the trunk of this 8-year-old boy. The lesions are firm and elastic, varying in color from yellow–pink to red–brown.

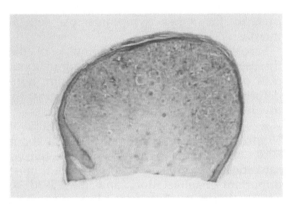

Figure 114.3

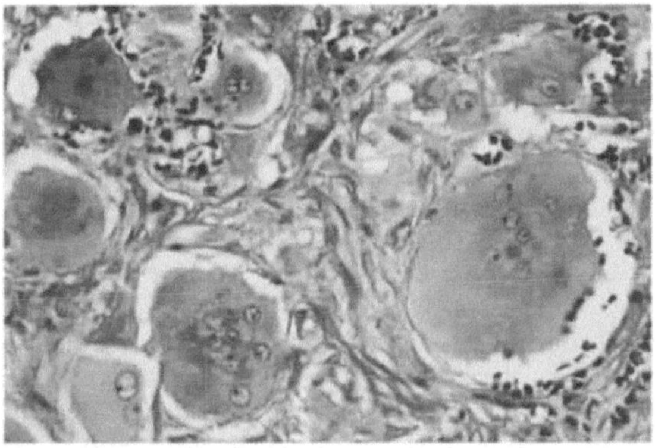

Figure 114.4

Figures 114.3 and 114.4

Reticulohistiocytosis. This nodular lesion of reticulohistiocytosis is constituted by a dense diffuse infiltrate of histiocytes with roundish nuclei and abundant granular cytoplasm. Most of the histocytes are multinucleate.

Sarcoidosis is a multisystem, granulomatous disorder of unknown cause that is uncommon in children.

EPIDEMIOLOGY

The disease occurs worldwide. Blacks are affected more often than whites. There is an equal incidence in males and females. In the majority (75% of cases) of young patients the disease appears between 8 and 15 years of age.

CLINICAL FINDINGS

Cutaneous manifestations are present in the 20–35% of patients with systemic sarcoidosis. Rarely, they are the only manifestation but more frequently they represent the first symptom. Skin sarcoidosis may manifest itself with a wide variety of skin lesions (papules, nodules or plaques). A papular rash is the commonest finding in young children and may have great diagnostic importance. It is characterized by yellow–brown, flat lesions that have a grayish–yellow color on diascopy (Figs 115.1 and 115.2). The condition begins peripherally, then becomes generalized. In children, the nodular and plaque variants are rare. These lesions consist of hard, asymptomatic, red–brown or violaceous patches, most often affecting the face and the proximal parts of the limbs.

Other types of sarcoidosis, such as angiolupoid sarcoidosis, lupus pernio, subcutaneous sarcoidosis and the erythrodermic, annular, and scar forms, are exceptional in the pediatric age group. In about 20% of adoles-

cent females, the early stage of the disease is characterized by the appearance of an erythema nodosum. This is a non-specific manifestation, but it is considered an important favorable prognostic sign.

When the disease occurs in children under 4 years of age, it preferentially affects the skin, the joints, the eyes, and the bones, but there is no pulmonary involvement. Skin lesions usually consist of a papular rash that may precede the other symptoms by several months.

Sarcoid arthritis is the hallmark of the disease in young children, occurring in about 60% of these patients. It is persistent, non-deforming and not painful; it predominantly involves the large joints.

Eye lesions are present in about 80% of children who have arthropathy and in about 50% of patients who have generalized sarcoidosis. Uveitis is the usual and most important manifestation, and may lead to severe disability with secondary glaucoma. Conjunctivitis, retinochoroiditis, optic nerve atrophy and decreased lacrimal gland secretion may all occur.

Skeletal changes, consisting of lysis with bone cysts, have been reported in about 50% of children with sarcoidosis under the age of 4 years. These lesions are often asymptomatic and mainly involve the hands and the feet.

In patients older than 5 years of age, sarcoidosis resembles the disease in adults and principally involves the lymph nodes, the lungs and the eyes. A bilateral hilar adenopathy with pulmonary infiltrates has been demonstrated in the vast majority of older children. Dyspnea and a progressive diminution of pulmonary function are common features. Peripheral adenopathy is present in about 50% of patients. Constitutional symptoms such as weight loss, fatigue, malaise and fever are also common. Less frequently there is hepatosplenomegaly.

The course of sarcoidosis may be acute, subacute or chronic. Acute forms are characterized by erythematopapular rashes, erythema nodosum, uveitis, arthralgias and lymphadenopathy. They usually last about 2 years and tend to resolve spontaneously. Subacute and chronic forms are dermatologically characterized by nodular lesions, lupus pernio and erythrodermic manifestations, and they are associated with pulmonary, ocular and bone involvement. Their course is prolonged and progressive. The prognosis of sarcoidosis in children seems to be more favorable than in adults.

LABORATORY FINDINGS

The most common abnormal laboratory findings are hyperglobulinemia (seen in 75% of cases) and eosinophilia (in 50%). Other possible laboratory abnormalities include hypercalcemia and hypercalciuria, an elevated erythrocyte sedimentation rate, elevated alkaline phosphatase levels and neutropenia. An elevation of serum angiotensin converting factor has been observed in active phases of the disease, although patients with only skin lesions have normal levels. Many patients present cutaneous anergy, demonstrated by lack of reactivity to tuberculin and other intradermal allergens. The Kveim test yields 80–90% positive results in patients with sarcoidosis. Radiological evidence of bilateral hilar lymphadenopathy is present in about 70% of adolescents but is rare in the younger children with sarcoidosis.

HISTOPATHOLOGICAL FINDINGS

In its stereotypical presentation, sarcoidosis consists of epithelioid histiocytes arranged in collections (tubercles) that are nearly devoid of a mantle of lymphocytes or plasma cells. These tubercles, known as 'naked' tubercles, are usually present in random array throughout the dermis and rarely within the subcutaneous tissue (Figs 115.3 and 115.4). A characteristic feature of sarcoidosis is the occasional presence of fibrin in the center of some epithelioid tubercles.

ETIOLOGY AND PATHOGENESIS

The etiology of sarcoidosis remains obscure despite extensive investigations. Sarcoidosis has been considered to be a reaction pattern to various infectious agents or allergens, probably in genetically predisposed people.

MANAGEMENT

Because sarcoidosis in children is potentially self-healing, the use of systemic therapy depends on the seriousness of the internal organ involvement (i.e. ocular, lung or liver disease or hypercalcemia). Corticosteroids are the drugs of choice. The usual dosage of oral prednisone is 1 mg/kg per day for several weeks. A very gradual reduction in corticosteroid dosage is suggested in order to avoid recurrence.

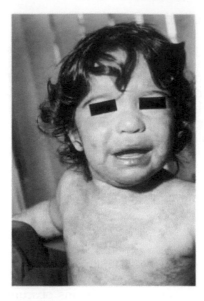

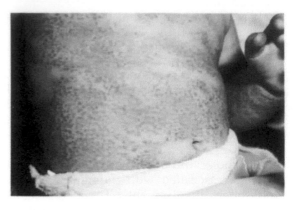

Figure 115.2
Sarcoidosis. The papules are red–brown, and some have shiny surfaces.

Figure 115.1
Sarcoidosis. There are numerous pink, smooth-surfaced papules, some of which tend to coalesce to form plaques.

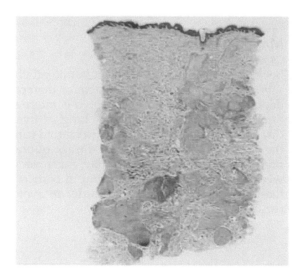

Figure 115.3

Figures 115.3 and 115.4
Sarcoidosis. Throughout the dermis are numerous, well-circumscribed, rounded or elongated aggregations of epithelioid histiocytes (tubercles), each of which is surrounded by a sprinkling of lymphocytes. Epithelioid histiocytes appear to have abundant, finely granular cytoplasm and round–oval vesicular nuclei with one or more small nucleoli.

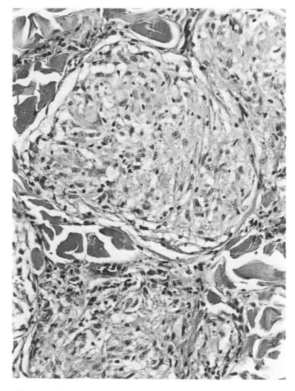

Figure 115.4

Scabies is an extremely contagious, epidemic disease that is characterized by severe itching. It is caused by the mite *Sarcoptes scabiei* var. *hominis*.

EPIDEMIOLOGY

Scabies is found universally and has epidemic outbursts that affect all races and social classes. The disease is commonest in children and young adults, but it may occur at any age.

CLINICAL FINDINGS

The pathognomonic skin lesions of scabies are burrows that appear as grayish-white, tortuous ridges several millimeters in length. The burrows are terminally capped by a small vesicle that is the resting place of the mite (Fig. 116.1). The lesions are usually found in areas with few or no hair follicles and where the stratum corneum is thin and soft. They occur most frequently in the finger webs, the volar aspects of the wrists, the axillae and, in infants, on the palms and soles. Itching is severe and intractable, particularly during the night and when the patient is warm. Secondary, non-pathognomonic lesions of scabies, caused by scratching, inappropriate treatments or hypersensitivity reactions, include papules, vesicles, pustules and excoriations that may be found all over the surface of the skin. When treatment is not undertaken early, children may have red–brown nodules (nodular scabies) that persist for a long time in spite of treatment (Fig. 116.2). Nodular lesions occur mainly on the covered parts of the body where the skin is thinnest, such as the genitalia and the axillary folds, and it is especially frequent in children aged less than 5 years.

Variants of the typical presentation of scabies include Norwegian scabies and neonatal scabies. Norwegian scabies (or crusted scabies) (Fig. 116.3) usually occurs in immunologically compromised people and is characterized by hyperkeratotic and crusted lesions of the palms and soles; these lesions are rich in parasites. This form may also involve the trunk, face, and scalp. The nails may be involved and appear dystrophic. Pruritus is mild and often absent. Neonatal scabies closely resembles Norwegian scabies and is characterized by a widespread eruption of vesicles, pustules and crusts involving all body areas, including the face. The neonates are not immunocompromised, and pruritus is absent. If not treated, the disease becomes chronic, and lichenification and nodular lesions occur. Pruritus often persists up to several weeks after eradication of mite infestation, an expression of a hypersensitivity phenomenon to mite antigens.

Complications

In infants and young children, secondary infections, such as staphylococcal and streptococcal impetigo, and eczematization are common. Streptococcal infections may give rise to acute glomerulonephritis.

LABORATORY FINDINGS

The diagnosis must be confirmed from a skin scraping of a burrow. Three findings are diagnostic – mites, their eggs and their fecal pellets. In infants, eosinophilia is frequently seen.

HISTOPATHOLOGICAL FINDINGS

The papular or nodular lesions of scabies are characterized by a superficial and deep, perivascular and interstitial, mixed cell infiltrate composed almost entirely of lymphocytes and eosinophils.

Papulovesicular lesions of scabies are marked by focal spongiosis and, at times, by spongiotic vesicles. In both papules and papulovesicles of scabies, the female mite, her ova and her progeny, in the form of nymphs and larvae, may be seen within tunnels (burrows) in the cornified layer (Fig. 116.4). Fecal nuggets may also be housed within the burrow.

Norwegian scabies, also known as hyperkeratotic crusted scabies, is typified by extreme orthokeratosis and parakeratosis, throughout which mites at all stages of evolution can be observed in quantity. The cornified layer of Norwegian scabies is peppered by ova, larvae, nymphs and adult mites, as well as by numerous egg shells and countless fecal nuggets.

ETIOLOGY AND PATHOGENESIS

Scabies is caused by the female of *Sarcoptes scabiei* var. *hominis*. The mite burrows deeply into the stratum corneum and deposits her eggs. She favors areas where the stratum corneum is thin, and this fact may explain the different distribution of the lesion in children and adults. Nodular lesions seem to be due to allergic sensitivity to the mite and its products. Transmission occurs especially from close personal contact (e.g. from mothers or baby-sitters to children). The incubation period is variable; pruritus usually begins within 1 month after exposure.

MANAGEMENT

After a cleaning bath, different scabicides may be applied (e.g. gamma-benzene hexachloride, mesulfene, benzylbenzoate, crotamiton, permethrin). Prolonged treatments should be avoided to prevent irritation and toxicity. Permethrin is recommended in scabies therapy in premature infants, small children, patients with neurological complications and nursing mothers. All members of a family or even an entire community should undergo treatment. Cloths and bedsheets should be sterilized. In nodular scabies, preparations of coal tars should be used.

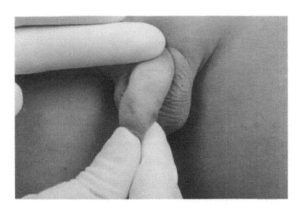

Figure 116.1
Scabies. Burrows are easily found in areas where the stratum corneum is thin and soft.

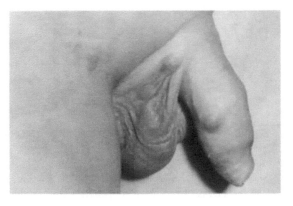

Figure 116.2
Scabies. These inflammatory, intensely itching nodules represent a variable diagnostic clue if burrows are absent or difficult to find.

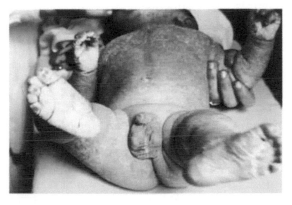

Figure 116.3
Norwegian scabies. In addition to widespread, reddish papules, some of which are scaly and which have become confluent; massive hyperkeratosis is also present on the sole.

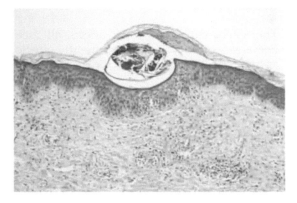

Figure 116.4
Scabies. This papular lesion of scabies shows a superficial and mid-dermal, perivascular and interstitial dermatitis constituted mostly of lymphocytes and eosinophils. The epidermis is slightly spongiotic, and the female scabies mite is housed in burrows within the cornified layer.

Scleroderma describes a group of diseases characterized by dermal hardening. These disorders range from solely cutaneous (morphea) to systemic forms (progressive systemic scleroderma).

MORPHEA

The solely cutaneous form affects all races. Females are three times as frequently affected as males. In 10–25% of cases the disease has its onset in childhood.

CLINICAL FINDINGS

Morphea includes several clinical subsets.

Plaque morphea is the most frequent type of localized scleroderma, accounting for approximately 70% of pediatric cases. It especially involves the trunk. Typically, lesions are oval in shape with a diameter of a few centimeters. The lesions are characterized by circumscribed, indurated, alopecic, ivory-colored patches (Fig. 117.1). The disease may consist of a single lesion or several asymmetrically distributed lesions. In active disease, the lesions may be prickly or slightly painful and are surrounded by a violaceous rim (lilac ring). Within the sclerodermic patches, telangiectasias can be occasionally seen and vesicobullous lesions may develop. Plaque morphea tends to show a spontaneous resolution in a few years. Healed lesions leave hyperpigmented, brownish patches that are not indurated.

Guttate morphea appears as multiple, round or oval, chalky-white lesions a few millimeters in diameter. They are characterized by minimal sclerosis and involve the shoulders, the neck and the chest. The lesions tend to remain stable.

Morphea profunda is a newly recognized subtype of localized scleroderma. It is characterized by multiple, non-tender, deep indurations. The lesions are localized in the deep dermis, the subcutaneous plane and the fascia. The overlying skin is usually brown in color. Typical patches of plaque morphea may coexist. The course is chronic and persistent.

Linear morphea accounts for approximately 18% of cases of localized scleroderma in pediatric patients. In about 20% of cases, one or more triggering factors, such as fever or trauma, can be identified. Linear morphea occurs as a hypopigmented, sclerotic, band-like lesion arising mainly on the lower extremities (Fig. 117.2). Less commonly it affects the anterior scalp, the frontal region of the head (Fig. 117.3), the arms and the anterior thorax. The disease tends to worsen and to involve the underlying tissues, and it therefore may produce severe deformities as a result of ankyloses and muscular contractures. These phenomena are especially common in children and result in impaired growth of the affected extremity. Patients with linear morphea may develop systemic autoimmune diseases.

Romberg's hemiatrophy is a segmental morphea that affects one side of the face (Fig. 117.4). As in linear morphea, the process affects not only the skin and subcutaneous fat, but also fascia, skeletal muscles and bones. Sometimes a linear morphea of the anterior scalp may coexist.

Generalized morphea is characterized by wide, hyperpigmented, sclerotic lesions diffusely involving the skin of the trunk and the thighs, while acral areas are usually spared. The disease spreads centrifugally. Sometimes the underlying muscles may be affected. Visceral involvement is rare. The disease tends to show improvement, but it persists for many years.

Disabling pansclerotic morphea of children is a recently recognized, severe variety of morphea, in which several types of localized scleroderma are combined. It accounts for approximately 2% of morphea varieties in childhood. The disease may start from a linear morphea. In this latter form, the lesions also involve subcutis, fascia, muscles and bones (Fig. 117.5). Extensor and acral areas are most commonly affected, with sparing of the fingertips and the toes, but the disease may affect also the scalp and the face. Arthralgia and severe pain caused by involvement of nerves may occur. Despite widespread and severe cutaneous involvement, Raynaud's phenomenon and signs of systemic scleroderma are usually absent. The course is progressive.

Eosinophilic fasciitis usually affects the distal area of a limb. It usually starts after physical exertion and is characterized by an area of tenderness and swelling with a cobblestone aspect on the overlying skin. The affected area subsequently becomes indurated. The disease usually regresses spontaneously or after corticosteroid treatment.

Pasini–Pierini atrophoderma usually appears on the trunk and is characterized by multiple atrophic lesions with a typical 'cliff-drop' border. The lesions are oval in shape with sizes ranging from a few millimeters to some centimeters in diameter. Concomitant lesions of typical plaque morphea have been described. The lesions are permanent.

LABORATORY FINDINGS

Eosinophilia has been reported in 30% of patients with localized scleroderma and in 80% of those with eosinophilic fasciitis. It is more common in linear morphea and in generalized morphea than in plaque morphea, and it seems to be related to the activity of the disease. Several serological findings typical of systemic autoimmune disorders have been reported. These include positivity for anti-nuclear antibodies, anti-ssDNA, anti-dsDNA, anti-centromere antibodies, anti-SCL 70 antibodies, and rheumatoid factors. These autoantibodies have been found in 31–57% of pediatric patients, with the highest percentage in linear morphea. Among children affected by linear morphea, the presence of ssDNA antibodies seems to define a subgroup with more severe and more extensive tissue involvement.

PROGRESSIVE SYSTEMIC SCLERODERMA

Progressive systemic scleroderma is a multi-systemic disease with wide variations in its clinical appearance. It is very rare in children. Females are affected at a rate five times higher than males. In less than 2% of patients is the onset under 9 years of age. Two major subtypes can be identified according to the cutaneous involvement – acroscleroderma and diffuse cutaneous systemic scleroderma.

In acroscleroderma, the skin involvement starts from the fingers, the hands and the face. Raynaud's phenomenon is usually present and may precede the skin lesions by years. In the early phases of the disease, the skin of the hands is slightly swollen, owing to a non-pitting edema, and this causes reduced mobility of the fingers. A new, recently described cutaneous marker of early acroscleroderma is represented by the 'round fingerpad' sign. This consists of the disappearance of the usual contour on fingerpads, which is replaced by a hemispheric contour. Gradually, skin hardening and sclerosis with hair loss and anhidrosis develop. Later, skin atrophy and telangiectases are evident and subsequently areas of calcinosis and painful ulcers on the fingertips may develop (Fig. 117.6). Ungual lesions consist of pronounced nail fold hyperkeratosis, spots of nail fold bleeding, and telangiectasia of nail fold capillaries. A particular variant of acroscleroderma is the 'CREST' syndrome (extensive Calcinosis cutis, Raynaud's phenomenon, dysphagia caused by Esophageal involvement, Sclerodactyly and widespread Telangiectasias). This variety of progressive systemic sclerosis is seen mainly in adults.

Diffuse cutaneous systemic scleroderma accounts for only 5% of cases of progressive systemic sclerosis. It usually starts from the trunk, sparing the acral portion of the body. Raynaud's phenomenon is usually absent. Sclerosis soon involves the whole integument.

From these two extreme grades of cutaneous involvement, transitional forms of progressive systemic scleroderma exist in which the early acral scleroderma soon extends to proximal areas of the body.

Pigmentary abnormalities are commonly seen. They consist of:

- focal patches of hypopigmentation and hyperpigmentation within sclerotic areas;
- generalized brown hyperpigmentation that resembles the skin discoloration seen in adrenal insufficiency;
- perifollicular pigmentation within patches of complete pigment loss, which mimics a repigmenting vitiligo.

Joint involvement with arthralgias is common, and sometimes ankylosis may develop. Multivisceral involvement is frequent.

To summarize – the gastrointestinal tract is frequently involved in childhood progressive systemic scleroderma, and dysphagia is present in about 20% of cases and may cause chronic aspiration pneumonia; diverticula of the colon are common. Primary pulmonary involvement may be asymptomatic; it consists of restrictive changes and impaired diffusion capacity. Myocardial and pericardial involvement may be severe and may be heralded by chest pain, angina pectoris, dyspnea and syncope. Hypertension is suggestive of renal involvement. A wide spectrum of renal involvement may occur, ranging from chronic, slowly progressive renal disease to the life-threatening renal crisis of acute scleroderma. This is usually preceded by a rapid worsening and extension of the skin involvement and is characterized by severe hypertension, convulsions and oligouria or anuria. In childhood the clinical manifestations of progressive systemic scleroderma are frequently atypical and the clinical aspects are extremely variable; sometimes there are features that overlap with other autoimmune connective tissue disorders. The course is chronic. Patients with skin hardening confined to the hands have a milder course than patients with extensive skin involvement. The prognosis is determined by cardiac and renal involvement.

LABORATORY FINDINGS

The main laboratory findings in scleroderma are:

- antinuclear antibodies, which are detected in the serum of 80% of patients with acrosclerosis and in 95% of patients with diffuse scleroderma;
- antinucleolar antibodies, which are present in fewer patients;
- anticentromere antibodies, which occur in 20% of patients with diffuse scleroderma and in 70% with CREST syndrome;
- anti-scleroderma 70 antibodies, which are detected in about 30% of patients.

Several circulating antibodies directed against a wide variety of nuclear and nucleolar antigens have been found in the serum of more than 95% of patients. Non-specific laboratory abnormalities consist mainly of an increased erythrocyte sedimentation rate, raised gammaglobulin levels and mild normochromic normocytic anemia. Hemolytic anemia and thrombocytopenia may also be found. Renal involvement is revealed by increased blood urea nitrogen, high levels of plasma creatinine and mild proteinuria. In children, the commonest radiographic abnormalities are dermal and subcutaneous calcifications in periarticular areas of the fingers.

HISTOPATHOLOGICAL FINDINGS

The histological findings are similar in all forms of scleroderma. The early changes are characterized by perivascular and interstitial infiltrate that affects the dermis, the septa in the subcutaneous fat and the fascia. The infiltrate often spares the upper half of the dermis and consists of lymphocytes, plasma cells, eosinophils and sometimes neutrophils.

In fully developed lesions, there is superficial and deep perivascular lymphoplasmocytic infiltrate within the dermis, aggregations of lymphocytes and plasma cells that are contiguous with septa of the subcutaneous fat, and the presence of these cells in the fascia. Collagen bundles are thickened, packed closely and parallel to one another (Fig. 117.7).

The late stage shows a thin dermis with thinned bundles of collagen, separated from one another by prominent spaces. The so-called eosinophilic fasciitis is simply an expression of morphea that favors the subcutaneous fat and fascia. Eosinophils are present in variable number.

ETIOLOGY AND PATHOGENESIS

Scleroderma is a disease of unknown origin. In genetically predisposed patients several environmental factors may play a role in inducing the abnormalities of scleroderma. These lesions, both in localized and systemic scleroderma, may be the consequence of immune dysfunctions, endothelial cell injury in blood vessel and connective and fibroblast alterations.

MANAGEMENT

For the localized forms of morphea, often no treatment is needed because of their tendency to heal slowly. Treatment with corticosteroid creams may be tried, but results are usually disappointing and the corticosteroids may cause skin atrophy. Intralesional corticosteroids may be helpful, but this treatment is painful and difficult to perform, owing to skin hardening, and may represent a problem in children. Skin atrophy may result. In morphea profunda antimalarials, systemic corticosteroids and several anti-inflammatory agents have been used. In eosinophilic fasciitis, systemic corticosteroid therapy is usually successful.

In more severe varieties of morphea, such as the linear and generalized forms, treatment is usually disappointing. However, psychological support is important, and physiotherapy helps to delay the onset of contractures.

Because progressive systemic scleroderma is an incurable, chronic, progressively disabling disorder that changes the body image, family counseling, patient education and psychological support are important preliminaries to any treatment. Non-pharmacologic treatment aims mainly at preventing Raynaud's phenomenon and consists of avoiding exposure to cold, keeping the whole body warm, and reducing emotional stress. There is no treatment that can change the natural course of the disease. However, a large variety of vasoactive, antifibrotic and immunosuppressive agents have been used. Among antifibrotic agents, D-penicillamine is the most commonly used drug, and it seems helpful in reducing skin hardening; moreover, it also has some immunosuppressive actions. Administration of intravenous factor XIII seems to improve skin lesions. Factor XIII acts by inhibiting the excessive collagen production by fibroblasts. The results from immunosuppressive and cytotoxic drugs are disappointing. Systemic corticosteroids have been shown to be of little benefit, except for overlap syndromes. Moreover, corticosteroid therapy requires caution, because it may precipitate a renal crisis; therefore, it must be avoided in patients with renal involvement. Cyclosporin-A, gamma-interferon and extracorporeal photochemotherapy have shown beneficial effects.

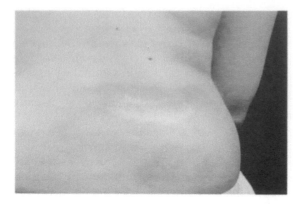

Figure 117.1
Plaque morphea. An irregularly shaped ivory-colored plaque surrounded by a violaceous ring.

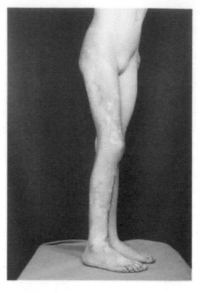

Figure 117.2
Linear morphea. There is a band of hyperpigmented and sclerotic skin. The lower extremities are a site of predilection.

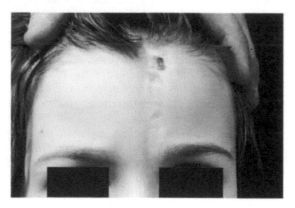

Figure 117.3
Linear morphea. This band of sclerotic skin is depressed beneath the skin surface.

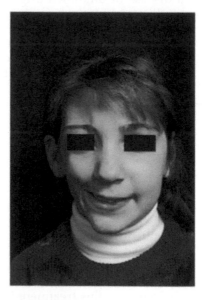

Figure 117.4
Romberg's hemiatrophy. This process is seen here on the right side of the face, affecting not only the skin and the subcutaneous fat, but also skeletal muscles and bones.

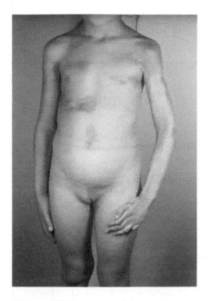

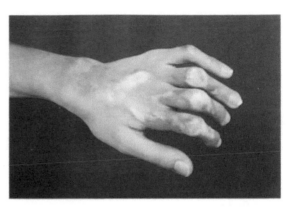

Figure 117.6
Acrosclerosis. This form of scleroderma is characterized by marked tightening of the skin with contractures of the fingers. The process is progressive and, in time, mutilating.

Figure 117.5
Disabling pansclerotic morphea. Severe sclerosis with muscoloskeletal atrophy of the left arm. Plaque-type lesions are present on the trunk.

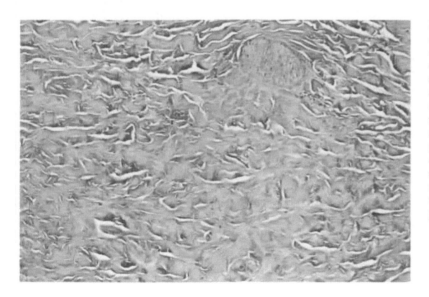

Figure 117.7
Scleroderma. At scanning magnification, the dominant pathological process is seen to be a marked sclerosis of the reticular dermis and of the upper part of the subcutaneous tissue. At higher magnification, collagen bundles are notably thickened, closely packed and parallel to one another. Among the adnexal structures, only the smooth muscles of hair erection appear to have been preserved by the pathological process.

Seborrheic dermatitis of infancy is a frequent eruption of the first weeks of life. It consists of red–yellow plaques covered by scales and it affects the scalp, the face and the large proximal flexures.

CLINICAL FINDINGS

Seborrheic dermatitis (Fig. 118.1) may begin with yellow, greasy scales on reddish papules on the scalp and then on the forehead, the ears, the retroauricular skin and, eventually, on the eyebrows and cheeks and in the nasolabial fold. Frequently the eruption starts from the diaper area (Fig. 118.2), but in many cases lesions appear more or less simultaneously in both sites, giving origin to the typical bipolar appearance of seborrheic dermatitis. On the scalp the hairs are amalgamated by a variable quantity of scales, whose presence and removal may cause minimal and transient alopecia. Seborrheic dermatitis in infants usually clears in a few weeks and does not recur. Pruritus, if present, is slight.

The erythrodermic form of seborrheic dermatitis (Fig. 118.3) is often known as Leiner's erythroderma, Leiner's syndrome or Leiner's disease. It generally begins with a progressive increase in the severity of a seborrheic dermatitis. The entire skin surface becomes red and edematous.

In the form due to inherited complement (C5) dysfunction, diarrhea together with failure to thrive supervene with compromise of the infant's general health.

Complications

Candidiasis occurs in about one-third of patients.

LABORATORY FINDINGS

Extensive investigations of the immune system should also always be carried out in all patients with diffuse, erythrodermic forms.

HISTOPATHOLOGICAL FINDINGS

Stereotypical fully developed lesions of seborrheic dermatitis are characterized by mounds of parakeratosis that contain lobules of plasma and, often, neutrophils (Fig. 118.4). The granular zone is focally decreased, and there are foci of spongiosis in psoriasiform rete ridges. Around very widely dilated venules of the superficial plexus, a sparse, moderately dense, predominantly lymphocytic infiltrate can be seen.

ETIOLOGY AND PATHOGENESIS

The cause of seborrheic dermatitis is unknown. Many factors (genetic, endocrine, infective, nutritional and emotional) seem to play roles. The causative role of *Pityrosporum orbicolaris*, well demonstrated in adult forms of seborrheic dermatitis, is not clear in infants.

MANAGEMENT

Because classic seborrheic dermatitis fades spontaneously after a few months, treatment is symptomatic and depends on the severity and localization of the disease. Emollients, ointments, and, more recently, ketoconazole shampoos may be useful to clear the scalp lesions. Mild, non-fluorinated topical corticosteroids may be used on limited surfaces for a few days, while antibacterial and anticandidal preparations should be used only in presence of superinfections. In Leiner's syndrome admission to hospital and treatment of the underlying biological defect by infusions of fresh plasma are mandatory.

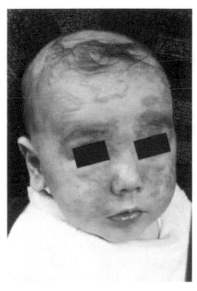

Figure 118.1
Seborrheic dermatitis. There are reddish papules, patches and plaques covered by slight scales on seborrheic areas (the forehead, the eyebrows, the malar eminences and the paranasal and nasolabial folds). The process also extensively involves the scalp.

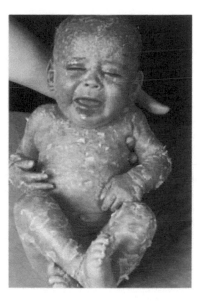

Figure 118.3
Leiner's disease. Universal erythema covered by large scales and scaly crusts is characteristic of this condition, which has been considered to be a peculiarly severe form of seborrheic dermatitis.

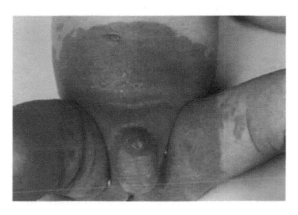

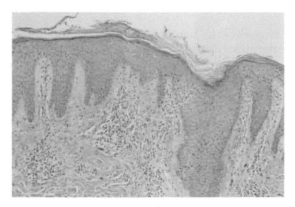

Figure 118.2
Seborrheic dermatitis. The eruption frequently starts from the diaper area with sharply demarcated, erythematous, scaly patches.

Figure 118.4
Seborrheic dermatitis. This lesion on the face is characterized by slight spongiosis, psoriasiform hyperplasia, focal hypogranulosis and mounds of parakeratosis that house lobules of plasma and neutrophils at their summit adjacent to follicular ostia. A moderately dense lymphohistiocytic infiltrate is present in the papillary dermis.

SCHÖNLEIN–HENOCH PURPURA

Schönlein–Henoch purpura (or anaphylactoid purpura) is a normothrombocytic purpura that occurs mainly in children. Clinically, it is characterized by a distinctive rash that begins in the lower extremities, and it is associated with gastrointestinal, joint and renal symptoms. It shows the histological features of a leukocytoclastic vasculitis.

EPIDEMIOLOGY

The disease has a worldwide distribution and affects both sexes. It occurs mostly in children under 10 years of age, most commonly during winter.

CLINICAL FINDINGS

The skin is usually the site of the initial manifestations. The main eruption consists of palpable purpura symmetrically distributed over the legs and the buttocks (Fig. 119.1), but the upper limbs (Fig. 119.2) and the face may be successively involved, while the trunk is usually spared. Individual lesions occur in crops and first appear as erythematous– edematous macules, which rapidly turn to hemorrhagic papules; they are often surrounded by erythematous rings. Blistering or ulceration may occasionally develop, mainly in areas with extensive involvement. The lesions gradually regress, becoming brown macules and then fading. The eruption is pleomorphic, and lesions at several stages of evolution are usually present at the same time. Single episodes last for a few weeks, but recurrences are described in one-half of cases. Gastrointestinal symptoms are present in 40–85% of children, and consist of colicky abdominal pain, vomiting and diarrhea. Gastrointestinal bleeding is not infrequent, but hematemesis occurs in less than 10% of patients. The abdominal pain may be the presenting symptom. Joint manifestations are reported with variable frequency in 50–75% of cases, and they are the initial symptoms of the disease in about one-quarter of patients. They consist of non-migratory arthralgia and periarticular swelling. The large joints, such as the ankles and the knees, are the ones most commonly affected. Usually the disease affects several joints simultaneously, but only one joint may be involved. Renal manifestations are rare and are the same as seen in glomerulonephritis (hematuria, oliguria, hypertension and edema). Renal involvement is the main factor determining prognosis.

Complications

Neurological symptoms, intestinal intussusception and stenosising uretritis may occur.

LABORATORY FINDINGS

Urinary abnormalities consist mainly of a hematuria and mild proteinuria with or without erythrocyte and granular casts. The anti-streptolysin-O titer may be elevated. Raised serum levels of immunoglobulin A levels and immunoglobulin A rheumatoid factor are described as being characteristic. Moreover, circulating immunocomplexes, cryoglobulins, a severe hypoprothrombine-mia and a decrease in factor XIII activity have been reported.

HISTOPATHOLOGICAL FINDINGS

The histological features are those of a leuko-cytoclastic vasculitis characterized by a perivascular and interstitial, predominantly neutrophilic infiltrate, together with evidence of neutrophilic 'nuclear dust' (Fig. 119.3). Extravased erythrocytes are evident in the upper part of the often edematous dermis (Fig. 119.4). Usually only developed lesions exhibit fibrin within the walls of venules.

ETIOLOGY AND PATHOGENESIS

The etiology is not yet known. A variety of antigenic stimuli, mainly of an infective nature, lead some genetically predisposed patients to synthesize high amounts of dimeric immunoglobulin A, owing to an abnormal T-cell control of immunoglobulin production. This excess of immunoglobulin A interacts with other immunoglobulins to form macromolecular complexes. The subsequent complement activation and the impairment in the clearance mechanisms of immune complexes lead to a failure of the coagulation pathway and causes vasculitis.

MANAGEMENT

Mild cases do not need any specific anti-inflammatory treatment, only supportive measures. Bed rest is mandatory, and antibiotic therapy is indicated when a bacterial infection is the triggering event. Oral prednisolone (0.5 mg/kg per day) should be administered when gastrointestinal symptoms are present. Intravenous methylprednisolone pulse therapy and plasma exchange have recently been recommended in children with severe renal involvement on renal biopsy or with deterio-rating renal function.

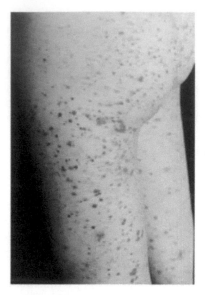

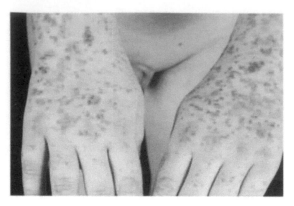

Figure 119.2
Schönlein–Henoch purpura. On the dorsum of the hands there are purpuric macules and papules, some of which have become confluent to form plaques. Some of the lesions are covered by scales.

Figure 119.1
Schönlein–Henoch purpura. The buttocks and the thighs are covered by reddish–purple macules, papules and small plaques.

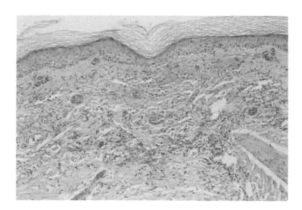

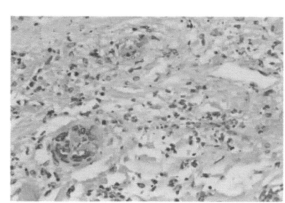

Figure 119.3   **Figure 119.4**

Figures 119.3 and 119.4
Schönlein–Henoch purpura. This purpuric papule of Schönlein–Henoch purpura shows a superficial perivascular and interstitial infiltrate of lymphocytes and neutrophils associated with abundant nuclear 'dust' and extravasated erythrocytes. Deposits of fibrin can be observed within the walls of most of the small vessels, and some lumens appear to be occluded by thrombi.

120   SINUS HISTIOCYTOSIS WITH MASSIVE LYMPHADENOPATHY

Sinus histiocytosis with massive lymphadenopathy (Rosai–Dorfman disease) is a benign, generally self-limited disease characterized by cervical lymphadenopathy. It is usually accompanied by fever, elevated erythrocyte sedimentation rate, leukocytosis with neutrophilia, and polyclonal hypergammaglobulinemia. Skin manifestations are observed in 10% of patients.

EPIDEMIOLOGY

Sinus histiocytosis is a relatively rare disease. About 450 cases have been studied. Of these, only 10% exhibited cutaneous lesions. Onset is in the first 20 years of life in approximately 80% of patients.

CLINICAL FINDINGS

Cutaneous lesions are not characteristic and consist of asymptomatic, usually numerous, yellowish macules and patches, reddish-brown papules, plaques and nodules that may become eroded or ulcerated (Figs 120.1 and 120.2). The variety of cutaneous lesions may precede the lymph node enlargement and may constitute the sole presenting feature of the disease. Massive bilateral cervical lymphadenopathy, usually painless, is the hallmark of the condition, occurring in 95% of cases. Periocular involvement resulting in a lobulated induration of the eyelids is a typical manifestation and is usually accompanied by preauricular adenopathy. The course is characterized by exacerbations and remissions and tends toward spontaneous resolu-

tion over several years. Usually the extranodal manifestations regress first, while adenopathy may persist for years.

LABORATORY FINDINGS

An elevated erythrocyte sedimentation rate, leukocytosis with neutrophilia, and polyclonal hypergammaglobulinemia are commonly found (in about 90% of tested patients).

HISTOPATHOLOGICAL FINDINGS

Within the dermis and lobules of the subcutaneous fat is a nodular infiltrate composed, in large part, of foamy histiocytes. These cells have roundish nuclei and abundant foamy cytoplasm with spidery outlines (Figs 120.3 and 120.4). Most of those cells are mononuclear , but some are binucleate and multinucleate. In addition to foamy histiocytes of variable countenances, there is a patchy lymphoplasmacytic infiltrate. In some lesions, the infiltrate of lymphocytes and plasma cells may predominate in many foci. Tiny collections of neutrophils may pepper the infiltrate, and erythrocytes are frequently extravasated. A particular finding in sinus histiocytosis with massive lymphadenopathy is ingestion of erythrocytes and leukocytes, both neutrophils and lymphocytes, by foamy histiocytes. This phenomenon is known as emperipolesis. A further specific histological feature of the disease is the presence of foamy histiocytes within the lumens of dermal lymphatic spaces. Most of the histiocytes forming the infiltrate are S100+ and CD1a-.

ETIOLOGY AND PATHOGENESIS

The cause is unknown. There are two main theories – a specific infection process and an immunological disorder.

MANAGEMENT

Because the vast majority of lesions of sinus histiocytosis heal completely, no treatment is necessary as a rule.

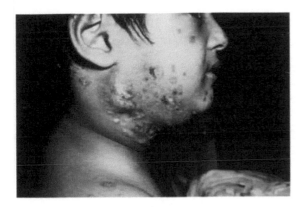

Figure 120.1
Sinus histiocytosis. There are reddish papules and nodules, some of them with central dells and others covered by hemorrhagic crusts. Cervical lymphadenopathy is evident.

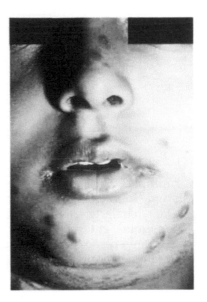

Figure 120.2
Sinus histiocytosis. There are discrete reddish-brown papules and papulopustules in this patient, who also has perleche.

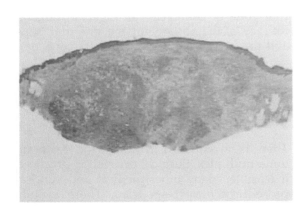

Figure 120.3

Figure 120.3 and 120.4
Sinus histiocytosis with massive lymphadenopathy. Throughout the dermis and the upper subcutaneous tissue is a proliferation of foamy histiocytes intermingled with lymphocytes, plasma cells, and neutrophils. Lymphocytes tend to be arranged in lymphoid follicle-like structures at the periphery of the lesion. Histiocytes have large round–oval nuclei and abundant foamy cytoplasm with spidery configuration. Some histiocytes appear to have ingested leukocytes (emperipolesis).

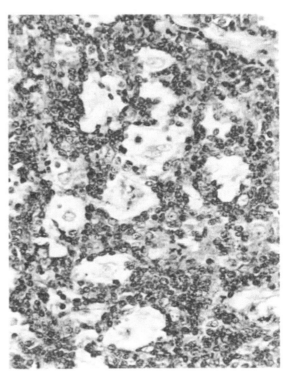

Figure 120.4

121

STEATOCYSTOMA MULTIPLEX

Steatocystoma multiplex, also known as sebocystomatosis and Gunther's disease, is an uncommon disorder characterized by the formation of numerous cutaneous cysts. Autosomal-dominant inheritance is usual, but sporadic cases have been reported.

CLINICAL FINDINGS

The disorder usually begins in infancy or adolescence but can be present at birth. The cysts are numerous and vary in size from a few millimeters to 2 mm or more in diameter (Figs 121.1 and 121.2). The smaller lesions are often firm, whereas the larger lesions may be soft. They are filled with an oily, odorless fluid or a gel-like material. The cysts are usually asymptomatic, and the overlying skin is normal or yellowish in appearance. The cysts of steatocystoma multiplex are usually situated on the anterior aspect of the chest (Fig. 121.1), the face, the neck and the axillae. Less frequently they are located on the scalp (see Fig. 121.2), the back (see Fig. 121.2), the abdomen, the genitalia and the extremities. Males tend to have more cysts on the anterior chest and back, whereas females have more in the axillary and groin area. The number and size of lesions increase slowly and become more evident at puberty.

Complications

In steatocystoma multiplex, bacterial infections may occur, and the cysts, usually asymptomatic, become painful.

HISTOPATHOLOGICAL FINDINGS

Within the dermis or the subcutaneous fat (or both) is a cystic hamartoma (Fig. 121.3), the cystic component of which is lined by epithelium just like that of a sebaceous duct (i.e. it is marked by a crenulated surface covered by a thin zone of compactly arranged orthokeratotic cells, the absence of the granular zone and the presence of a thin spinous zone, and the presence of a basal layer).

MANAGEMENT

There is no standard treatment for steatocystoma multiplex. Surgical excision is practiced if feasible. Many other medical and surgical procedures have been tried. These include prolonged courses of antibiotics, dermabrasion, cryosurgery, and carbon dioxide laser therapy. Isotretinoin has been used with contradictory results. Its beneficial effect is limited to the inflammatory forms of the condition.

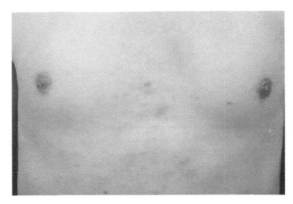

Figure 121.1
Steatocystoma multiplex. These firm asymptomatic cysts are covered by normal skin. The anterior chest is a site of predilection.

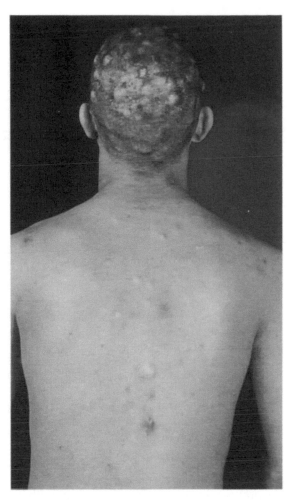

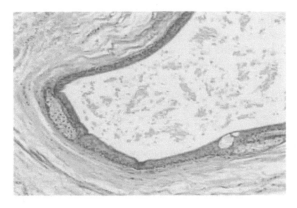

Figure 121.3
Steatocystoma. A large cystic hamartoma is situated in the dermis and subcutaneous tissue. The cyst wall is thin and is characterized by a crenulated, orthokeratotic cornified layer and the absence of the granular zone. Small sebaceous lobules connect with the cystic cavity by a sebaceous duct. Note that the cystic cavity contains sebum.

Figure 121.2
Steatocystoma multiplex. There are multiple, dome-shaped, papular lesions on the trunk that represent cysts of steatocystoma multiplex. The scalp is also extensively involved by the process.

122

SUBCUTANEOUS FAT NECROSIS OF THE NEWBORN

Subcutaneous fat necrosis is a rare disease affecting the panniculus of the newborn.

CLINICAL FINDINGS

Subcutaneous fat necrosis is generally noted during the 1st week of life in full-term newborns as a hardening and thickening of some areas of the skin. A careful examination reveals several painless nodules, frequently coalescent in plaques, covered by normal or erythematous skin. They are usually located on the upper part of the back (Figs 122.1 and 122.2), and the deltoids, the buttocks, the arms or the thighs, and sometimes the cheeks may be involved. The nodules are freely movable over the muscles and bones. The lesions appear rapidly but develop gradually. The indurated plaques disappear spontaneously in several weeks to months and usually without problems. Patients appear well and afebrile.

Complications

Complications occur in those cases in which nodules undergo colliquation and drain spontaneously.

HISTOPATHOLOGICAL FINDINGS

Subcutaneous fat necrosis is characterized, at scanning magnification, by a patchy infiltrate of inflammatory cells throughout lobules in the subcutaneous fat (Figs 122.3 and 122.4). At higher magnification, the infiltrate is seen to consist mostly of histiocytes, many of which possess foamy cytoplasm. Often, these foamy cells are multinucleate. Lymphocytes in variable numbers accompany the histiocytes. The crucial finding is the presence of needle-like clefts in occasional foamy histiocytes and, less commonly, in adipocytes themselves.

ETIOLOGY AND PATHOGENESIS

The etiopathogenesis is obscure. Many factors may trigger the process, including cold, trauma *in utero*, obstetrical trauma, poor nutrition, infections and biochemical defects.

MANAGEMENT

No treatment is required.

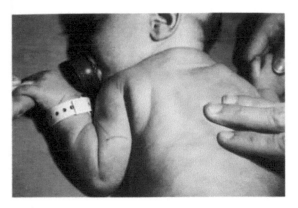

Figure 122.1
Subcutaneous fat necrosis. Numerous, non-scaly, reddish patches and plaques are a consequence of involvement by subcutaneous fat necrosis, mostly of the subcutaneous fat.

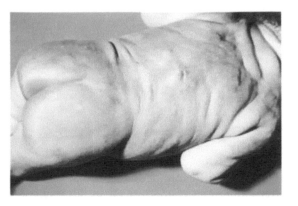

Figure 122.2
Subcutaneous fat necrosis. There is a diffuse nodularity of the skin surface, and the skin overlying the nodules is hyperpigmented.

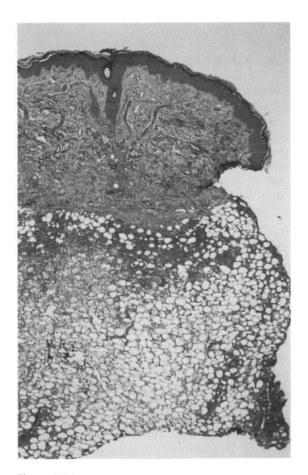

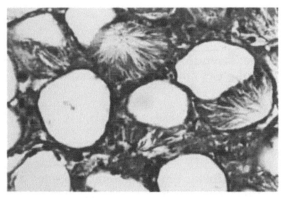

Figure 122.4

Figures 122.3 and 122.4
Subcutaneous fat necrosis. At scanning magnification, areas of necrosis and a scant inflammatory infiltrate diffusely involves fat lobules. At higher magnification (Fig. 122.4), the infiltrate consists of histiocytes, some of which contain crystals within the cytoplasm.

Figure 122.3

123

SWEET'S SYNDROME

Sweet's syndrome (acute febrile neutrophilic dermatosis) is characterized by an explosive onset of painful, dark red macules that quickly evolve into papules and plaques, especially on the limbs, as well as fever, arthralgia and neutrophilia, all of which follow a viral syndrome.

EPIDEMIOLOGY

Sweet's syndrome is rare in childhood. The age of onset ranges between 3 months and 12 years.

CLINICAL FINDINGS

Painful dusky pink violaceous papules and nodules coalesce to form sharply demarcated plaques (Figs 123.1 and 123.2). The plaques expand centrifugally to form rings and leave postinflammatory hyperpigmentation in their centers. Advanced lesions may show tiny vesicles or pustules at their margins. There is no ulceration or scarring. Plaques tend to be asymmetrical; they may occur at any site but show a predilection for the face (see Fig. 123.1), the neck and the upper extremities (see Fig. 123.2). Patients commonly complain of high fever, malaise, headaches, arthralgias, conjunctivitis and episcleritis. On occasion, Sweet's syndrome is not accompanied by an acute onset of fever or peripheral neutrophilia. Untreated skin lesions resolve spontaneously, although resolution may take up to a few months. More than one-half of patients have recurrences, which often affect previously involved sites.

Associations

An upper respiratory infection (including tonsillitis and epiglossitis) and high fever precede the skin lesions by several days. Between 10 and 15% of adults with Sweet's syndrome have malignant neoplastic diseases, most commonly acute myelogenous leukemia.

LABORATORY FINDINGS

Peripheral leukocytosis with neutrophilia ($15,000$–$25,000/mm^3$ with 90% neutrophils) is a common feature, but peripheral eosinophilia (greater than $500/mm^3$) and thrombocytosis (occasionally exceeding $10/mm^3$) may be seen. An elevated erythrocyte sedimentation rate is the most consistent laboratory abnormality.

HISTOPATHOLOGICAL FINDINGS

The most striking findings are a dense, nodular or diffuse, predominantly neutrophilic infiltrate within the reticular dermis and marked edema of the papillary dermis (Figs 123.3 and 123.4). The infiltrate, which may also contain eosinophils and be associated with extravasated erythrocytes, first presents in the upper half of the dermis and then extends throughout the dermis. Although there may be abundant nuclear 'dust', no fibrin is present in the walls of venules, an indication that there is no vasculitis. The papillary dermis often is so markedly edematous that subepidermal vesiculation seems incipient.

Etiology and pathogenesis

The cause is not known and the pathogenesis of Sweet's syndrome is not understood. An abnormal chemotactic stimulus or an abnormal chemotactic neutrophilic response has been suggested as being responsible. Sweet's syndrome has been thought by some to represent a hypersensitive reaction to antigens of bacteria, viruses or neoplastic cells.

Management

Corticosteroids given orally (2 mg/kg per day) for 10 days and then slowly tapered, achieve a dramatic response. Because Sweet's syndrome tends to recur, therapy must be long-term, so dapsone would appear to be more desirable than systemic corticosteroids as a maintenance drug.

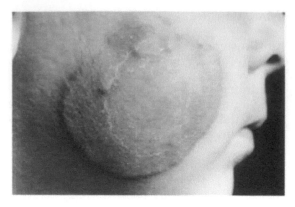

Figure 123.1
Sweet's syndrome. The annular plaque shows an erythematous, edematous, raised border and a depressed center with post-inflammatory scaling.

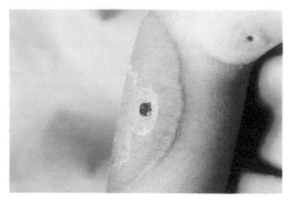

Figure 123.2
Sweet's syndrome. In the same patient as in Fig. 123.1, other typical plaques were present on the limbs. The roundish crust was the consequence of punch biopsies.

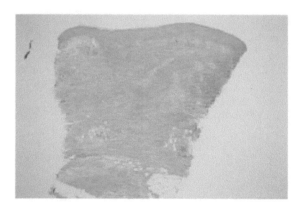

Figure 123.3

Figure 123.4

Figures 123.3 and 123.4
Sweet's syndrome. A dense, diffuse, mostly neutrophilic infiltrate in the reticular dermis, marked edema of the papillary dermis, the presence of nuclear 'dust' and the lack of deposits of fibrin within the vessel walls are typical histological features of Sweet's syndrome. Note that lymphocytes, histiocytes and some eosinophils join the neutrophils in the infiltrate.

124 SWIMMING POOL GRANULOMA

Swimming pool granuloma (or fish tank granuloma) is caused by *Mycobacterium marinum* and is the commonest atypical mycobacterial infection in pediatric patients.

CLINICAL FINDINGS

The penetration of *M. marium* is favored if there are small cutaneous wounds. The incubation period is variable, ranging from 1 week to 2 months, but it is usually 2–3 weeks. The initial lesion appears at the site of inoculation as a purplish-red papule that evolves quickly into a verrucoid nodule (Fig. 124.1). The commonest sites of infection are the hands, the elbows, the feet and the knees. The nodule may ulcerate, giving rise to a torpid ulcer with undermined borders (Fig. 124.2). The lesion generally remains solitary, but in some instances secondary lesions may develop proximally along cutaneous lymphatic vessels (sporotricoid form). Regional lymph nodes are generally not involved. The lesions usually undergo spontaneous resolution to heal with scarring after 1–3 years.

HISTOPATHOLOGICAL FINDINGS

Fully developed lesion consists of a suppurative, granulomatous dermatitis and panniculitis, often accompanied by pseudo-carcinomatous hyperplasia (Figs 124.3 and 124.4).

MANAGEMENT

Several chemotherapeutic regimens have proved effective, including tetracycline, minocycline, rifampicin (rifampin) and co-trimoxazole (trimethoprim–sulfamethoxazole). Preventive measures, such as the use of gloves, may reduce the incidence of this disease.

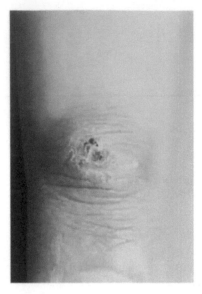

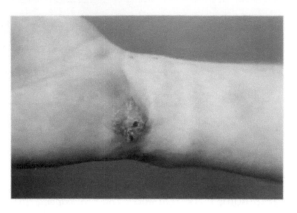

Figure 124.2
Swimming pool granuloma. This ulcerated and crusted pinkish-purple nodule is typical of cutaneous infection caused by atypical mycobacteria.

Figure 124.1
Swimming pool granuloma. Overlying an interphalangeal joint is a plaque that has a pink base and is covered by scales and scaly crusts.

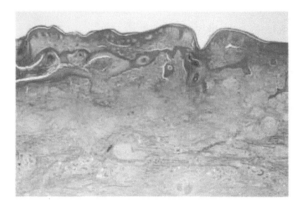

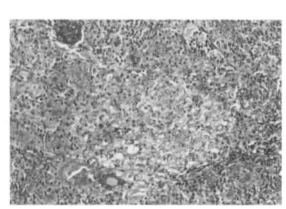

Figure 124.3   **Figure 124.4**

Figures 124.3 and 124.4
Swimming pool granuloma. This lesion of swimming pool granuloma is characterized by dense suppurative granulomatous inflammation and hyperplasia of follicular infundibula that house collections of neutrophils. At higher magnification (Fig. 124.4), note the mixture of neutrophils, lymphocytes, epithelioid histiocytes and giant cells within the reticular dermis.

Syphilis is an infectious disease caused by *Treponema pallidum*. In pediatric patients syphilis may be acquired by transplacental infection or as a consequence of sexual abuse. The clinical features of infection caused by sexual abuse are exactly the same as those observed in adults. Therefore, this chapter illustrates only congenital syphilis.

Congenital syphilis occurs when the fetus is infected *in utero* by a mother who has syphilis. The disease is referred to as 'early congenital syphilis' when it appears under 2 years of age and 'late congenital syphilis' when it is not symptomatic until late childhood.

EPIDEMIOLOGY

Because the time of appearance of the disease depends on the time of maternal fetal infection, in early severe syphilis spontaneous abortions and stillbirth deaths are common events. When the child is born alive the onset of clinical signs is at birth in about 35% of cases or during the first 4 weeks of life in about 65% of cases.

In late congenital syphilis clinical signs generally appear in patients from 5 to 16 years of age.

The world incidence of congenital syphilis is variable. The disease occurs in about 0.05% of live-born children in the USA.

CLINICAL FINDINGS

Early congenital syphilis

Mucocutaneous lesions are present in about 50% of cases and resemble those observed in acquired secondary syphilis. The skin rash consists mostly of maculopapular or papular scaling and copper–red lesions that appear chiefly on the extremities (Fig. 125.1), the diaper area and the face. Bullous and eroded lesions (syphilitic pemphigus) are rare, but distinctive manifestations of this disease and are more commonly found on the extremities. The palms and soles are the sites of predilection (Fig. 125.2). Blisters vary in size from 10 to 50 mm in diameter; their content may be serous or it may be turbid and rich in treponemes. A diffuse desquamation or a desquamation subsequent to the bullous eruption is another characteristic finding. Perioral and perianal fissures are present in about 70% of cases. Purpura and petechiae may appear when thrombocytopenia is severe. Syphilitic coryza is generally the first sign of the disease, occurring 1–2 weeks before the cutaneous rash. The discharge is initially watery, becoming progressively purulent and then hemorrhagic. Mucous patches and condylomata lata are more rarely present. Hepatosplenomegaly is present in about 65% of cases. It may be associated with jaundice and it induces a bloated aspect to the abdomen. Osteochondritis is an early and common sign; it preferentially involves the ends of the long bones and induces swelling and pain. Pseudoparalysis of the limbs (Parrot's pseudoparalysis) may result from bone pain. Later, in the 1st year of life, a periostitis may be radiographically detected. Lymphadenopathy, anemia, thrombocytopenia, meningitis, choroiditis and uveitis are less frequent features.

Late congenital syphilis

Skin and mucous membranes lesions are observed in 2–17% of cases and consist of nodules and gummas like those observed in acquired tertiary syphilis. The distinctive lesions of late congenital syphilis may be caused by persistent local infection, by immunologically mediated conditions and by malformations that occur because of previous infections at a critical period of growth and development (stigmata). Interstitial keratitis, eighth-nerve deafness and bilateral hydrarthrosis are the most common active expressions of late disease. Among stigmata, frontal bossae, saddle nose, short maxillae and high arched palate are present in over 70% of patients. Dental deformities, noted in about 60% of cases, are highly diagnostic. They consist of Hutchinson's teeth and mulberry molars. Hutchinson's teeth are permanent incisors with a barrel shape and a degree of notching at the free edge. Mulberry molars are dome-shaped with more numerous, poorly developed cusps. Other stigmata, such as clavicular malformations, rhagades and sabre shin, are less common. The so-called Hutchinson's triad (Hutchinson's teeth, interstitial keratitis and eighth-nerve deafness) is considered pathognomonic of late congenital syphilis.

LABORATORY FINDINGS

The demonstration of treponemas in a lesion by dark field examination is the simplest method of confirming the diagnosis. When patients are asymptomatic the diagnosis is based essentially on serology. The fluorescent treponema antibody–absorption test (for immunoglobulin M) has been used for this purpose. The positivity of this test must be judged with caution.

HISTOPATHOLOGICAL FINDINGS

Primary syphilis is characterized by a mixed cell infiltrate that contains plasma cells in an edematous stroma associated with prominent blood vessels.

Secondary syphilis shows a psoriasiform lichenoid dermatitis in which histiocytes and plasma cells predominate (Figs 125.3 and 125.4).

In tertiary syphilis there is a caseation necrosis within a granulomatous dermatitis or panniculitis.

MANAGEMENT

Penicillin is the drug of choice for syphilis in all its stages. In congenital syphilis the major problem is whether the infected infant has central nervous system involvement, since the conventional treatment with benzathine penicillin G does not produce detectable penicillin levels in cerebrospinal fluid. Therefore, infants with congenital syphilis should have an examination of cerebrospinal fluid before treatment.

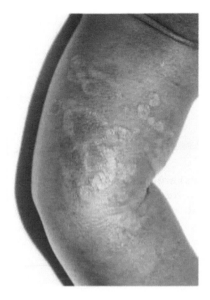

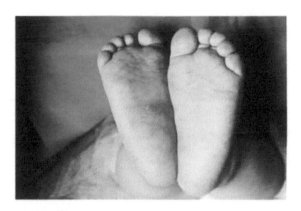

Figure 125.2
Early congenital syphilis. On the soles of this child there are coppery-red papules and roundish areas of desquamation subsequent to bullous lesions.

Figure 125.1
Early congenital syphilis. The limbs are the site of predilection for the papular rash. The figurate pattern is due to confluence of single papule.

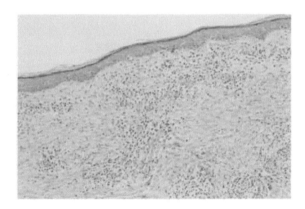

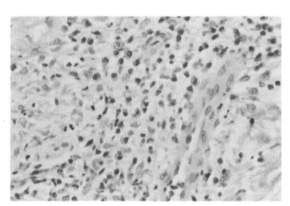

Figure 125.3   **Figure 125.4**

Figures 125.3 and 125.4
Secondary syphilis. An early papule of secondary syphilis, such as the one here, is characterized by a superficial and deep, focally band-like infiltrate composed of plasma cells, histiocytes and lymphocytes. At higher magnification, plasma cells are seen to predominate overwhelmingly in the infiltrate.

126 SYRINGOCYSTADENOMA PAPILLIFERUM

Syringocystadenoma papilliferum is an uncommon, asymptomatic, proliferating lesion that is characterized histologically by being an apocrine papillated cystadenoma.

EPIDEMIOLOGY

Fifty per cent of the tumors of syringocystadenoma papilliferum are reportedly present at birth, and the remainder are usually seen during infancy or childhood.

CLINICAL FINDINGS

Syringocystadenoma papilliferum may occur as a solitary plaque or as multiple papules, usually arranged in a linear configuration. The plaque form consists of a digitated or papillated alopecic lesion, skin-colored to dark brown, often covered by a blistering crust (Fig. 126.1). The less common papular form presents as skin-colored to pink papules that frequently show central umbilication, through which small fistulae may discharge fluid. The majority of the lesions (in 75% of cases) are located on the head and neck, 20% on the trunk and 5% on the extremities. If untreated, the condition persists for life.

Associations

Syringocystadenoma papilliferum may occur independently; in about 40% of cases it appears in association with nevus sebaceus (Fig. 126.2).

HISTOPATHOLOGICAL FINDINGS

Syringocystadenoma papilliferum consists of papillated structures lined by apocrine epithelium that is contiguous with the infindibular epithelium (Fig. 126.3).

MANAGEMENT

The only effective treatment is complete surgical excision of the lesions.

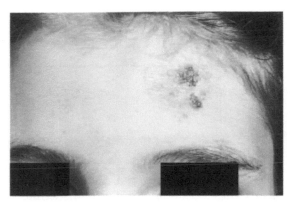

Figure 126.1
Syringocystadenoma papilliferum. This partially treated lesion (as evidenced by the healing ulcers) consists of a plaque upon which there are numerous papillations.

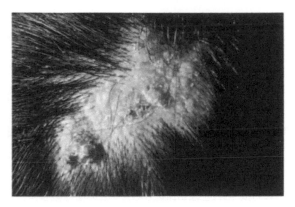

Figure 126.2
Syringocystadenoma papilliferum in association with a nevus sebaceus. The area of the tumor consists of the papillomatous and crusted lesion located on the left part of the nevus sebaceus.

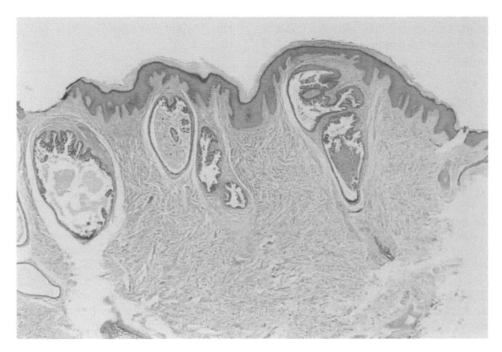

Figure 126.3
Syringocystadenoma papilliferum. This papillated lesion exhibits some cystic structures lined by apocrine epithelium, which forms numerous papillae that project into the lumens.

127

SYRINGOMA

Syringoma is a common benign tumor of the eccrine sweat gland ducts.

EPIDEMIOLOGY

Syringomas begin to appear during late adolescence; only the eruptive variant generally appears before puberty. Approximately 75% of patients are women.

CLINICAL FINDINGS

Syringomas are asymptomatic, firm papules, varying in size from 1 to 5 mm in diameter; rarely papules may be as large as 10 mm. They have round, oval or polygonal shapes, and their long axes often run parallel to Langer's lines (Figs 127.1 and 127.2). The surface of syringomas is low-domed or flat-topped. Although they are usually skin-colored, syringomas may also assume shades of yellow, red–brown and even bluish-purple (the last in dark-skinned people). Syringomas are usually numerous, and they may be found in localized areas or they may be widespread. The commonest localized site is the periorbital area (see Fig. 127.1), which is involved in more than 50% of patients. Widespread syringomas tend to involve concurrently the anterior trunk, including the anterior neck and chest, the upper extremities, the axillae, the volar forearms and the periumbilical and genital regions. Eruptive syringoma is a peculiar clinical variant in which the lesions appear in successive crops in these regions over short periods of time during the early teenage years and in the 20s. Eruptive

syringomas generally spare the periorbital area. These lesions do not demonstrate a tendency to resolve.

Associations

Syringomas seem to be common in patients with Down's syndrome, 39% of whom are affected.

HISTOPATHOLOGICAL FINDINGS

Within the upper half of the dermis there are nests, cords, strands and duct-like structures composed of epithelial cells. The duct-like structures are generally lined by two layers of cells – an outer, more basaloid layer, and an inner, more squamoid layer (Figs 127.3 and 127.4). The epithelial cells often have pale or even clear cytoplasm. The lumens may be filled with pale, homogeneous, eosinophilic material. Characteristically, the basaloid cells of duct-like structures and nests form 'tails' of epithelium, prompting comparison to the appearance of tadpoles or commas (see Fig. 127.4). These epithelial structures are surrounded by a stroma with thickened bundles of collagen.

MANAGEMENT

No treatment is necessary except for cosmetic reasons. Complete excision, cryotherapy, electrodesiccation and application of trichloroacetic acid have all been used with some success.

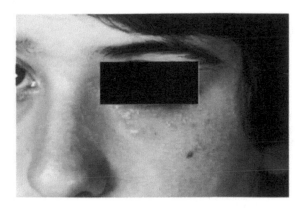

Figure 127.1
Syringoma. Discrete whitish and skin-colored papules are present on the eyelids, the nose and the malar eminence.

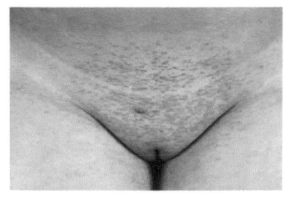

Figure 127.2
Syringoma. Brownish, ovoid papules following Langer's lines are characteristic of syringomas. The genitalia are one site of predilection.

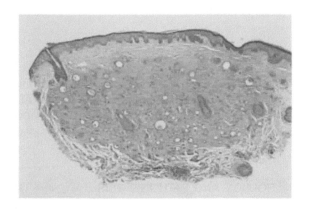

Figure 127.3

Figure 127.4

Figures 127.3 and 127.4
Syringoma. In the dermis, there is a nodular, sharply demarcated neoplasm constituted of both epithelial and stromal components. Epithelial cells are arranged in nests, cords, strands and duct-like structures, the walls of which are lined by two rows of cells. The outer row exhibits more basaloid cells, the inner row more squamoid cells. Note that some of the ductal structures have small, comma-like tails of epithelial cells, giving them the appearance of tadpoles. The stroma is composed of thickened collagen bundles that are separated from normal dermis by clefts.

128

TINEA VERSICOLOR

Tinea versicolor is a superficial fungal infection characterized by fine scaling and a disturbance of skin pigmentation. It is observed most commonly in young adults of either sex, and less commonly in children.

EPIDEMIOLOGY

The distribution of tinea versicolor is worldwide. However, in tropical and subtropical regions where temperature and humidity are high, the incidence in children is close to 40% according to some experts. The ages of affected young patients range from a few months to 12 years.

CLINICAL FINDINGS

The clinical features of tinea versicolor in children are similar to those in adults. Hyperchromic (yellow–brown), hypochromic or achromic patches can be seen (Figs 128.1 and 128.2). The color varies according to the patient's degree of pigmentation, sun exposure and the severity of the disease. In chronic disease, both hyperchromic and hypochromic lesions can be found in the same patient. Early lesions are small (lentil-sized), asymptomatic and multiple; later they may merge to form large patches. The margins are irregular. Typical desquamation can be revealed upon slight scratching. Tinea versicolor in children may affect the same regions as in adults (the neck, the trunk and the shoulders), but often the lesions affect the face (which is rarely affected in adults). If not treated, the lesions are chronic and relapsing.

LABORATORY FINDINGS

In children, microscopic examination of a potassium hydroxide preparation of scales from lesions is necessary to confirm the diagnosis. If spores (known colloquially as 'spaghetti and meatballs' or as 'frankfurters and beans') are seen in the cornified layer, the diagnosis is tinea versicolor.

HISTOPATHOLOGICAL FINDINGS

The lesions are characterized by short, stubby hyphae and round spores that stain basophilic with hematoxylin and eosin ('spaghetti and meatball' pattern) and that are situated in the cornified layer (Fig. 128.3).

ETIOLOGY AND PATHOGENESIS

The etiological agent is *Malassezia furfur*. Dicarboxylic acid produced by the yeast directly inhibits the synthesis of melanin; this is the cause of the typical hypopigmentation of the patches.

MANAGEMENT

In children, the treatment is topical only. Most available topical antimycotics (mainly imidazole derivatives) are extremely active against *M. furfur*. Since the lesions are often limited to the face, creams are generally used. When applied for 10–15 days, creams usually allow the sterilization of lesions to be obtained. If the patches are spread and involve the trunk, it is preferable to resort to shampoo or foam, which can be applied more easily.

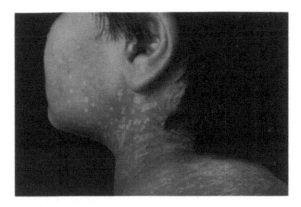

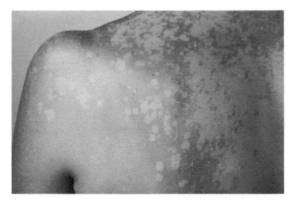

Figure 128.1
Tinea versicolor. Hypopigmented patches extend to the face, which is rarely affected in adults. Many of the spores and hyphae of *M. furfur*, the causative organism of tinea versicolor, are present in the cornified layers of the hypopigmented zones.

Figure 128.2
Tinea versicolor. There are numerous, hypopigmented macules and patches that tend to coalesce.

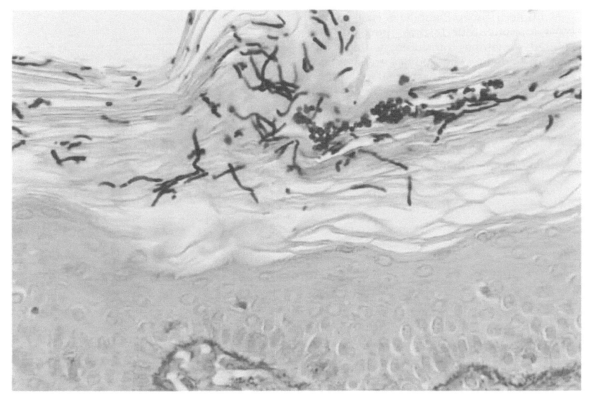

Figure 128.3
Tinea versicolor. At scanning magnification this lesion is typified by laminar hyperkeratosis and a sparse lymphocytic infiltrate around the vessels of the superficial plexus. Within the cornified layer there are short, broad hyphae and collections of round basophilic spores, a combination that has been named 'spaghetti and meatballs'. Fungal elements are better seen with periodic acid–Schiff stain.

129

TRICHOEPITHELIOMA

Trichoepithelioma is an uncommon, benign neoplasm of hair follicle differentiation. It affects mainly females.

CLINICAL FINDINGS

Trichoepithelioma in children occurs either as a multiple form or as a solitary form.

Multiple trichoepithelioma is characterized by numerous round, firm, pink or skin-colored, sometimes translucent nodules of 2–5 mm in diameter. The nodules are symmetrically distributed in the nasolabial folds, on the cheeks and on the eyelids (Figs 129.1 and 129.2). The number of tumors may increase over the years.

Solitary trichoepithelioma consists of a skin-colored, round, smooth, firm, asymptomatic nodule usually not more than 10 mm in diameter. The face is the most usual site.

HISTOPATHOLOGICAL FINDINGS

Trichoepitheliomas are symmetrical, well-circumscribed dermal neoplasms composed mostly of follicular germinative cells that are usually arranged in a cribriform pattern (Figs 129.3 and 129.4).

MANAGEMENT

In multiple trichoepithelioma, cryotherapy, electrodesiccation and carbon dioxide laser therapy give variable cosmetic results. In solitary trichoepithelioma, surgical excision is recommended.

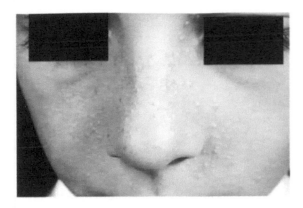

Figure 129.1

Trichoepithelioma. Numerous, discrete, skin-colored papules are present over the nose and malar eminences and near the eyelids.

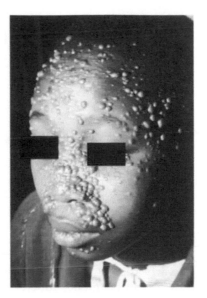

Figure 129.2

Trichoepithelioma. Numerous smooth-surfaced, skin-colored papules and nodules, many of which have become confluent, are heaped on the face.

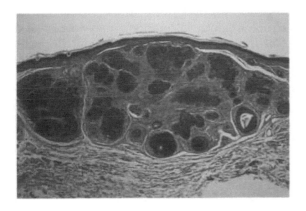

Figure 129.3

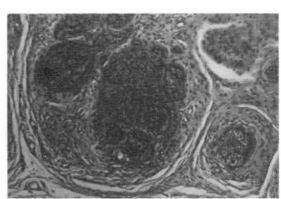

Figure 129.4

Figures 129.3 and 129.4

Trichoepithelioma. This small, well-circumscribed, superficial neoplasm is a trichoepithelioma because aggregations of follicular germinative cells form cribriform and retiform patterns and because the connective tissue is an exaggeration of the embryonic perifollicular sheath, being composed of numerous thin and wavy fibrocytes and delicate fibrillary bundles of collagen. Germ-like structures and follicular papillae are seen at the periphery of the cribriform elements in the foci.

Cutaneous tuberculosis is either the result of the inoculation of *Mycobacterium tuberculosis* into the skin of previously unaffected persons (congenital tuberculosis, tuberculous chancre), or it results from exogenous infection in subjects with some degree of immunity (lupus vulgaris, warty tuberculosis, scrofuloderma, orificial tuberculosis, miliary tuberculosis). Tuberculids represent an allergic reaction to components of *M. tuberculosis* reaching highly immune skin and spread from an internal focus. Nowadays, only papulonecrotic tuberculids occur in developed countries.

EPIDEMIOLOGY

Nowadays only sporadic cases occur in the developed countries, but cutaneous tuberculosis has a worldwide distribution. Lupus vulgaris is the most frequent form of cutaneous tuberculosis in children. Skin tuberculosis may appear at any age during childhood. Primary cutaneous tuberculosis usually occurs in infants.

CLINICAL FINDINGS

Tuberculous chancre (cutaneous primary complex) appears at sites of primary inoculation within 2–4 weeks. A minor form of skin injury is necessary for the bacillus to penetrate into the skin. The early lesion is a small, brownish-red papule that may subsequently enlarge and ulcerate. The ulcer is indolent, crateriform and crusted (Fig. 130.1). A regional lymphadenopathy develops 3–8

weeks after the infection. The glands slowly enlarge and after weeks or months may soften and become cold abscesses. Most cases are contracted on the extremities or on the face through common injuries. Primary tuberculous infection of the penis subsequent to ritual circumcision is very characteristic.

Lupus vulgaris is the most frequently observed form of cutaneous tuberculosis in children. The characteristic lesion is a well-demarcated plaque consisting of small, soft, reddish-brown papules (Fig. 130.2). They are asymptomatic and have an apple-jelly color on diascopy. The plaque grows by peripheral extension and is often accompanied by central atrophy. Fresh lesions may appear in the atrophic area. Ulcerations may occur and scarring may result. The head and the neck are involved in about 90% of patients. Mucous membranes and cartilages may be involved, too.

Warty tuberculosis is usually caused by exogenous re-infection. In children, the sites of predilection are the lower extremities and the buttocks, because they are the areas most subject to trauma (Fig. 130.3). Clinically, the disease starts as small, firm, hyperkeratotic, indolent papules with a purple inflammatory halo. Progressive peripheral expansion leads to the development of a verrucous plaque. Spontaneous involution may be seen in the center of the plaque, and activity may be observed in the borders. The lymph nodes are usually not affected.

Scrofuloderma (tuberculosis colliquativa cutis) results from direct extension into the skin of an underlying tuberculous focus, most commonly from lymph nodes and bones. It usually appears in the submandibular and supraclavicular regions and on the lateral aspects of the neck (Fig. 130.4). Initially the lesion presents as a bluish-red induration overlying an infected lymph node. Through liquefaction, ulceration with bluish under-lined borders and draining fistular sinuses develop. Cord-like scars and localized recur-rences are characteristic.

Orificial tuberculosis is a rare form of autoinoculation tuberculosis that occurs at mucocutaneous junctions in anergic patients with advanced internal infection. The tongue, the area on and around the anus, and the vulva are the most commonly affected sites. Lesions appear as shallow, painful ulcers with undermined bluish edges, the lesions tend not to heal spontaneously. Ulcers may be covered by pseudomembranous material.

Acute miliary tuberculosis occurs in infants from hematogenous dissemination of mycobacteria. The skin lesions are in the form of a profuse eruption, particularly on the trunk, of minute reddish-brown papules or vesicles. These lesions may become necrotic and may heal with the formation of small, white, depressed scars.

Papulonecrotic tuberculid is characterized by recurring eruptions of necrotizing papules affecting the limbs and buttocks symmetri-cally. These lesions are asymptomatic and leave varioloid scars.

LABORATORY FINDINGS

The intradermal tuberculin test, using purified protein derivative, is presently the test of choice, and it is positive in patients who have or have had a tubercular infection. In cases of tuberculous chancre, the test is initially negative but becomes positive during the course of the disease.

HISTOPATHOLOGICAL FINDINGS

There are several common denominators to nearly all cutaneous forms of tuberculosis –

caseation necrosis, granulomatous inflamma-tion and a lymphocytic infiltrate of varying density. These components are present to different degrees in the different manifesta-tions of cutaneous tuberculosis. In summary, the histopathological findings of the most important clinical variants are:

* in tuberculous chancre, cutaneous ulcera-tion with neutrophils and tuberculoid granulomas that contain numerous tuber-cle bacilli;
* in lupus vulgaris, dermal collections of epithelioid cells and giant cells surrounded by many lymphocytes and plasma cells; rarely caseation necrosis is seen within granulomas (Figs 130.5 and 130.6);
* in warty tuberculosis, pseudocarcinoma-tous epidermal hyperplasia, neutrophilic intraepidermal microabscesses and collec-tions of neutrophils and tuberculoid granu-loma in the dermis;
* in scrofuloderma, extensive areas of caseation necrosis surrounded by tubercu-loid granulomas;
* in orificial tuberculosis, ulcerative nodules with necrosis, tuberculoid granulomas and many tubercle bacilli;
* in acute miliary tuberculosis, neutrophilic microabscess containing many bacilli.
* in papulonecrotic tuberculid, vasculitis associated with necrosis surrounded by lymphocytes, epithelioid cells and giant cells.

MANAGEMENT

The treatment of all forms of cutaneous tuberculosis in children is the same as the treatment of systemic tuberculosis: a combi-nation of isoniazid (10–20 mg/kg per day) and rifampicin (rifampin; 10–20 mg/kg per day) both for 9 months. Streptomycin and ethambutol are not recommended for young children.

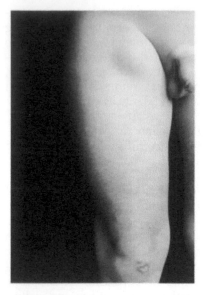

Figure 130.1
Tuberculous chancre. A papule and plaque of primary tuberculosis are present on the knee, and there is swelling in the inguinal region as a consequence of a lymphadenopathy.

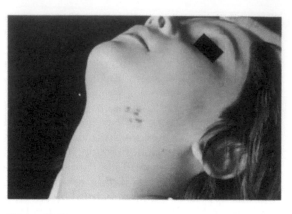

Figure 130.2
Lupus vulgaris. Several reddish-brown papules covered by slight scales are early lesions in the neck.

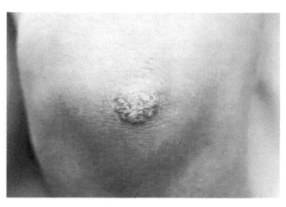

Figure 130.3
Warty tuberculosis. This solitary nodule on a knee is reddish-brown and covered by scaly crusts. The cause of this lesion is *Mycobacterium bovis* rather than *Mycobacterium tuberculosis.*

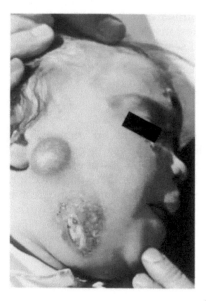

Figure 130.4
Scrofuloderma. Near the jaw line is an ulcer covered by purulent crusts and surrounded by erosions, scaly crusts and slight scarring. The lesion in the preauricular region, a consequence of marked lymphadenopathy, is reddish-brown and covered by scales.

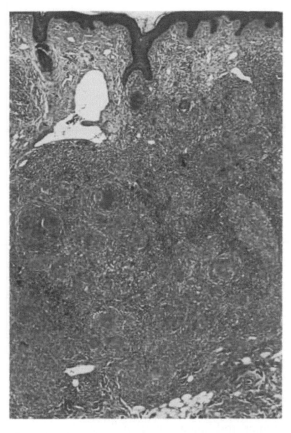

Figure 130.5

Figures 130.5 and 130.6
Lupus vulgaris. This lesion is characterized by many granulomas situated in the reticular dermis. These granulomas are constituted of collections of epithelioid cells and numerous giant cells. Note that each granuloma is surrounded by a dense infiltrate of lymphocytes. The epidermis is unaffected.

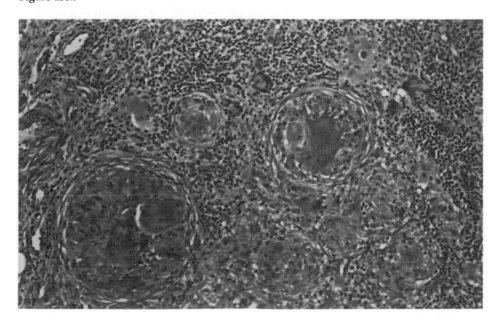

Figure 130.6

Tuberous sclerosis (epiloia, Pringle–Bourneville's disease) is a multisystemic hamartomatosis that involves the skin, the central nervous system, the eyes, the heart, the kidneys and the bones. The most characteristic features of this disorder are skin lesions, epilepsy and mental retardation.

EPIDEMIOLOGY

Tuberous sclerosis occurs in all races. Its incidence has been estimated to be 1 in 10,000.

CLINICAL FINDINGS

The skin lesions that are pathognomonic of tuberous sclerosis are angiofibromas, periungual fibromas, shagreen patches, and ash-leaf white spots. Facial angiofibromas, the so-called adenoma sebaceum of Pringle, usually become evident during childhood and are present in 80% of cases as pink–red, smooth, firm papules, 1–10 mm in diameter and symmetrically situated on the nasolabial folds, the cheeks and the chin (Fig. 131.1). Such lesions grow steadily in number and size with age. Periungual fibromas (Koenen's tumors) appear at puberty in 50% of patients as flesh-colored, elongated excrescences that emerge from the nailbed and folds (Fig. 131.2). Shagreen patches are connective tissue nevi of the collagen type; in 20–40% of cases they occur on the lumbosacral region during early childhood as yellowish orange, soft, irregular plaques, 10–100 mm in diameter (Fig. 131.3). Hypopigmented lance–ovate

macules (ash-leaf spots) are found in 90% of patients at birth and represent an early diagnostic marker of this disorder. They are variable in size and number, are usually situated on the trunk (Fig. 131.4) and the limbs, and are most easily detectable by examination under Wood's light. These lesions do not alter their shapes and size with age.

Nervous system involvement occurs in about 70% of patients and consists mostly of mental retardation and epilepsy. Epilepsy usually develops during infancy or childhood, thus preceding the skin lesions.

Ocular involvement occurs in about 50% of cases and is characterized by retinal hamartomas and hamartomas of the optic nerves.

Renal involvement consists of angiolipomas (occurring in 60% of patients) and cysts (occurring in 20%).

Cardiac rhabdomyomas are associated with tuberous sclerosis in over 50% of infants. These tumors are often asymptomatic and may be self-healing. Frequently they represent, at birth, the first manifestation of the disease and are detectable by echocardiography.

Skeletal involvement, detectable in about 50% of patients using routine radiography and computed tomography, is represented by sclerotic patches, pseudocysts and periosteal new bone.

LABORATORY FINDINGS

Sclerotic calcifications in the brain are visible by computed tomography in about 50% of patients.

HISTOPATHOLOGICAL FINDINGS

Adenoma sebaceum is a hamartoma composed of fibrocytic, follicular, vascular and sometimes melanocytic elements (Figs 131.5 and 131.6).

Periungual and subungual fibromas consist of polypoid lesions in an epidermis of normal volar skin. The lesions are composed of thick bundles of collagen in vertical array in concert with an increased number of venules.

Shagreen patches are collagenous nevi marked by a papillated surface and thick bundles of collagen in the reticular dermis that are oriented perpendicular to the skin surface.

Ash-leaf spots are characterized by a normal complement of melanocytes with a decreased amount of melanin within the epidermis.

ETIOLOGY AND PATHOGENESIS

Tuberous sclerosis is inherited as an autosomal-dominant trait that shows great variability. The genes for tuberous sclerosis have been located in chromosomes 16p13 and 9q34.

MANAGEMENT

Facial angiofibromas may be treated with diathermy, dermabrasion or argon laser therapy for cosmetic reasons. Anticonvulsive drugs are moderately useful. Genetic counseling of affected patients and their families should be undertaken with care in order to identify any minimal sign of the disease in apparently unaffected parents and relatives.

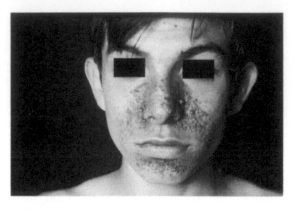

Figure 131.1
Facial angiofibromas. There are many smooth-surfaced, skin-colored and slightly brownish papules.

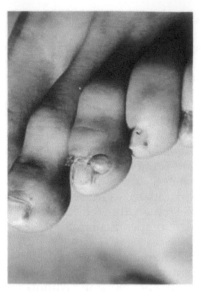

Figure 131.2
Periungual fibromas (Koenen's tumors). These somewhat warty, firm papules may be present at the sides of nail plates, as shown here, or beneath them. Because of their shape, they have also been called 'garlic clove' tumors.

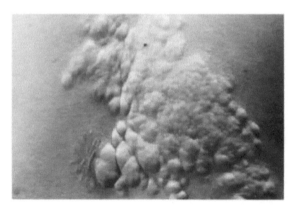

Figure 131.3
Shagreen plaque of tuberous sclerosis. This plaque, with a bumpy surface, consists of numerous, closely crowded, skin-colored papules.

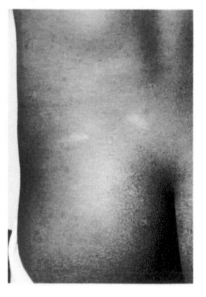

Figure 131.4
Ash-leaf spots of tuberous sclerosis. The elongated hypopigmented patches are diagnostic and are usually the first cutaneous sign of tuberous sclerosis.

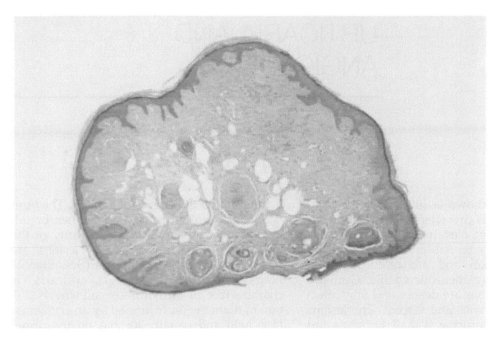

Figure 131.5

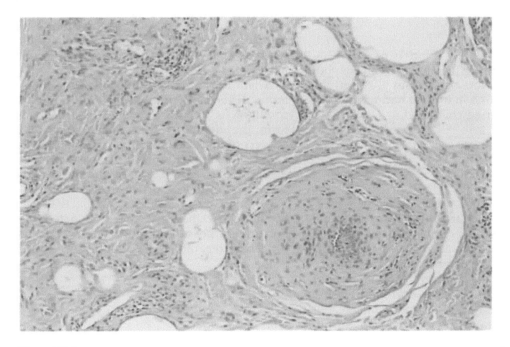

Figure 131.6

Figures 131.5 and 131.6
Adenoma sebaceum. This dome-shaped papule, which comes from a patient with tuberous sclerosis, is characterized by numerous dilated vessels, an increased number of oval and multinucleate fibrocytes, and thickened collagen bundles that are arranged in lamellae around vellus follicles.

URTICARIA AND ANGIOEDEMA

Urticaria (also known as hives or nettle rash) is any rash that is characterized by the appearance of transient elevated patches (wheals). The wheals may be redder or paler than the surrounding skin and are often itchy. In angioedema (angioneurotic edema, Quinke's edema), the lesions are deeper and may affect mucous membranes and viscera. The lesions are only mildly pruritic, if at all. Urticaria and angioedema may coexist.

EPIDEMIOLOGY

Urticaria is relatively common in children but angioedema is less so. About 10% of the general population may have had urticaria or angioedema during childhood.

CLINICAL FINDINGS

Urticaria usually presents as elevated, edematous papules of variable dimensions and redness. The shape of the lesions may be round–oval, annular, arciform or polycyclic (Fig. 132.1); their disposition is, as a rule, irregular or bizarre, except for special forms of urticaria (e.g. light urticaria, dermographism). The erythema may vary from case to case, but when the edema of the lesions is intense, it provokes a pallor in the central area of the wheal. The characteristic hard elastic consistency of the wheal may be felt easily only in large, well-elevated lesions. The number of lesions may change greatly, not only from patient to patient but also in the same patient,

depending on the degree of activity. The term 'giant urticaria' is usually used when broad, elevated patches involve the majority of the tegument. Individual urticarial lesions are relatively evanescent and last for less than 24 hours. So-called cholinergic urticaria is characterized by numerous, small wheals (2–5 mm in diameter) surrounded by an erythematous halo and usually located on the upper trunk. This form of urticaria occurs most commonly after physical or psychological stress or ingestion of spicy food or hot beverages. The course of urticaria in children is usually short (acute urticaria), but in some cases it may last for months (chronic urticaria).

When the process involves the deeper, more distensible portions of the skin, the condition is known as angioedema. In this form the depth of the edema makes the borders of the lesions, which are usually large and easily confluent (Fig. 132.2), less defined. Angioedema may be accompanied by systemic symptoms, such as fever, arthralgias, abdominal pain, vomiting, diarrhea, headache, dizziness and shock. To date it has not proved possible to suspect the cause of urticaria from the clinical appearance of the lesions.

Complications

There are no major complications from urticaria that is confined to the skin. More serious is the involvement of vital structures by angioedema. When angioedema involves the tongue and the larynx, respiratory compromise may be sufficiently severe to cause death.

HISTOPATHOLOGICAL FINDINGS

Fully developed lesions of urticaria are typified by sparse, superficial, and often superficial and deep, perivascular and interstitial infiltrates composed mostly of neutrophils and eosinophils (Figs 132.3 and 132.4). The epidermis is entirely unaffected, as is the dermoepidermal junction. Edema in urticaria forms mostly in the reticular dermis.

ETIOLOGY AND PATHOGENESIS

Although urticarial lesions can be provoked by either immune or non-immune mechanisms, urticaria is usually allergic in cause, as is angioedema. Type I hypersensitivity reactions (immunoglobulin E or immunoglobulin G_4 reagin-mediated immunity) and type III hypersensitivity reactions (immune-complex reaction) are both involved in allergic urticaria. Allergens that can be identified include inhalants, ingestants, injectants, infections or infestations, and contactants. In addition to immune-mediated urticaria, there are non-allergic forms provoked by many substances. via direct liberation of vasoactive substances. Physical urticarias, such as those that are consequences of pressure, heat, cold, ultraviolet light, and cholinergic and adrenergic stimuli, also need to be considered. Hereditary angioedema results from a deficiency of C1 esterase inhibitor.

MANAGEMENT

Management of urticaria must be tailored to the cause of the urticaria, trying to eliminate the triggering factors. Allergic urticaria may be managed by antihistamines and by systemic corticosteroids. Systemic anti-H_1 antihistamines are the drugs of choice in all the forms of non-severe urticaria to control itching. The use of anti-H_2 antihistamines, such as cimetidine, which could be considered useful for a better control of the disease, is sometimes frustrating, probably because histamine is able to act, via H_2 receptors, on mast cells and basophils to stop their degranulation. The blockage of H_2 receptors would inhibit the feedback that self-regulates the histamine liberation. Among systemic anti-H_1 antihistamines, the authors prefer to use, in children, hydroxizine, ciproeptadine, or chlorpheniramine by mouth. In chronic forms, more recent, non-sedating antihistamines (e.g. terfenadine, astemizole, cetirizine, loratadine) can also be considered.

Systemic corticosteroids should be given only in severe forms that are unresponsive to antihistamines. They should be used for a limited period to avoid side effects, some of which (e.g. growth arrest) can be particularly critical in childhood.

Hereditary angioedema may be treated with danazol, which induces increased production of C1 esterase inhibitors.

Systemic corticosteroids should be administered during the flare-ups of the disease, while severe episodes must be treated in hospital with subcutaneous administration of 0.1–0.5 ml of adrenaline (epinephrine) (1:1000), forced ventilation and, if necessary, tracheostomy.

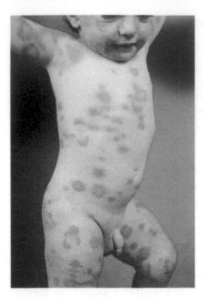

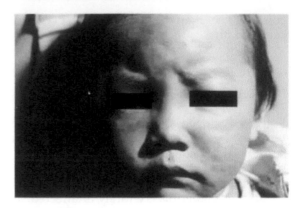

Figure 132.2
Angioedema. The eyelids, the forehead and the cheeks are markedly swollen as a consequence of edema. It is an exaggeration of urticaria at skin sites that are highly distensible.

Figure 132.1
Urticaria. The arciform or figurate arrangement of the wheals is a very characteristic pattern in infants and children.

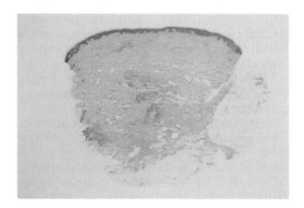

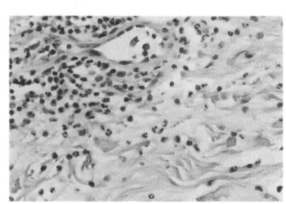

Figure 132.3   **Figure 133.4**

Figures 132.3 and 132.4
Urticaria. The specimen from which these sections were cut was taken from a child with papular and plaque lesions of urticaria. Note the superficial and deep perivascular and interstitial infiltrate composed of lymphocytes, neutrophils and some eosinophils. The epidermis is completely unaffected by the pathological process.

Varicella (chickenpox) and zoster (shingles) are common, acute infectious diseases. Although they are two distinct clinical entities they are caused by the same virus. Varicella is the primary infection; zoster is a recurrence of varicella after a variable period of time and in a limited area.

EPIDEMIOLOGY

Varicella has a worldwide distribution. About 3 million cases are reported in the USA each year. The disease can develop at any age. The peak of incidence occurs from 5–9 years of age. Herpes zoster is unusual in children and exceptional in neonates.

CLINICAL FINDINGS

After a short prodromal period characterized by low fever and malaise, the disease is heralded by the appearance of a macular, pruritic rash. The lesions rapidly progress, over a few days, from macules to papules, and then to the typical 'tear-drop' vesicles on an erythematous base (Fig. 133.1). In 2–3 days the vesicles turn into pustules and the drying process begins in the center, producing an umbilicated appearance and then a crust. Lesions occur in successive crops, so that the various stages of the rash can be observed concomitantly. Characteristically the eruption is concentrated on the trunk and the head, whereas the lesions are distributed more sparsely on the face and the extremities (Fig. 133.2). Lesions also develop on the mucous membranes, especially on the palate. Itching is almost a constant feature, although it can be very variable. Healing is complete in 2–3 weeks, usually with minimal scarring. Varicella is one of the most highly communicable diseases. The average period of incubation is 15 days, and epidemics are frequent in pre-school children communities. The infectiveness of the disease is higher in the first stage of the symptoms.

Zoster in children has the same clinical features as in adults. The typical erythematovesicular rash is unilateral and limited to an area of the skin innervated by the affected sensory nerve, but usually there is no or little neuralgia. Also, fever and local lymphadenopathy are rarely encountered in children. The favorite affected area is controversial – rare on the head (Fig. 133.3), herpes zoster has a predilection for cervical (Fig. 133.4) and lumbosacral localizations, but some experts claim a high frequency on the trunk. Recovery is rapid and without sequelae in 1–2 weeks.

Complications

The most common complication of varicella is secondary bacterial infection that causes scarring of the skin. Post-zoster neuralgia is a rare occurrence in children.

LABORATORY FINDINGS

The detection of the virus can be easily obtained by Tzank's smear, which shows the typical alteration of the epithelial cells affected by the herpesvirus.

HISTOPATHOLOGICAL FINDINGS

Cutaneous infection by herpesvirus, either varicella–zoster virus or herpes simplex virus, produces predictable changes within the epidermis and epithelial structures of the adnexae – ballooned keratinocytes marked by abundant pale cytoplasm, steel–gray nuclei with margination of nucleoplasm, and the tendency to multinucleation of keratinocytes (Figs 133.5 and 133.6).

ETIOLOGY AND PATHOGENESIS

Varicella and zoster are distinct clinical entities caused by the same virus, the varicella–zoster virus.

MANAGEMENT

In normal children the treatment of both diseases is merely symptomatic with wet dressings and oral antihistamines to relieve the pruritus. Secondary bacterial infections must be prevented. In immunosuppressed patients, administration of acyclovir is useful.

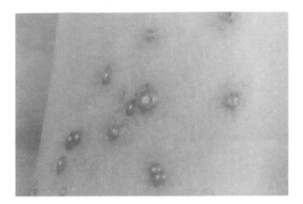

Figure 133.1
Varicella. A close view of the typical 'tear-drop' vesicles.
Some of these tense vesicles, situated on slightly reddish
bases, have hints of umbilication in their centers.

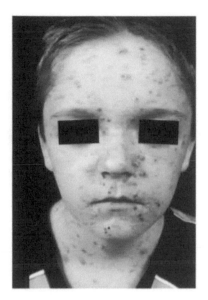

Figure 133.2
Varicella. An adolescent with a severe form of varicella.
The different stages of the lesions (vesicles, pustules and
crusts) are clearly visible.

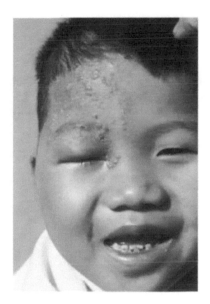

Figure 133.3
Zoster. Many tense vesicles sit on top of a broad reddish
base, and the vesicles follow a dermatomal distribution
limited to one side of the face. Note the marked periorbital swelling.

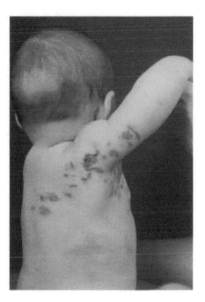

Figure 133.4
Zoster. Many vesicles and hemorrhagic crusts can be seen
on an erythematous base in an infant. The lesions are
distributed in a linear pattern.

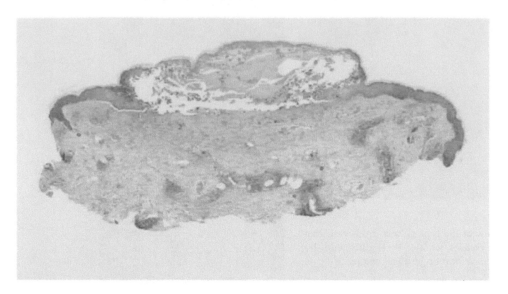

Figure 133.5

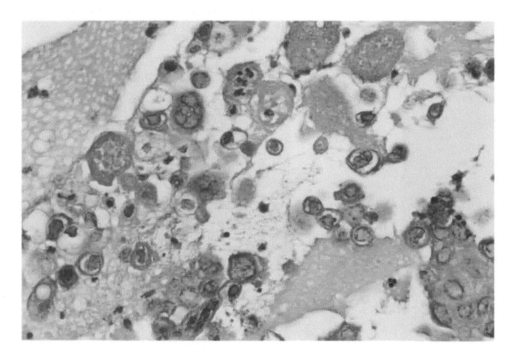

Figure 133.6

Figures 133.5 and 133.6
Herpes zoster. An intraepidermal acantholytic vesicle has become subepidermal because of the rupture of the bottom of the blister. Within the vesicle, numerous acantholytic keratinocytes with characteristic steel–gray nuclei and accentuation of the peripheral nucleoplasm, multinucleate cells and necrotic keratinocytes can be seen at higher magnification.

Vascular birthmarks are lesions that occur at birth or during the first months of life that are formed by abnormal vessels. They can be divided into two categories – vascular malformations and vascular tumors. Vascular malformations are caused by errors in the morphogenesis of the vessels during embryogenesis; thus, they are almost always visible from birth and are substantially stable or modify only slowly over years or decades. Vascular malformations can be formed by a single type of vessel or by different types of vessels giving rise to combined malformation; thus, the variety of clinical presentation is great. Vascular malformations never regress. Vascular tumors are, in the great majority, capillary hemangiomas (benign tumors composed of immature capillaries). The differences in clinical presentation are due to differences in the extent and depth of the lesions. Hemangiomas, after a fast-growing period of a few months, involute before the first decade of life. This chapter illustrates the two most common vascular birthmarks – the capillary malformations and capillary hemangiomas.

CAPILLARY MALFORMATIONS

Capillary malformations are also known as vascular nevi, naevi flammei and flat angiomas.

EPIDEMIOLOGY

Capillary malformations of the midline are almost the rule in Caucasian children. They have a familial tendency and can be observed in more than 70% of newborns. They have an equal sex distribution. Lateral or mosaic capillary malformations are relatively uncommon.

CLINICAL FINDINGS

Two types are seen – salmon patches and port-wine stain. Salmon patches are those common lesions that are localized in the midline. They are found at the nape of the neck (nevus of Unna, stork bite, nevus flammeus nuchae) (Fig. 134.1), on the forehead (angel's kiss) (Fig. 134.2), on the upper eyelids and above the glabella; the interscapular and sacral areas are rarely involved. They appear as a flat, rose-red, irregular geographical area of a few centimeters in diameter. Salmon patches spare mucous membranes, fade with age and are asymptomatic.

Port-wine stains are an uncommon type of malformation variously localized unilaterally or in a mosaic pattern. The size is variable, from few millimeters to a complete dermatomere; the color is pink at the beginning but turns to red or red–purple with time. The lesions are usually localized on the head (Fig. 134.3) and may involve mucous surfaces (Fig. 134.4). They never regress spontaneously. Unlike salmon patches, the texture of the affected areas may change and the skin become darker and irregular. For this reason and because of their usual location, port-wine stains are usually a severe cosmetic problem.

Associations and complications

Because vascular malformations are embryogenic errors, any type of associated anomaly is possible. Complications are dependent on the localization, the extent and association with other malformations. When vascular nevi are localized on one side along the distribution of the first branch of the trigeminal nerve, they can be associated with ipsilateral meningeal and retinal angiomatosis (Sturge–Weber syndrome) (Fig. 134.5). Visual disturbances include glaucoma and bouphthalmos, while neurologic symptoms include seizures, hemiplegia and mental retardation. Nevi flammei, when associated with venous malformation of the limbs, may cause a hypertrophy of the affected limb with orthopedic deformity (Klippel–Trenaunay syndrome) (Fig. 134.6).

LABORATORY FINDINGS

Skull X-rays may reveal calcifications in Sturge–Weber syndrome. Computed tomography scanning or magnetic resonance imaging are useful, especially to rule out the existence of intracranial or orbital malformations. Thermography is of little help. Single photon emission computed tomography and positron emission tomography are newer techniques that can give early information.

HISTOPATHOLOGICAL FINDINGS

Salmon patches and port-wine stains are characterized by a dilatation of capillaries and small venules in the superficial dermis that is not accompanied by endothelial cell proliferation (Fig. 134.7). In port-wine stain the vascular ectasia may gradually involve deep dermal blood vessels and may sometimes develop into changes such as those of hemangioma.

ETIOLOGY AND PATHOGENESIS

The pathogenesis of vascular nevi is unknown, even though it has to be stressed that perinatal traumas play no role, as demonstrated by children born by Cesarean delivery.

MANAGEMENT

The management of vascular nevi is mainly with vascular laser therapy (pulsed-dye at 585 or 595 nm), with results ranging from good to excellent. In venous and arteriovenous malformations, the treatment is surgical.

CAPILLARY HEMANGIOMAS

Capillary hemangiomas are also known as infantile hemangiomas.

EPIDEMIOLOGY

Hemangioma is the most common benign tumor of infancy (affecting up to 10% of newborns). They have a marked female preponderance, with three times as many girls as boys affected.

CLINICAL FINDINGS

All hemangiomas have the same structure, but their localization at different levels produces different presentations. They can occupy all skin layers, but more frequently they are superficial, just below a thinned epidermis; occasionally they are deep and covered by normal skin. Hemangiomas appear as circumscribed nodules that may be found anywhere on the skin or mucous membranes, but they are most commonly located on the head. They can be solitary or several but rarely multiple. They can be of variable dimensions, but the great majority do not exceed a few centimeters in diameter. The distinction between superficial and deep hemangiomas is justified only to facilitate the diagnostic approach.

Superficial hemangioma

Superficial hemangiomas are also known as strawberry hemangiomas. In the first few days after birth, a superficial hemangioma can be seen as a round or oval, pale area (herald patch) that rapidly turns into a flat erythematous patch, which, within a few days or weeks, enlarges and elevates from the skin surface. In a few months it reaches its maximum size; the tumor has a bright red color and a hard elastic consistency. It is hyperthermic and not fully compressible (Fig. 134.8). In the following months, generally after the 1st year of life, involution starts – consistency and temperature fade and small pale areas appear in the center, which becomes flatter. This spontaneous regression is usually complete by the 5th to 7th year of life, even though small areas of telangiectasias may persist at the periphery. Because the location of these hemangiomas is very superficial, the texture of the skin, except in small lesions, becomes altered and does not revert completely to normal after the involution of the lesion (Figs 134.9 and 134.10).

Deep hemangiomas

Deep hemangiomas are also known as cavernous hemangiomas. They usually appear as round or oval, poorly defined nodules that are characterized by elastic consistency and are covered by normal-appearing skin, which shows a tendency to a blue hue (see Fig. 134.10). Because of their localization, deep hemangiomas are usually noted later than superficial hemangiomas. In addition, they seem to regress more slowly, so that they can represent a disturbing problem for cosmetic reasons. The deep location does not generally affect the superficial epidermal texture.

Associations and complications

No constant associations are recorded with hemangiomas. Complications particularly arise in lesions located on the orifices, the head and the neck; ulceration with hemorrhage and aerodigestive tract obstruction may occur. In periocular lesions, amblyopia and astigmatism may occur (Fig. 134.11). In hemangiomas that are undergoing rapid regression, eschars lead to scars. Infections are rare, as are hemodynamic changes. Hepatomegaly, anemia and congestive heart failure can complicate diffuse or huge lesions. Skeletal distortions have been very rarely reported.

LABORATORY FINDINGS

Echo Doppler is the most useful investigation. It shows increasing blood flow with multiple arteriovenous pseudoshunts during the growing phase. Thermography shows an increase in skin temperature during the growing phase. New ultrasound devices may be of great diagnostic help in some cases and thus make other hazardous investigations unnecessary (e.g. conventional arteriography). Computed tomography and magnetic resonance imaging are sometimes indispensable.

HISTOPATHOLOGICAL FINDINGS

The feature common to all hemangiomas is a marked proliferation of dilated endothelium-lined spaces separated by fibrous trabeculae, which may be situated in the dermis or in the subcutaneous fat. Usually, early lesions consist of a proliferation of plump endothelial cells arranged in solid, sharply demarcated aggregations that occasionally tend to circumscribe small capillary lumens (Fig. 134.12). In fully developed lesions, the vascular lumens become wider and are lined by a single layer of plump endothelial cells, and most of them are filled with erythrocytes. Regressing hemangiomas show progressive occlusion and replacement of small and large vessels by fibrosis.

ETIOLOGY AND PATHOGENESIS

Although numerous angiogenic factors have been identified, the cause of hemangiomas remains unknown.

MANAGEMENT

For small hemangiomas (with the exception of periorificial lesions) the best therapy is to wait for spontaneous remission, explaining to parents the natural history of the disease. For this purpose, pictures illustrating the benign self-healing course of a typical lesion are very helpful. In the first months of life, elastic compression, whenever possible, is suggested. When the lesions grow dramatically, pulse corticosteroid therapy gives the best results. It consists of a cycle of 20–30 days of oral corticosteroids (prednisone 2–4 mg/kg per day), which can be repeated every other month. This treatment has minimal side effects and allows vaccinations in the period between treatments. Interferon-alpha can be considered for alarming hemangiomas that are unresponsive to systemic corticosteroids. When hemangiomas have stopped their growth, elastic compression may also be used to speed up the regression. For large hemangiomas that show a slow tendency to involute, the suggested treatment consists of intralesional injection of triamcinolone acetonide; beneficial effects should be seen after 1 month. Finally, plastic surgery is indicated where other treatments have proven unsatisfactory and in all cases in which the fibroadipose tissue remnants are conspicuous.

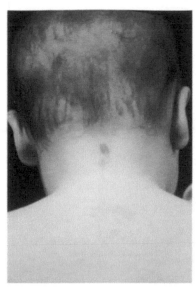

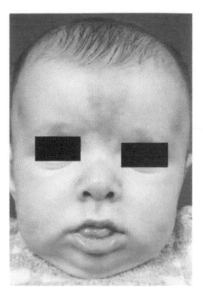

Figure 134.1
Salmon patch. This flat, rose-red irregular geographical area is localized at the nape of the neck and can be considered a normal occurrence in a Caucasian newborn.

Figure 134.2
Salmon patch. This flat, rose, V-shaped patch located on the forehead can be considered normal in a Caucasian newborn. It will fade with age.

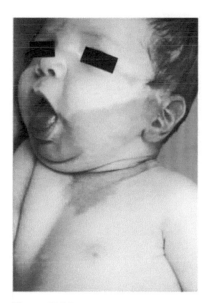

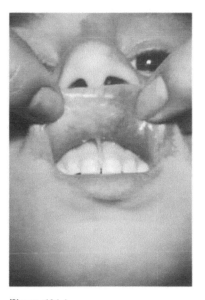

Figure 134.3
Port-wine stain. This lesion, localized unilaterally on the third branch of the trigeminal nerve, is pink–red but, unless treated, it will turn red–purple with time.

Figure 134.4
Port-wine stain. This vascular patch affects the second branch of the trigeminal nerve and not only involves the skin but also the mucosal surface.

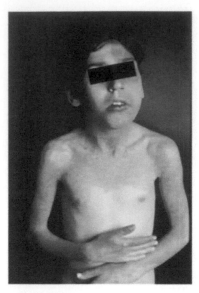

Figure 134.5
Sturge–Weber syndrome. Glaucoma and seizures are the consequences of meningeal and retinal angiomatosis in this child affected by a large capillary malformation.

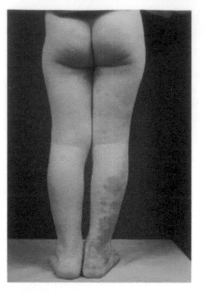

Figure 134.6
Klippel–Trenaunay syndrome. In this young girl the symmetrical involvement of the lower limbs is evident, this is due to venous malformation in association with the capillary patch of the leg.

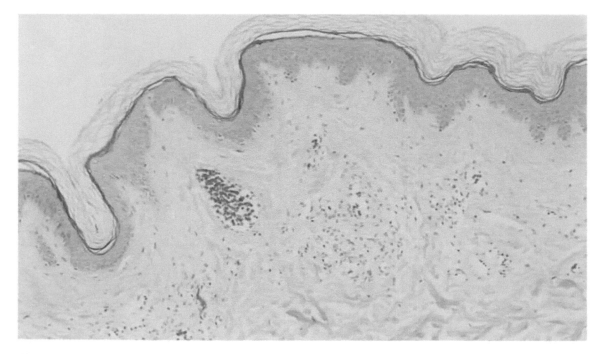

Figure 134.7
Port-wine stains. A dilation of capillaries and small venules in the superficial dermis not accompanied by endothelial cell proliferation is the histological hallmark of this malformation.

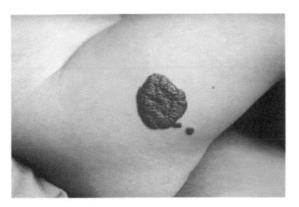

Figure 134.8
Capillary hemangioma. This well-defined vascular tumor, which has a vivid red color and a hard elastic consistency, was not present at birth. It is a superficial capillary hemangioma.

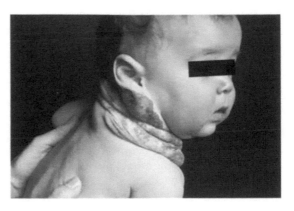

Figure 134.9
Capillary hemangioma. Huge lesions may regress but the texture of the skin is permanently altered; plastic surgery should be advised.

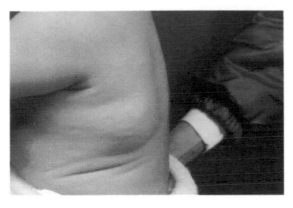

Figure 134.10
Capillary hemangioma. This round, elastic, poorly defined nodule is covered by normal skin, which has a tendency to a blue hue. Echo Doppler reveals a clear pattern of vascularization.

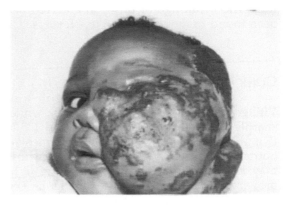

Figure 134.11
Capillary hemangioma. In this patient, this disfiguring mass is dangerous because of the risk of ulceration and visual impairment.

Figure 134.12
Capillary hemangioma. In this fully developed lesion, the vascular lumens are wide and lined by a single layer of plump endothelial cells; most of them are filled with erythrocytes.

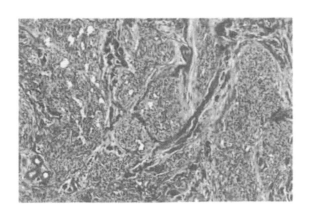

135

VITILIGO

Vitiligo is a common, acquired, circumscribed loss of cutaneous pigment caused by destruction of melanocytes.

EPIDEMIOLOGY

Vitiligo affects all races and both sexes equally and occurs in about 1% of the world's population. The mean age of onset in children has been found to range from 4.6 to 4.8 years.

CLINICAL FINDINGS

Vitiligo is characterized by chalk-white, sharply outlined patches (Fig 135.1 and 135.2) that are often surrounded by hyperpigmented borders. In the early stages the pigment loss may be partial, with various stages of light brown coloration (trichrome vitiligo). The sizes, shapes and number of lesions are very variable, but initial lesions are almost always round or oval and tend to grow centrifugally with typical convex margins. It is possible to distinguish a localized form, which involves one region of the skin, sometimes with a unilateral dermatomal array (segmental vitiligo) (see Fig. 135.2) and a generalized form, which often has a symmetrical distribution (see Fig. 135.1). Sites of predilection are the face, particularly around the eyes and the mouth, the dorsum of the hands, the axillae, the groin and the genitalia. Involvement of the palms and soles is common but evident only by Wood's lamp examination. A halo of depigmentation around a pigmented nevus (vitiligo perinevica) may be the initial symptom of the disease. Leukotrichia is relatively common in these patients and their relatives. Mucosae may also be involved, especially the genitalia,

the nipples, the lips and the gingivae. The course of vitiligo is unpredictable. The disease may remain stationary, extend or progress rapidly. Spontaneous repigmentation may occur; however, such repigmentation is almost never homogeneous and presents a perifollicular distribution.

Associations

Vitiligo may be associated with other skin disorders (e.g. alopecia areata, morphea, lichen sclerosus et atrophicus, psoriasis, melanoma). Several extracutaneous conditions, mostly characterized by an autoimmune pathogenesis, may be observed in patients with vitiligo.

HISTOPATHOLOGICAL FINDINGS

Early lesions of vitiligo show a sparse superficial perivascular infiltrate of lymphocytes associated with a normal complement of melanocytes at the dermoepidermal junction and normal amounts of melanin within the epidermis. Fully developed lesions have no melanocytes and no melanin within the epidermis (Fig. 135.3).

ETIOLOGY AND PATHOGENESIS

The etiopathogenesis of vitiligo is unknown. About 30–40% of patients have a positive family history of the condition. Three major theories have been put forward to explain the cause of the disease – the autodestructive theory, the neurogenic theory, and the autoimmune theory. The autoimmune theory, the most favored, is based on the frequent association of vitiligo with other autoimmune diseases and the detection of 'vitiligo antibodies' to normal human melanocytes.

MANAGEMENT

Treatment of vitiligo is frequently unsatisfactory. Patients older than 12 years of age are generally treated with oral psoralen compounds or khellin followed by gradual exposure to sunlight or psoralen and ultraviolet-A therapy. For localized lesions in children, a topical treatment (psoralen lotion at very low concentrations) followed by short, well-controlled ultraviolet-B or ultraviolet-A exposure twice a week may be useful. Hydrocortisone has been used for repigmenting isolated small macules. Sunscreen may be useful for avoiding sunburn.

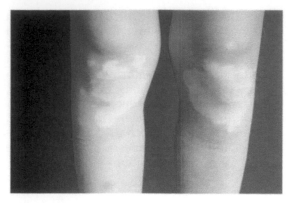

Figure 135.1
Vitiligo. Symmetrical, achromic lesions are present on the knees. A Koebner phenomenon may occur at this site after trauma.

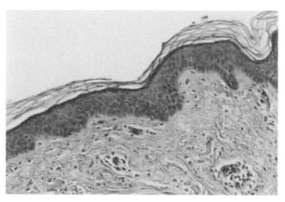

Figure 135.3
Vitiligo. In sections stained by hematoxylin and eosin, fully developed lesions of vitiligo are characterized by complete absence of melanocytes and melanin within the epidermis. A sparse perivascular lymphocytic infiltrate is present around the vessels of the superficial plexus.

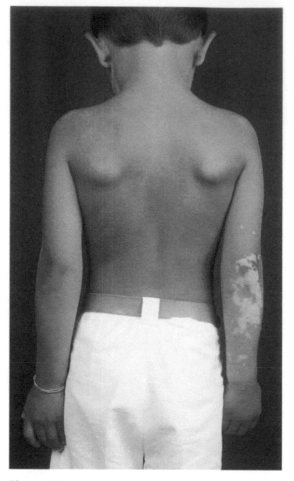

Figure 135.2
Vitiligo. The localized variant is characterized by achromic patches that involve one region of the skin, sometimes with a dermatomal distribution (segmental vitiligo).

136

WARTS

Warts are proliferative, chronic, benign lesions of the skin and adjacent mucous membranes that are caused by epidermotropic DNA viruses of the papova goup (human papillomaviruses). Each particular type of wart has been found to be associated with an individual papillomavirus or group of papillomaviruses.

EPIDEMIOLOGY

Warts are one of the commonest dermatological disorders throughout the world. In children, warts represent 3–5% of all skin problems and generally occur during the school year.

CLINICAL FINDINGS

Common warts are typically exophytic (ie elevated) neoplasms. Their surface is hyperkeratotic and rough because of minute papillary projections, and their size varies from a few millimeters to few centimeters (Fig. 136.1). Not infrequently they are confluent and hypertrophic, especially in periungual locations. They are gray, brownish or flesh-colored, and early warts may have a smooth surface. Common warts are localized mainly on the dorsum of the hands, but they can also be palmar or plantar or can appear elsewhere on the skin, on the semimucosa (e.g. on the red of the lips), or very rarely, on mucous membranes.

Plane warts are slightly raised above the skin level, are smaller than common warts and have flatter, smoother surfaces (Fig. 136.2). More frequently they are multiple, irregularly disseminated or grouped and confluent; they are sometimes distributed in lines because of the Koebner phenomenon. They are mainly localized on the face, especially the forehead, and less commonly on the forearms.

Filiform warts are elongated and digitated excrescences that usually occur on the eyelids and around the lips and the nose (Fig. 136.3).

Plantar warts are endophytic, firm, round, painful lesions surrounded by smooth keratotic rings. They occur on the plantar surfaces of the feet. When pared they reveal small black points that represent thrombosed capillaries of dermal papillae.

Genital warts (condylomata acuminata) appear as soft, pink, elongated excrescences that tend to cornification. They occur on the genitalia and in the perianal region (Fig. 136.4). They are not common in infants and children.

Approximately two-thirds of warts resolve spontaneously within 2 years.

HISTOPATHOLOGICAL FINDINGS

Verruca vulgaris consists of papillated or digitated epidermal hyperplasia; hypergranulosis; collarettes of adnexal epithelium; and dilated, tortuous capillaries in the dermal papillae (Fig. 136.5).

Condylomata acuminata is characterized by papillated, epidermal hyperplasia; focal parakeratosis; focal hypergranulosis; and dilated, tortuous blood vessels in dermal papillae.

Verruca plana shows mammillated epidermal hyperplasia, halos around nuclei in the granular zone or vacuolated gray–blue cytoplasm in cells in the upper part of the viable epidermis; and a cornified layer marked by basket-weave configuration (Fig. 136.6)

MANAGEMENT

Wart therapy, although always challenging, presents additional dilemmas in young chidren. As in all therapeutic decisions, the risk–benefit ratio must be carefully consid-ered. Since treatment is always painful and young children usually have no desire to be treated, the situation can be traumatic for the patients, parents and doctors. One must keep in mind the great tendency for spontaneous resolution of warts and better long-term cosmetic results when that occurs. The decision regarding therapy depends on the patient's age, the type of wart, the likelihood of its spontaneous resolution, the symptoma-tology, the discomfort of the therapy, the risk of scarring and the desires of the patient's parents. A non-aggressive treatment is usually the best solution.

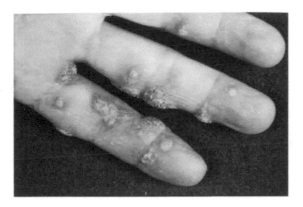

Figure 136.1
Common warts. These discrete papules are slightly papillated and hyperkeratotic.

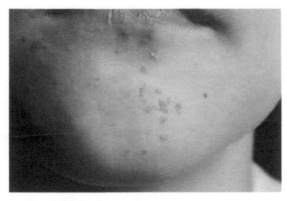

Figure 136.2
Plane warts. Numerous tan papules, some of which have become confluent, tend to be aligned in linear fashion.

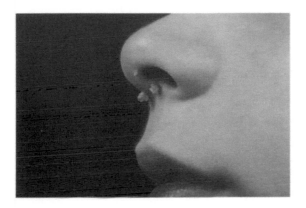

Figure 136.3
Filiform warts. Elongated and digitated excrescences on the nose.

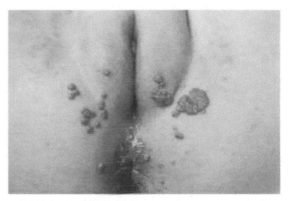

Figure 136.4
Condylomata acuminata. In this early stage in the evolution of condylomata acuminata, papules are both discrete and confluent, slightly reddish and devoid of marked hyperkeratosis. Some warty lesions are present in the perianal region.

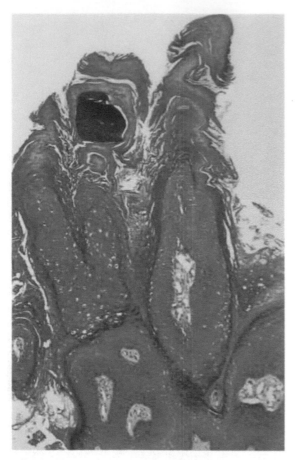

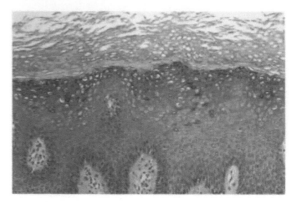

Figure 136.6
Verruca plana. Mammillated epidermal hyperplasia, orthokeratotic hyperkeratosis, hypergranulosis, and keratinocytes of the upper spinous zone and of the granular zone with blue–gray cytoplasm are characteristic histological features of plane warts.

Figure 136.5
Verruca vulgaris. A fully developed lesion of verruca vulgaris is characterized by marked digitated epidermal hyperplasia, collarettes of adnexal epithelium, prominent tortuosity of the capillaries in dermal papillae, and hypergranulosis. Parakeratosis can be seen at the tips of digitations together with collections of red cells, whereas corneocytes between these digitations are orthokeratotic. Note that keratinocytes of the granular layer have clear spaces around nuclei.

137

Xanthoma disseminatum or (Montgomery's syndrome) is a rare, benign, normolipemic form of histiocytoxanthomatosis. It affects the skin and mucous membranes and is frequently associated with diabetes insipidus.

EPIDEMIOLOGY

About 60% of cases of xanthoma disseminatum have their onset between the ages of 5 and 25 years.

CLINICAL FINDINGS

The cutaneous manifestations are marked by the eruption of hundreds of papules that are red–brown at first and then become yellowish. They show a predilection for the flexural surfaces and the intertriginous areas such as the axillae (Fig. 137.1), the groin, the neck, the antecubital and the popliteal fossae, the periorbital regions (Fig. 137.2) and the genitalia. The lesions, particularly those in flexures and folds, tend to merge quickly to form verrucous plaques. In about 50% of cases, xanthomatous lesions may also be observed on the mucous membranes of the mouth, the pharynx and the larynx and on the conjunctiva and the cornea. Symptoms of dyspnea and dysphagia are not uncommon. Vasopressin-sensitive transitory diabetes insipidus is present in about 40% of the cases. Polyuria and polydypsia are generally mild. Xanthoma disseminatum is essentially a self-limited disease. The skin lesions and the diabetes insipidus resolve spontaneously after several years. Only a few cases have demonstrated a progressive course.

LABORATORY FINDINGS

A normal lipid profile is a dogma of this disease.

HISTOPATHOLOGICAL FINDINGS

The papulonodular lesions are characterized by an infiltrate of large mononuclear or multinucleate foamy histiocytes intermingled with lymphocytes, plasma cells and neutrophils (Figs 137.3 and 137.4).

MANAGEMENT

Treatment is usually not helpful. Systemic corticosteroids and antimitotic agents have been used in the more disfiguring forms. Pitressin is necessary to check the diabetes insipidus.

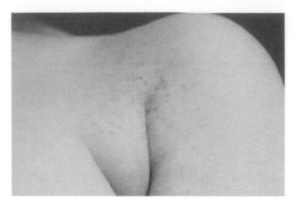

Figure 137.1
Xanthoma disseminatum. Yellow–brown papules concentrated on the axillary folds in a 5-year-old patient with diabetes insipidus.

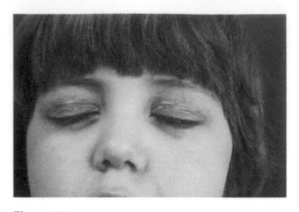

Figure 137.2
Xanthoma disseminatum. Yellow–brown papules merging into plaques are present on the eyelids of the same patient.

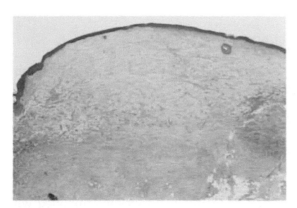

Figure 137.3

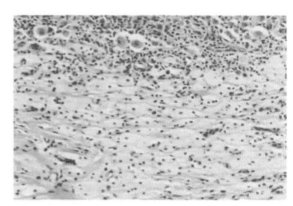

Figure 137.4

Figures 137.3 and 137.4
Xanthoma disseminatum. The majority of the cells constituting this fully developed lesion of xanthoma disseminatum are large histiocytes with vesicular nuclei and abundant foamy cytoplasm. Other cells in the infiltrate include large histiocytes with eosinophilic cytoplasm, lymphocytes, plasma cells and neutrophils.

138

XERODERMA PIGMENTOSUM

Xeroderma pigmentosum is a rare, hereditary disorder. It is characterized by hypersensitivity to sunlight, the early development of freckle-like lesions on photoexposed areas, skin atrophies and a high incidence of skin cancers.

EPIDEMIOLOGY

Xeroderma pigmentosum is a rare disease, occurring in about 1 in 250,000 births.

CLINICAL FINDINGS

The disease manifests itself as soon as exposure to light takes place. It is progressive, causing photophobia in newborns, the first skin changes at 1–5 years of age and skin tumors during adolescence. Neurological signs, when present, appear in early infancy. Cutaneous lesions occur predominantly, but not exclusively, on photoexposed areas, and it is possible to recognize three successive stages. At first, the skin becomes dry and erythematous, with or without blisters after sunburn. Pigmented, bizarrely shaped freckles appear and are intermingled with hypopigmented areas and telangiectasias (Fig. 138.1). In the second stage, continuous sun exposure and subsequent sunburns induce atrophy of the skin and may leave scars (e.g. mutilation of the fingertips or the ears, and ectropion). The third stage is characterized by the development of basal cell carcinomas (Fig. 138.2), squamous cell carcinomas (Fig. 138.3), keratoacanthomas, malignant melanomas and, rarely, sarcomas. The first tumors appear in childhood or adolescence and then increase in size and number. Precancerous lesions, appearing as verrucosities, cutaneous horns, bizarrely shaped lentigo maligna or even scars, arise on large areas and give the skin a characteristic reticular appearance. Ophthalmological symptoms are found in about 80% of cases and are extremely variable – photophobia and conjunctivitis are early symptoms, and corneal opacities, ulcerations, and symblepharon and ectropion occur later. Mouth lesions, such as cheilitis and freckle-like hyperpigmentation, and basal and squamous cell carcinomas of the lips may be observed. True mucous membrane lesions, such as buccal mucosa and tongue erosions and papillomas or gingivostomatitis, have been reported.

The variable degree of severity of the disease is related to the presence of different molecular defects. In the De Sanctis–Cacchione syndrome, the clinical picture of xeroderma pigmentosum is associated with neurological symptoms including microcephaly, progressive mental deterioration, low intelligence, hyporeflexia or areflexia, choreoathetosis, ataxia, spasticity and Achilles tendon shortening with eventual tetraparesis. Markedly retarded growth and hypogonadism may also occur.

LABORATORY FINDINGS

Routine laboratory tests are usually normal. Cultured cells show higher sensitivity to ultraviolet radiation-induced damage, the growth rate is reduced and the cellular recovery is delayed. There is a reduced rate of DNA synthesis. Mutations in the genes that encode for the DNA repair proteins can be detected.

HISTOPATHOLOGICAL FINDINGS

Early histological skin changes in children with xeroderma pigmentosum include evidence of premature solar elastosis, hyperkeratosis, focal atrophy of the epidermis, and a sparse lymphohistiocytic infiltrate in the papillary dermis. In some areas there is hyperpigmentation of the basal layer of the epidermis with or without an increase in the concentration of melanocytes. In time these features become more pronounced, and focally basal keratinocytes exhibit large and hyperchromatic atypical nuclei (Fig. 138.4).

ETIOLOGY AND PATHOGENESIS

Xeroderma pigmentosum is a genetically inherited disease, caused by an autosomal-recessive mutation. The clinical features result from a genetically determined defect of the enzyme system, which normally repairs the ultraviolet radiation-induced DNA damage. Complementation studies using heterokaryons have shown that at least nine complementation groups of xeroderma pigmentosum exist (from A to I), with one variant group.

MANAGEMENT

Treatment consists of life-long avoidance of exposure to the sun by using adequate protection (clothes, sunglasses and sunscreens) in order to delay the onset of the clinical symptoms and tumors. Some patients have been treated with oral retinoids for months to years in order to provide protection against tumors. Beta-carotene per os is another effective treatment in association with retinoids. In affected families, prenatal diagnosis can be performed. Precancerous lesions and skin tumors should be excised.

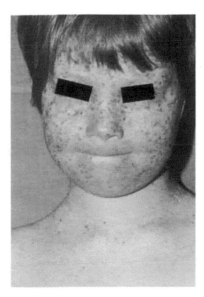

Figure 138.1
Xeroderma pigmentosum. The skin of the neck and shoulders is thin, dry and scaly with many hypopigmented and hyperpigmented macules. The combination of dyschromia, atrophy and telangiectasia is called poikiloderma.

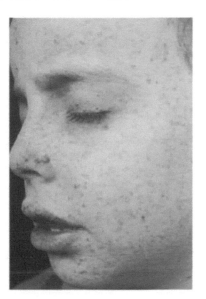

Figure 138.2
Xeroderma pigmentosum. The nodular lesion on the nose is a basal cell carcinoma.

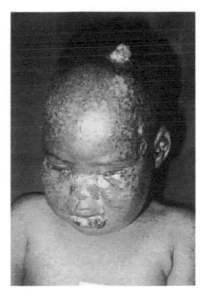

Figure 138.3
Xeroderma pigmentosum. The reticulated hypopigmentation and hyperpigmentation on the chest and the arms is typical of sun-exposed skin in xeroderma pigmentosum. On the lips, the cheeks and the forehead there are squamous cell carcinomas.

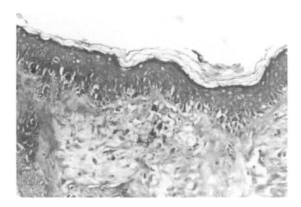

Figure 138.4
Xeroderma pigmentosum. This melanoma *in situ* developed on the face a 21-year-old patient with xeroderma pigmentosum. There are an increased number of atypical melanocytes arranged as solitary units and small nests within the epidermis. The atypical melanocytes arranged as solitary units predominate markedly over melanocytes disposed in nests. A few of the atypical melanocytes lie above the dermoepidermal junction. Note the severe solar elastosis in this section.

INDEX

Page numbers in *italics* refer to illustrations.

T - #0474 - 071024 - C432 - 246/189/20 - PB - 9780367396756 - Gloss Lamination